Nathaniel Collins, DVM

Nathaniel Collins, DVM

Diagnostic Cytology
of the Dog and Cat

Technical Editors

Rick L. Cowell, DVM, MS, Dipl ACVP
Ronald D. Tyler, DVM, PhD, Dipl ACVP

Book Editor: Paul W. Pratt, VMD
Associate Editor: Robert C. Brady, DVM
Production Manager: Elisabeth S. Stein
Cover Design: Elizabeth R. Mason
Illustrations: Sherl A. Holesko

American Veterinary Publications, Inc.
5782 Thornwood Drive
Goleta, California 93117
© **1989**

© **1989** by Rick L. Cowell and Ronald D. Tyler. Copyright under the International Copyright Union. All rights reserved. This book is protected by copyright. No part of it may be reproduced, stored in a retrieval system, or transmitted in any form or by any means, electronic, mechanical, photocopying, recording or otherwise, without written permission from the publisher.

While every effort has been made to ensure the accuracy of information contained herein, the publisher and authors are not legally responsible for errors or omissions.

Revised and Reprinted, 1993.

Library of Congress Catalog Card Number: 88-83423

ISBN 0-939674-25-4

Printed and Bound in the United States of America

Contents

Chapter		Page
1	Introduction	1
2	Cutaneous and Subcutaneous Lesions: Masses, Cysts, Ulcers and Fistulous Tracts	21
3	Nasal Exudates	47
4	The Oropharynx and Tonsils	55
5	The Eyes and Associated Structures	63
6	The External Ear Canal	77
7	Subcutaneous Glandular Tissue: Mammary, Salivary, Thyroid and Parathyroid Glands	83
8	The Lymph Nodes	93
9	Bone Marrow	99
10	Synovial Fluid	121
11	The Musculoskeletal System	137
12	Cerebrospinal Fluid	141
13	Abdominal and Thoracic Fluid	151
14	Transtracheal and Bronchial Washes	167
15	The Lung Parenchyma	179
16	The Liver	189
17	The Splenic Parenchyma	199
18	The Renal Parenchyma	207
19	Urinary Sediment	213
20	The Male Reproductive Tract: Prostate, Testes, Semen	217
21	The Vagina	225
22	Rectal Mucosal Scrapings	235
	Color Plate Section	240
	Index	256

Authors

Claire B. Andreasen, DVM, MS
Resident
Department of Veterinary Pathology
College of Veterinary Medicine
University of Georgia
Athens, GA 30602

Claudia J. Baldwin, DVM, MS
Diplomate ACVIM
Assistant Professor
Veterinary Clinical Sciences
College of Veterinary Medicine
Iowa State University
Ames, IA 50011

Duane F. Brobst, DVM, PhD
Diplomate ACVP
Professor
Department of Veterinary Clinical Medicine
and Surgery
Washington State University
Pullman, WA 99164

Gary Bryan, DVM, MS
Diplomate ACVO
Professor
Department of Veterinary Clinical Medicine
and Surgery
Washington State University
Pullman, WA 99164

Rick L. Cowell, DVM, MS
Diplomate ACVP
Associate Professor
Department of Veterinary Pathology
College of Veterinary Medicine
Oklahoma State University
Stillwater, OK 74078

J. Robert Duncan, DVM, PhD
Diplomate ACVP
Professor
Department of Veterinary Pathology
College of Veterinary Medicine
University of Georgia
Athens, GA 30602

Bernard F. Feldman, DVM, PhD
Professor
Department of Pathobiology
Virginia-Maryland Regional College of
Veterinary Medicine
Virginia Polytechnic Institute
Blacksburg, VA 24061-0442

Tracy W. French, DVM
Diplomate ACVP
Assistant Professor
Department of Pathology
New York State College of Veterinary
Medicine
Cornell University
Ithaca, NY 14853

Kenneth S. Latimer, DVM, PhD
Diplomate ACVP
Associate Professor
Department of Veterinary Pathology
College of Veterinary Medicine
University of Georgia
Athens, GA 30602

Peter S. MacWilliams, DVM, PhD
Diplomate ACVP
Clinical Associate Professor
Department of Pathobiological Sciences
School of Veterinary Medicine
University of Wisconsin
Madison, WI 53706

Jeanne M. Maddux, DVM, PhD
Diplomate ACVP
541 Roberts Roost Road
Fairbanks, AK 99712

Edward A. Mahaffey, DVM, PhD
Diplomate ACVP
Associate Professor
Department of Veterinary Pathology
University of Georgia
Athens, GA 30602

James H. Meinkoth, DVM, MS
Assistant Professor
Department of Veterinary Pathology
College of Veterinary Medicine
Oklahoma State University
Stillwater, OK 74078

D.J. Meyer, DVM
Diplomate ACVIM, ACVP
Associate Professor
Department of Pathology
College of Veterinary Medicine and
Biomedical Sciences
Colorado State University
Fort Collins, CO 80523

Rebecca B. Morton, DVM, MS
Diplomate ACVM
Assistant Professor
Department of Veterinary Parasitology,
Microbiology and Public Health
College of Veterinary Medicine
Oklahoma State University
Stillwater, OK 74078

Patricia N. Olson, DVM, PhD
Diplomate ACT
Associate Professor
Department of Clinical Sciences
College of Veterinary Medicine and
Biomedical Sciences
Colorado State University
Fort Collins, CO 80523

Bruce W. Parry, BVSc, PhD
Diplomate ACVP
Lecturer, Clinical Pathology
Department of Veterinary Paraclinical
Sciences
University of Melbourne
Werribee, Victoria 3030, Australia

Keith W. Prasse, DVM, PhD
Diplomate ACVP
Professor
Department of Pathology
College of Veterinary Medicine
University of Georgia
Athens, GA 30602

Pauline M. Rakich, DVM, PhD
Temporary Instructor
Athens Diagnostic Laboratory
College of Veterinary Medicine
University of Georgia
Athens, GA 30602

Robert M. Shull, DVM
Diplomate ACVP
Associate Professor
Department of Pathobiology
University of Tennessee
P.O. Box 1071
Knoxville, TN 37901

Mary Anna Thrall, DVM, MS
Diplomate ACVP
Associate Professor
Department of Pathology
College of Veterinary Medicine and
Biomedical Sciences
Colorado State University
Fort Collins, CO 80523

Ronald D. Tyler, DVM, PhD
Diplomate ACVP
Associate Professor
Department of Veterinary Pathology
College of Veterinary Medicine
Oklahoma State University
Stillwater, OK 74078

Susan M. Winston, DVM
Diplomate ACVO
Veterinary Ophthalmology Clinic
6004 Goshen Springs Road
Norcross, GA 30071

Joseph G. Zinkl, DVM, PhD
Diplomate ACVP
Professor
Department of Clinical Pathology
School of Veterinary Medicine
University of California
Davis, CA 95616

1

Introduction

R.D. Tyler, R.L. Cowell, C.J. Baldwin and R.J. Morton

Cytologic examination has become recognized as a very useful tool for practicing veterinarians.[1-11] In most situations, cytologic samples can be collected quickly, easily and inexpensively, with little or no risk to the patient. Frequently, the samples can be prepared, stained and interpreted while the client waits in the exam room. The cytologic interpretation often is valuable in establishing a diagnosis, identifying the disease process (neoplasia vs inflammation), directing therapy, forming a prognosis, and/or determining what diagnostic procedure should be performed next. As a result, the patient receives better and/or more expeditious care, and the client is more satisfied.

Risk vs Value

The accuracy of cytologic examination as a diagnostic tool has been studied and reviewed in the human and veterinary literature.[5,12-17] Most studies have compared cytologic results to histopathologic results and/or biologic behavior of the lesion. Some studies indicate that fine-needle aspiration biopsy (FNAB) is more accurate than conventional core needle biopsy or fine aspirate core biopsy.[12,13,16] Fine-needle aspiration poses very little risk to the patient. Complications subsequent to fine-needle aspiration of abdominal organs (*eg,* liver, spleen, pancreas, prostate) or abdominal masses are much less than those expected for conventional core biopsy techniques.[17,19] In a study of 11,700 human patients, Livraghi *et al* concluded that "some serious complications (peritonitis through the crossing of the digestive tract, fistula formation, bacteremia, tumor seeding) theoretically possible in most FNABs have either never occurred or have occurred in such a tiny percentage of cases as to be regarded as negligible for practical purposes."[19]

Implantation of malignant cells along the aspiration tract and induction of hematologic metastasis subsequent to FNAB of malignant tumors are extremely rare and pose no practical danger to the patient, especially when the aspiration tract is removed during excision of the malignant tumor.[12,14,19,20] However, in some instances, contraindications exist and will be discussed in their respective chapters.

Terminology

To facilitate the following discussions, some of the terms used throughout the text are briefly discussed below.

Hypertrophy refers to an increase in cell size and/or functional activity in response to a stimulus.

Hyperplasia refers to an increase in cell numbers, via increased mitotic activity, in response to a stimulus. If a tissue is capable of mitotic division, hyperplasia will occur in concert with hypertrophy.

Neoplasia refers to increased cell growth and multiplication that is not dependent on a stimulus external to the neoplastic tissue.

Metaplasia refers to a reversible process in which one mature cell type is replaced by another mature cell type. It often represents the adaptive replacement of cells sensitive to a stimulus by cells less sensitive to the stimulus. For example, chronic irritation of the ciliated columnar epithelial cells of the trachea and bronchi results in their focal or widespread replacement by stratified squamous epithelial cells.

Dysplasia, in common medical usage, refers to reversible, irregular, atypical, proliferative cellular changes in response to irritation or inflammation.

Anaplasia refers to a lack of differentiation of tissue cells. The less differentiated a tumor is, the more anaplastic it is and, generally, the greater its malignant potential.

Dyscrasia refers to an increase or decrease in the numbers of one or more cell components or maturational stages of a tissue out of proportion to the other cell components or maturational stages.

Chromatin pattern refers to the microscopic appearance of the nuclear chromatin. In general, the chromatin pattern coarsens as malignant potential increases. Some commonly used terms for chromatin patterns are listed, briefly described, and schematically depicted in Table 1.

Romanowsky-type stains, in this text, refers to hematologic stains (Wright's, Giemsa, Diff-Quik, etc) commonly used to perform differential WBC counts on peripheral blood smears.

Hematologic stains can refer to those stains commonly used in hematologic examination and include Romanowsky-type stains and supravital stains, such as new methylene blue, or may refer only to Romanowsky-type stains. The context of the discussion in which it is used generally makes its meaning obvious.

Collection and Smear Preparation

Cytologic samples can be collected by swabbing, scraping and/or aspirating the lesion. The technique(s) used to collect cytologic samples and prepare slides vary, depending on the anatomic location and characteristics of the tissue being sampled and characteristics of the patient (*eg,* tractability).

When possible, several smears should be prepared, leaving some unstained, so smears are available for special stains if necessary. Specific techniques and preparation procedures will be discussed in the chapter dealing with the tissue for which they are used. General considerations for collection and preparation of cytologic samples are discussed below.

Imprints

Imprints for cytologic evaluation can be prepared from external lesions on the living animal or from tissues removed during surgery or necropsy. They are easy to collect and require minimal restraint, but collect fewer cells than scrapings and contain greater contamination (bacterial and cellular) than FNABs. As a result, imprints from superficial lesions often only reflect a secondary bacterial infection and/or inflammation-induced tissue dysplasia. This markedly hinders their use in diagnosis of neoplasia.

Ulcers should be imprinted before they are cleaned. The lesion should then be cleaned with a saline-moistened surgical sponge and reimprinted and/or scraped. A fine-needle aspirate of the tissue underlying the surface of the lesion should be collected also. In some conditions, such as *Dermatophilus congolensis* infection (streptothricosis) and *Coccidioides immitis* infection, impressions from the uncleaned lesion often contain far more organisms than impressions from cleaned lesions and samples collected by FNAB. Imprints of the underside of the scabs from *Dermatophilus congolensis*-produced lesions are usually most rewarding. Other conditions may yield more information on the imprints from cleaned lesions than the imprints from uncleaned lesions.

To collect imprints from cleaned cutaneous lesions or tissues collected during surgery or necropsy, blood and tissue fluid should first be removed from the surface of the lesion being imprinted by blotting with a clean absorbent material. Excessive blood and tissue fluids inhibit tissue cells from adhering to the glass slide, producing a poor cellular preparation. Also, excessive fluid inhibits cells from spreading and assuming the size and shape they usually have in air-dried smears. The middle of a clean glass microscope slide is then touched against the blotted surface of the tissue to be imprinted. Though multiple imprints generally are made on each slide, one imprint per slide usually is sufficient. When possible, several slides are imprinted so slides are available for special stains if necessary.

Scrapings

Smears of scrapings can be prepared from tissues collected during necropsy or surgery or from external lesions on the living animal. Scraping has the advantage of collecting many cells from the tissue and, therefore, is advantageous when the lesion is firm and yields few cells. The major disadvantages are that they are more difficult to collect and they collect only superficial samples. As a result, scrapings from superficial lesions often only reflect a secondary bacterial infection and/or inflammation-induced tissue dysplasia. This markedly hinders their use in diagnosis of neoplasia.

Scrapings are prepared by holding a scalpel blade perpendicular to the lesion's cleaned and blotted surface, and pulling the blade toward

Introduction

Table 1. Selected chromatin patterns.

Pattern	Description	Schematic
Smooth (sometimes referred to as a "fine" chromatin pattern)	A finely etched uniform pattern of thin chromatin strands. Aggregates of chromatin are not present.	
Finely stippled	A smooth chromatin pattern with small discrete aggregates of chromatin scattered throughout the nucleus.	
Lacy (reticular)	A uniform pattern of medium-sized chromatin strands. Significant aggregates of chromatin are not present. Some people use "reticular" to imply a pattern with slightly thicker chromatin strands than in lacy patterns.	
Coarse (ropy or cord-like)	A pattern of very thick chromatin strands.	
Clumped	Large aggregates of chromatin are scattered throughout the nucleus. May occur with lacy or coarse chromatin patterns.	
Smudged	The chromatin pattern is not discrete. The outlines of chromatin strands and/or clumps are vague. The usual pattern for lymphocytes.	

Figure 1. Fine-needle aspiration from a solid mass. After the needle is within the mass (A), negative pressure is placed on the syringe by rapidly withdrawing the plunger (B), usually one-half to three-fourths the volume of the syringe barrel. The needle is redirected several times while negative pressure is maintained, if this can be accomplished without the needle's point leaving the mass. Before removing the needle from the mass, the plunger is released, relieving negative pressure on the syringe (C).

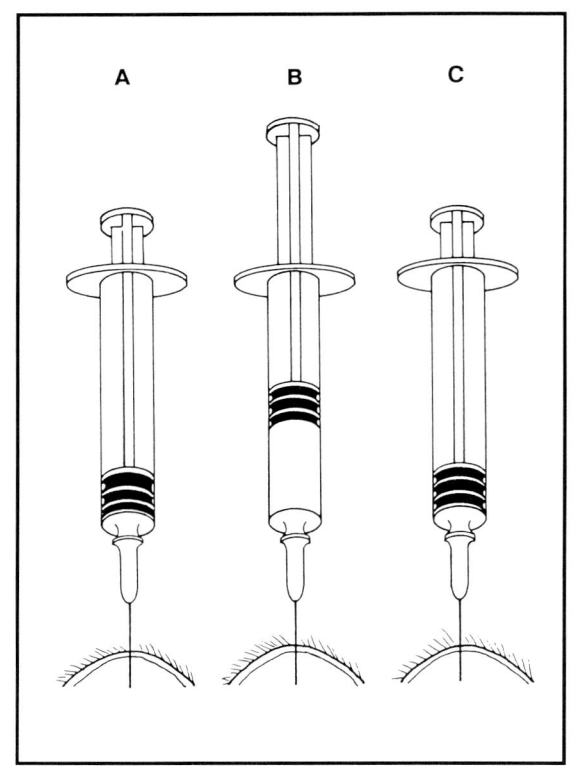

oneself several times. The material collected on the blade is transferred to the middle of a glass microscope slide and spread by one or more of the techniques described below for preparation of smears from aspirates of solid masses.

Swabs

Generally, swab smears are collected only when imprints, scrapings and aspirates cannot be made, as with fistulous tracts and vaginal collections. The lesion is swabbed with a moist, sterile cotton swab. Sterile isotonic fluid, such as 0.9% NaCl, should be used to moisten the swab. Moistening the swab helps minimize cell damage during sample collection and smear preparation. If the lesion is very moist, the swab need not be moistened. After sample collection, the swab is gently rolled along the flat surface of a clean glass microscope slide. *Do not rub the swab across the slide surface*, as this causes excessive cell damage.

Aspiration of Masses

Fine-needle aspiration biopsies can be collected from masses (including lymph nodes, nodular lesions and internal organs). For cutaneous lesions, they avoid superficial contamination (bacterial and cellular), but collect fewer cells than scrapings.

Selection of syringe and needle: Fine-needle aspiration biopsies are collected with a 21- to 25-ga needle and a 3- to 20-ml syringe. The softer the tissue being aspirated, the smaller the needle and syringe used. It is seldom advantageous, however, to use a needle larger than 21 ga for aspiration, even for firm tissues such as fibromas. When needles larger than 21 ga are used, tissue cores tend to be aspirated, resulting in a poor yield of free cells suitable for cytologic preparation. Also, larger needles tend to cause greater blood contamination.

The size of syringe used is influenced by the consistency of the tissue being aspirated. Softer tissues, such as lymph nodes, often can successfully be aspirated with a 3-ml syringe. Firm tissues, such as fibromas and squamous-cell carcinomas, require a larger syringe to maintain adequate suction for sufficient collection of cells from the tissue. Since the ideal size of syringe is not known for many masses before aspiration, a 12-ml syringe is a good all-around size.

Preparation of the site for aspiration: If microbiologic tests are to be performed on a portion of the sample collected, or a body cavity (peritoneal and thoracic cavities, joints, etc) is to be penetrated, the area of aspiration is surgically prepped. Otherwise, skin preparation is essentially that required for a vaccination or venipuncture. An alcohol swab can be used to clean the area.

Aspiration Procedure: The mass to be aspirated is held firmly to aid in penetration of the skin and mass and to control the direction of the needle. The needle, with syringe attached, is introduced into the center of the mass and strong negative pressure is applied by withdrawing the plunger to about three-fourths the volume of the syringe (Fig 1). Several areas of the mass should be sampled, but aspiration of the sample into the barrel of the syringe and contamination of the sample by aspiration of tissue surrounding the mass must be avoided. To accomplish this, when the mass is large enough to allow the needle to be redirected and moved to several areas in the mass without danger of the needle's leaving the mass, negative pressure is maintained during redirection and movement of the needle. However, when the mass is not large enough for the needle to be redirected and moved without danger of the needle's leaving the mass, negative pressure is relieved during redirection and movement of the needle. In this situation, negative pressure is applied only when the needle is static. Often, high-quality collections do not have aspirated material visible in the syringe and sometimes not even in the hub of the needle.

After several areas are sampled, the negative pressure is relieved from the syringe and the needle is removed from the mass and skin. Next, the needle is removed from the syringe and air is drawn into the syringe. Then, the needle is replaced onto the syringe and some of the tissue in the barrel and hub of the needle is expelled onto the middle of a glass microscope slide by rapidly depressing the plunger. When possible, several preparations should be made as described below.

Preparation of Smears from Aspirates of Solid Masses

Several methods can be used to prepare smears for cytologic evaluation of solid masses, including lymph nodes. The experience of the person preparing the smears and characteristics of the sample influence the choice of smear preparation technique. The authors suggest a combination of slide prep-

Figure 2. Combination cytologic preparation. A. A portion of the aspirate is expelled onto a glass microscope slide (prep slide). B. Another glass microscope slide is placed over about one-third of the preparation. If additional spreading of the aspirate is needed, gentle digital pressure can be used. Excessive pressure should be avoided. The spreader slide is smoothly slid forward. C. This makes a squash prep of about one-third of the aspirate (area 1). The spreader slide also contains a squash prep (not depicted).

Next, the edge of a tilted glass microscope slide (second spreader slide) is slid backward from the end opposite the squash prep until it contacts about one-third the expelled aspirate (D,E). Then, the second spreader slide is slid rapidly and smoothly forward. F. This produces an area (3) that is spread with mechanical forces like those of a blood smear preparation. The middle area (2) is left untouched and contains a high concentration of cells.

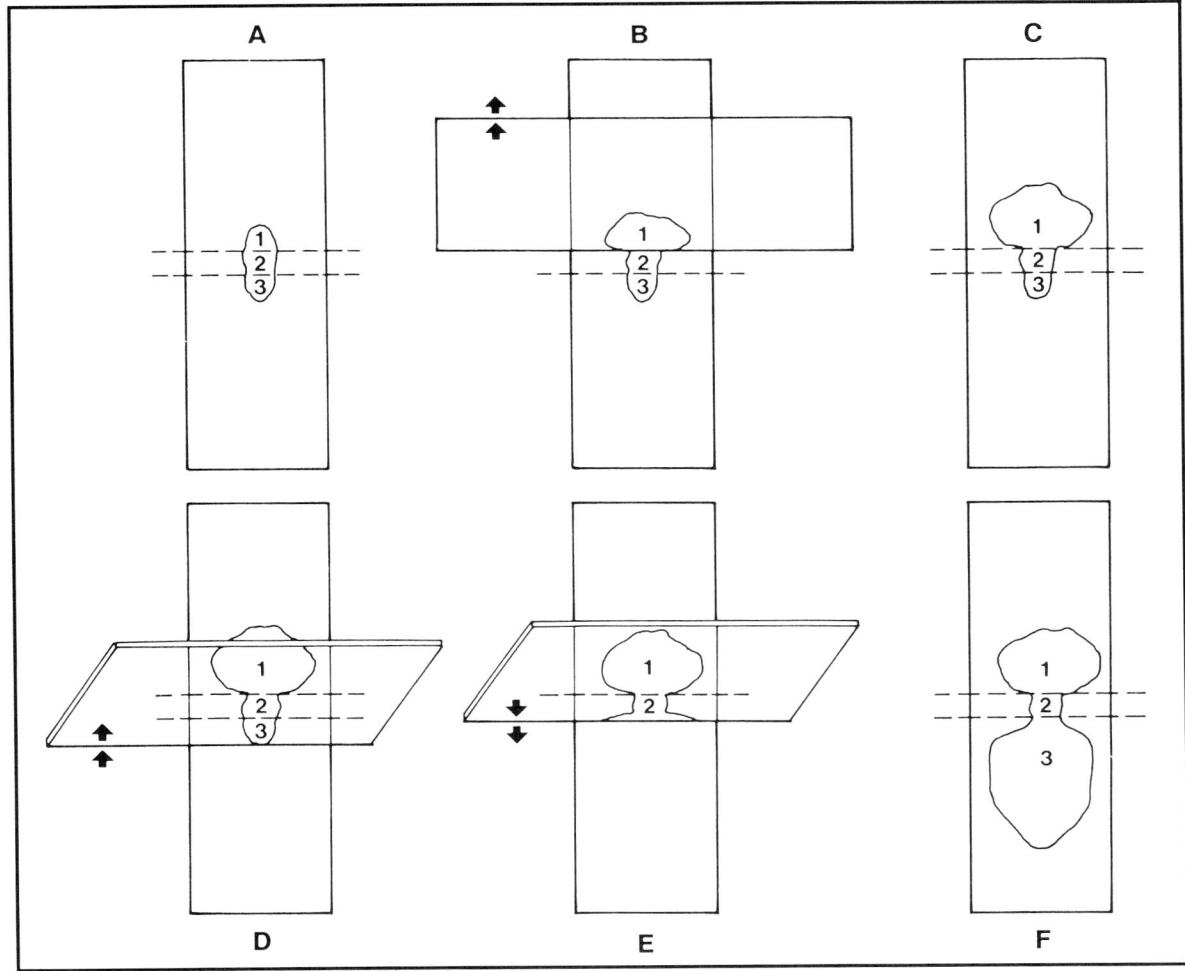

Figure 3. Squash preparation. A. A portion of the aspirate is expelled onto a glass microscope slide and another slide is placed over the sample. B. This spreads the sample. If the sample does not spread well, gentle digital pressure can be applied to the top slide. Care must be taken not to place excessive pressure on the slide, causing the cells to rupture. C. The slides are smoothly slid apart. D. This usually produces well-spread smears but may result in excessive cell rupture.

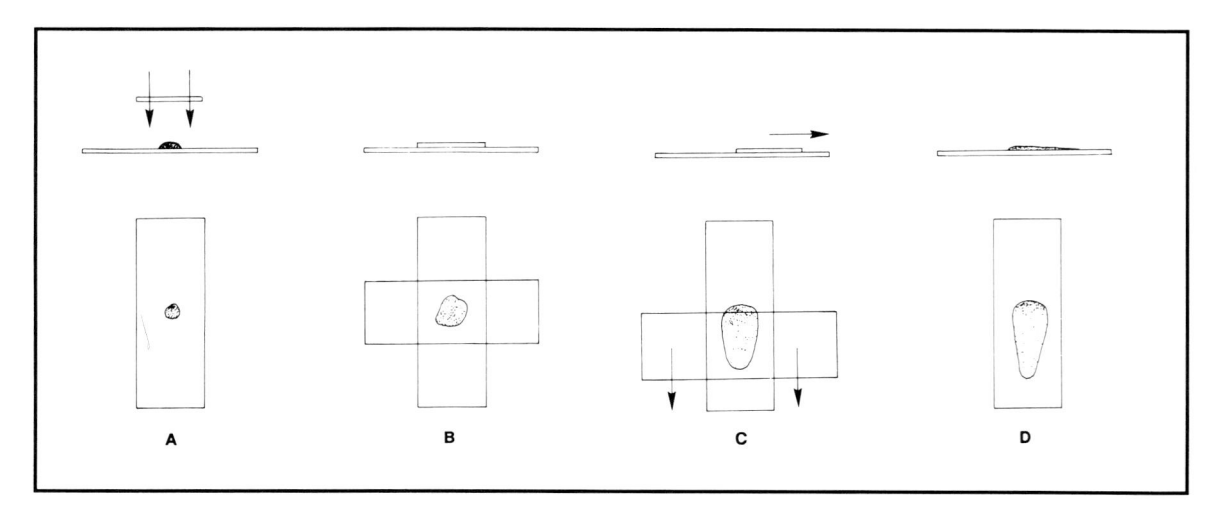

Figure 4. A modification of the squash preparation. A. A portion of the aspirate is expelled onto a glass microscope slide and another slide is placed over the sample. B. This causes the sample to spread. If necessary, gentle digital pressure can be applied to the top slide to spread the sample more. Care must be taken not to use excessive pressure and cause cell rupture. C. The top slide is rotated about 45° and lifted directly upward, producing a spread preparation with subtle ridges and valleys of cells (D).

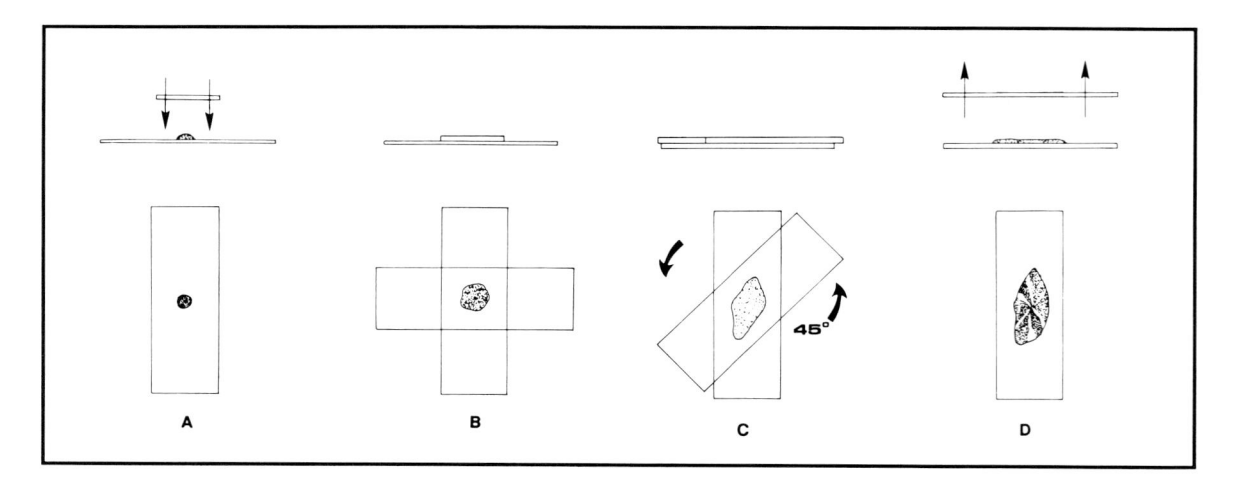

aration techniques. Some cytologic preparation techniques are described below.

Combination Technique: One combination procedure involves spraying the aspirate onto the middle of a clean glass microscope slide (prep slide). Keeping the prep slide on a flat, solid, horizontal surface, pull another slide (spreader slide) backward at a 45-degree angle to the first slide until it contacts about one-third of the aspirate (Fig 2). Then slide the spreader slide smoothly and rapidly forward, as if making a blood smear. Next, place the spreader slide horizontally over the back one-third of the aspirate at a right angle to the prep slide. Allow the weight of the spreader slide (top slide) to spread the material, resisting the temptation to compress the slides manually. Keeping the spreader slide flat and horizontal, quickly and smoothly slide it across the prep slide.

This makes a squash prep of the back third of the aspirate. The middle third of the aspi-

Introduction

Figure 5. Needle spread or "starfish" preparation. A. A portion of the aspirate is expelled onto a glass microscope slide. B. The tip of a needle is placed in the aspirate and moved peripherally, pulling a trail of the sample with it. This procedure is repeated in several directions, resulting in a preparation with multiple projections.

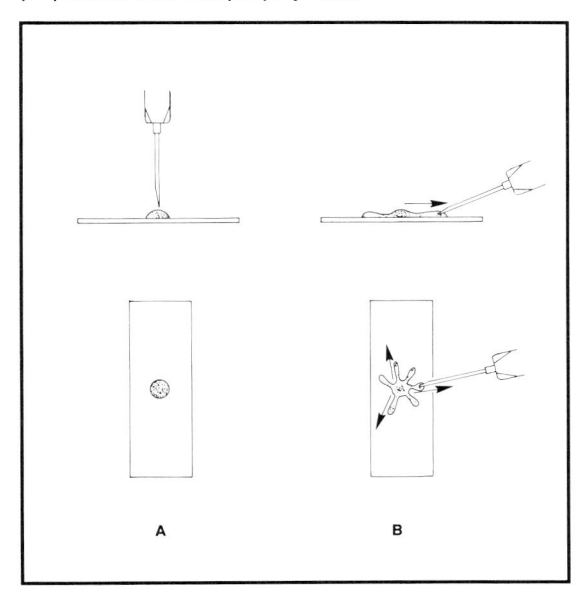

This makes a squash prep of the back third of the aspirate. The middle third of the aspirate is left untouched. This procedure leaves the front third of the aspirate gently spread. If the aspirate is of fragile tissue, this area should contain sufficient unruptured cells to evaluate. The back third of the aspirate has been spread with the shear forces of a squash prep. If the aspirate contains clumps of cells that are difficult to spread, there should be some clumps sufficiently spread in the back one-third of the preparation. If the aspirate is of very low cellularity, the middle third remains more concentrated and is the most efficient area to study.

Squash Preparation: In expert hands, the squash preparation can yield excellent cytologic smears. However, in less experienced hands, it often yields cytologic smears that are unreadable because too many cells are ruptured or the sample is not sufficiently spread. A squash preparation is made by expelling the aspirate onto the middle of one slide and then placing a second slide over the aspirate horizontal with and at right angles to the first slide (Fig 3). The second slide is then quickly and smoothly slid across the first slide.

Figure 6. Blood smear technique. A. A drop of fluid sample is placed on a glass microscope slide close to one end, then another slide is slid backward to contact the front of the drop. B. When the drop is contacted, it rapidly spreads along the juncture between the 2 slides. The spreader slide is then smoothly and rapidly slid forward the length of the slide, producing a smear with a feathered edge (C,D).

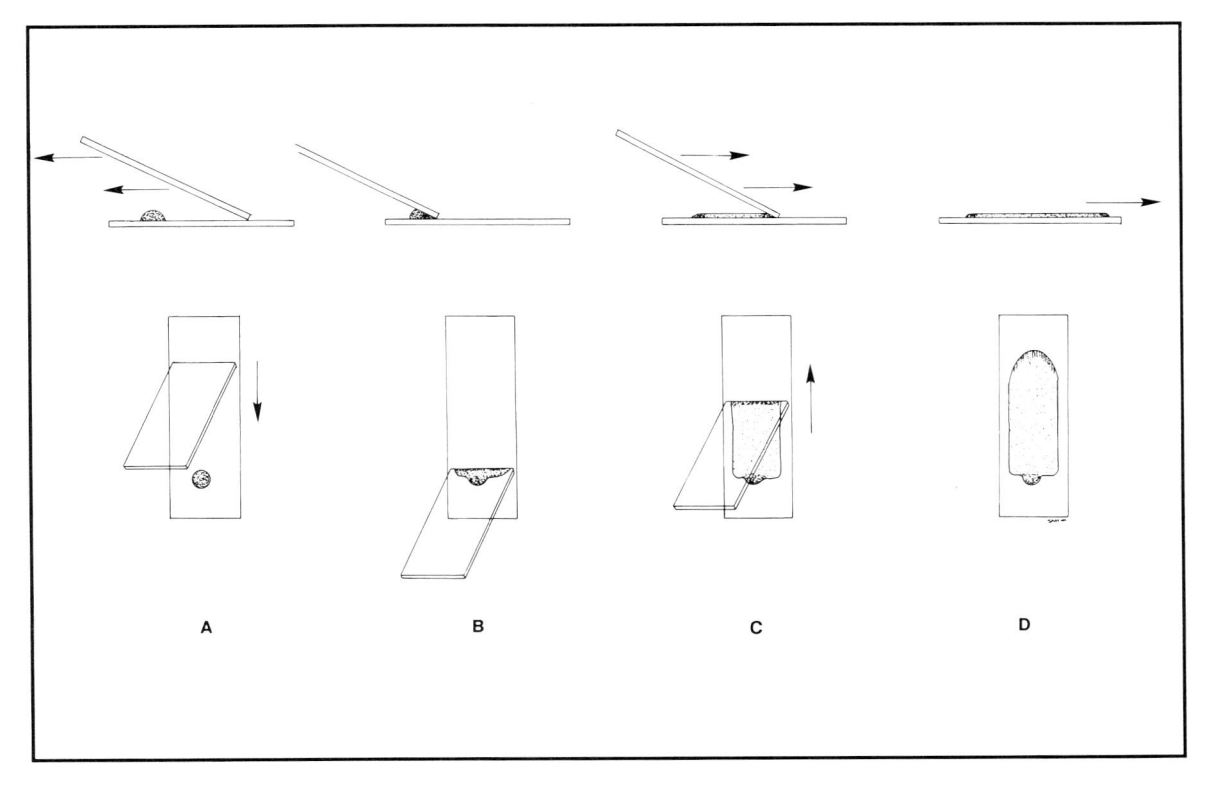

Chapter 1

Other Spreading Techniques: A modification of the squash preparation that has less tendency to rupture cells is to lay the second slide over the aspirate, then rotate the second slide 45 degrees and lift it upward (Fig 4).

Another technique for spreading aspirates is to drag the aspirate peripherally in several directions with the point of a syringe needle, producing a starfish shape (Fig 5). This technique tends not to damage fragile cells, but allows a thick layer of tissue fluid to remain around the cells. Sometimes, the thick layer of fluid prevents the cells from spreading well and interferes with evaluation of cell detail. Usually, however, some acceptable areas are present.

Preparation of Smears from Fluids

Cytologic smears should be prepared immediately after fluid collection. When possible, fluid samples for cytologic examination should be collected in ethylenediaminetetraacetic acid (EDTA) tubes. Smears can be prepared directly from fresh, well-mixed fluid or from the sediment of a centrifuged sample by blood smear (Fig 6), line smear (Fig 7) and squash prep (Fig 3) techniques. The cellularity, viscosity and homogeneity of the fluid influence the selection of smear technique.

The squash prep technique often spreads viscous samples and samples with flecks of particulate material better than the blood smear and line smear techniques. The blood smear technique usually produces well-spread smears of sufficient cellularity from homogeneous fluids containing ≥ 5000 cells/μl but often produces smears of insufficient cellularity from fluids containing <5000 cells/μl. The line smear technique can be used to concentrate fluids of low cellularity, but often does not sufficiently spread cells from highly cellular fluids. In general, translucent fluids are of low to moderate cellularity, whereas opaque fluids are usually highly cellular. Therefore, translucent fluids often require concentration, either by centrifugation or by the line smear technique. When possible, concentration by centrifugation is preferred.

To prepare a smear by the blood smear technique, place a small drop of the fluid on a glass slide about 1.0-1.5 cm from the end (Fig 6). Slide another slide backward at a 30- to 40-degree angle until it contacts the drop. When the fluid flows sideways along the crease

Figure 7. Line smear concentration technique. A. A drop of fluid sample is placed onto a glass microscope slide close to one end, and another slide is slid backward to contact the front of the drop. B. When the drop is contacted, it rapidly spreads along the juncture between the 2 slides. C. The spreader slide is then smoothly and rapidly slid forward. D. After the spreader slide has been advanced about two-thirds to three-fourths the distance required to make a smear with a feathered edge, the spreader slide is raised directly upward. This produces a smear with a line of concentrated cells at its end, instead of a feathered edge.

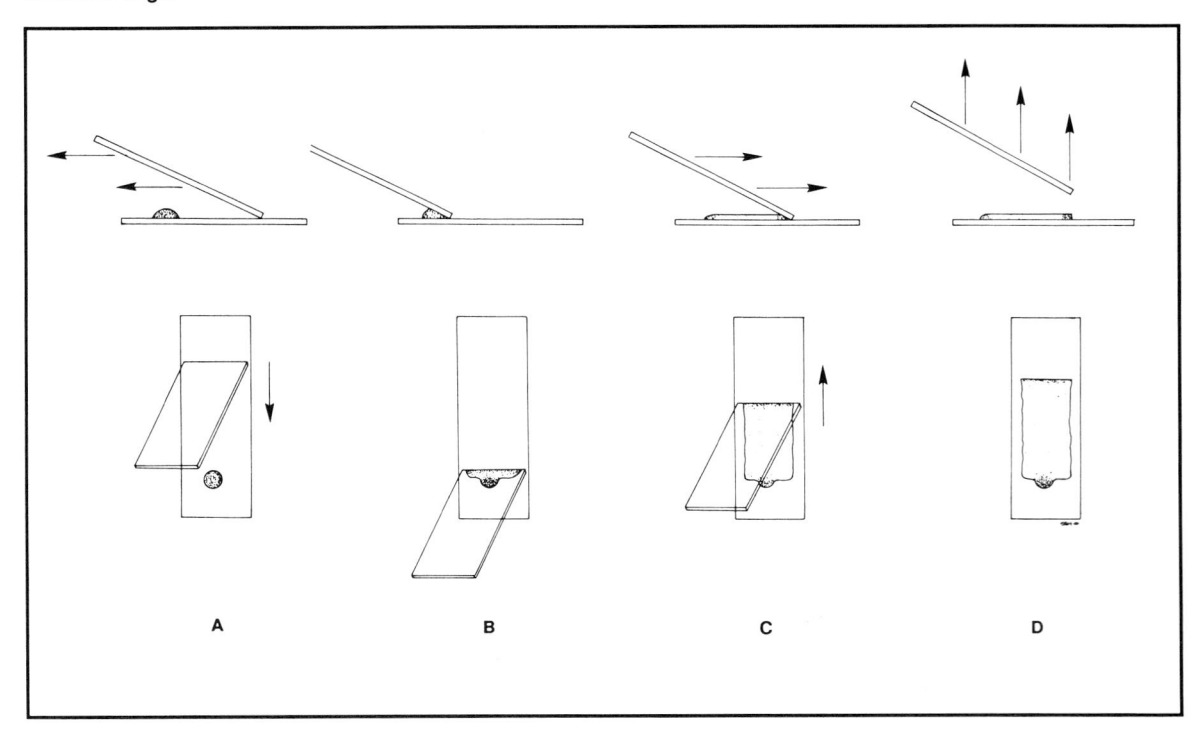

between the slides, quickly and smoothly slide the second slide forward until the fluid has all drained away from the second slide. This makes a smear with a feathered edge.

To concentrate fluids by centrifugation, the fluid is centrifuged 5 minutes at 165-360 G. This is achieved by operating a centrifuge with a radial arm length of 14.6 cm (the arm length of most urine centrifuges) at 1000-1500 rpm. After centrifugation, the supernatant is separated from the sediment and analyzed for total protein concentration. The sediment is resuspended in a few drops of supernatant by gently thumping the side of the tube. A drop of the resuspended sediment is placed on a slide and a smear is made by the blood smear or squash prep technique. When possible, several smears should be made by each technique.

When the fluid cannot be concentrated by centrifugation or the centrifuged sample is of low cellularity, the line smear technique (Fig 7) can be used to concentrate cells in the smear. A drop of fluid is placed on a clean glass slide and the blood smear technique is used, except the spreading slide is raised directly upward about three-fourths of the way through the smear, yielding a line containing a much higher concentration of cells than the rest of the slide. Unfortunately, an excessive amount of fluid may also remain in the "line" and prevent the cells from spreading well.

Staining

Types of Stains

Several types of stains have been used for cytologic preparations. The 2 general types most commonly used are the Romanowsky-type stains (Wright's stain, Giemsa stain, Diff-Quik) and Papanicolaou stain and its derivatives, such as Sano's trichrome. The advantages and disadvantages of both types of stains are discussed below. However, because the Romanowsky-type stains are more rewarding, practical and readily available in practice situations, the remainder of this discussion deals predominantly with Romanowsky-type stained preparations.

Romanowsky Stains: Romanowsky-type stains are inexpensive, readily available and easy to prepare, maintain and use. They stain organisms and the cytoplasm of cells excellently. Though nuclear and nucleolar detail cannot be perceived as well with Romanowsky-type stains as with Papanicolaou-type stains, nuclear and nucleolar detail usually is sufficient for differentiating neoplasia and inflammation, and for evaluating neoplastic cells for cytologic evidence of malignant potential (criteria of malignancy).

Smears to be stained with Romanowsky-type stains are first air dried. Air drying partially preserves ("fixes") the cells, and causes them to adhere to the slide so they do not fall off during the staining procedure.

There are many commercially available Romanowsky-type stains, including Diff-Quik, DipStat and other quick Wright's stains. Most, if not all, Romanowsky-type stains are acceptable for staining cytologic preparations. Diff-Quik stain does not undergo the metachromatic reaction. As a result, granules of some mast cells do not stain. When mast-cell granules do not stain, the mast cells may be misclassified as macrophages. This can lead to confusion in examination of some mast-cell tumors. The variation between different Romanowsky-type stains should not cause a problem once the evaluator has become familiar with the stain s/he uses routinely.

Each stain usually has its own unique recommended staining procedure. These procedures should be followed in general, but should be adapted to the type and thickness of smear being stained and to the evaluator's preference. The thinner the smear and the lower the total protein concentration of the fluid, the less time needed in the stain. The thicker the smear and the greater the total protein concentration of the fluid, the more time needed in the stain. As a result, fluid smears with low protein content and low cellularity, such as some abdominal fluid samples, may stain better using one-half or less of the recommended contact time. Thick smears, such as smears of neoplastic lymph nodes, may need to be stained twice the recommended time or longer. Each person tends to have a different staining technique s/he prefers. By trying variations in the recommended time intervals for stains, the evaluator can establish which times produce the preferred staining characteristics.

New Methylene Blue Stain: New methylene blue (NMB) stain is a useful adjunct to Romanowsky-type stains. It stains cytoplasm weakly, if at all, but gives excellent nuclear and nucleolar detail. Because NMB stains cytoplasm weakly, often the nuclear detail of cells in cell clumps can be visualized. Generally, RBCs do not stain but may develop a pale blue tint with NMB. As a result, marked RBC contamination does not obscure nucleated cells.

Papanicolaou Stains: The delicate Papanicolaou-type stains give excellent nuclear detail and delicate cytoplasmic detail. They allow the viewer to see through layers of cells in cell clumps and to evaluate nuclear and nucleolar changes very well. They do not stain cytoplasm as strongly as Romanowsky stains and, therefore, do not demonstrate cytoplasmic changes as well as Romanowsky stains. They also do not demonstrate bacteria and other organisms as well as Romanowsky stains.

Papanicolaou-type staining requires multiple steps and considerable time. Also, the reagents often are difficult to locate, prepare and maintain in practice. Papanicolaou stains and their derivatives require the specimen to be wet-fixed, *ie*, the smear must be fixed before the cells have dried. Usually this is achieved by spraying the smear with a cytologic fixative or placing it in ethanol immediately after preparation. When the smear is to be placed in ethanol, it should be made on a protein-coated slide. This prevents the cells from falling off the slide when it is immersed.

Staining Problems

Poor stain quality often perplexes both the novice and experienced cytologist. Most staining problems can be avoided if the following precautions are taken:

- Use new slides, fresh, well-filtered (if periodic filtration is required) stain(s), and fresh buffer solution (if a buffer is required).
- Stain cytologic preparations immediately after air drying.
- Take care not to touch the surface of the slide or smear at any time.

Occasionally a sample may be contaminated with a foreign substance, such as K-Y Jelly, that alters the specimen's staining. Table 2 gives some of the problems that can occur with Romanowsky-type stains and some proposed solutions to these problems.

Microscopic Evaluation

After the smear has been stained and dried, it is scanned at low magnification (4-10X objective) to determine if all areas of the smear are stained adequately and if there are any localized areas of increased cellularity or areas with unique staining features. If the smear is inadequately stained, it can be restained; however, not all areas of a slide need to be adequately stained. For example, only the edges of thick smears may stain adequately, and yet the slides may be adequately evaluated.

Any areas of increased and/or unique cellularity are mentally noted for future evaluation. Also, large objects, such as crystals, foreign bodies, parasites and fungal hyphae, may be seen while scanning the slide at low magnification. When proper staining is assured and all areas of increased and/or unique cellularity are recognized, magnification is increased to the 10X or 20X objective. An impression of the cellularity and cellular composition (inflammatory cells, epithelial cells, spindle cells, etc) of the smear and of cell size usually is developed at this magnification. Areas of increased cellularity and/or unique cellularity are evaluated.

Next, the smear is viewed with the 40X objective. To improve resolution by decreasing light diffraction, a drop of oil can be placed on the smear; then a coverslip is placed over the drop of oil. At this magnification, individual cells are evaluated and compared to other cells in the smear. Usually, nucleoli and the chromatin pattern can be discerned. With experience, one can see most organisms visible microscopically with the 40X objective. However, it may be necessary to use the 100X (oil-immersion) objective to identify some organisms and inclusions, and to confirm the identity of organisms seen with the 40X objective. Cell morphology (nuclear chromatin pattern, nucleoli, etc) is evaluated in detail with the 100X (oil-immersion) objective.

Interpretation

Cytologic examination can be a very useful tool for practicing veterinarians. While a definitive diagnosis is not always achieved, the general process (inflammation, etc) usually is recognized within a few minutes if a logical, methodical approach is used. Often definitive diagnosis is not necessary for practical management of the case. When a definitive diagnosis is necessary but cannot be achieved by cytologic examination, the cytologic results often help select the most rewarding procedure to perform next (*eg*, culture, biopsy, radiography). For example, a cytologic preparation containing only inflammatory cells, whether organisms are present or not, indicates that a culture might be helpful, whereas a preparation containing only tissue cells lead toward biopsy and away from culture.

Evaluation of a cytologic preparation should take only a few minutes once the evaluator has gained the basic skills of microscope

Introduction

Table 2. Some possible solutions to problems seen with common Romanowsky-type stains.

Excessive Blue Staining (RBC may be blue-green)

Problem	Solution
Prolonged stain contact	Decrease staining time
Inadequate wash	Wash longer
Specimen too thick	Make thinner smears if possible
Stain, diluent, buffer or wash water too alkaline	Check with pH paper and correct pH
Exposure to formalin vapors	Store and ship cytologic preps separate from formalin containers
Wet fixation in ethanol or formalin	Air dry smears before fixation
Delayed fixation	Fix smears sooner if possible
Surface of the slide was alkaline	Use new slides

Excessive Pink Staining

Problem	Solution
Insufficient staining time	Increase staining time
Prolonged washing	Decrease duration of wash
Stain or diluent too acidic	Check with pH paper and correct pH; fresh methanol may be needed
Excessive time in red stain solution	Decrease time in red solution
Inadequate time in blue stain solution	Increase time in blue stain solution
Mounting coverslip before preparation is dry	Allow preparation to dry completely before mounting coverslip

Weak Staining

Problem	Solution
Insufficient contact with one or more of the stain solutions	Increase staining time
Fatigued (old) stains	Change stains
Another slide covered specimen during staining	Keep slides separate

Uneven Staining

Problem	Solution
Variation of pH in different areas of slide surface (may be due to slide surface being touched or slide being poorly cleaned)	Use new slides and avoid touching their surface before and after preparation
Water allowed to stand on some areas of the slide after staining and washing	Tilt slides close to vertical to drain water from the surface or dry with a fan
Inadequate mixing of stain and buffer	Mix stain and buffer thoroughly

Precipitate on Preparation

Problem	Solution
Inadequate stain filtration	Filter or change the stain(s)
Inadequate washing of slide after staining	Rinse slides well after staining
Dirty slides used	Use clean new slides
Stain solution dries during staining	Use sufficient stain and do not leave it on slide too long

Miscellaneous

Problem	Solution
Overstained preparations	Destain with 95% methanol and restain; Diff-Quik-stained smears may have to be destained in the red Diff-Quik stain solution to remove the blue color; however, this damages the red stain solution
Refractile artifact on RBC with Diff-Quik stain (usually due to moisture in fixative)	Change the fixative

operation. If cytologic changes are sufficient to establish a reliable diagnosis, they should be sufficiently plentiful and prominent for recognition within several minutes of serious viewing. When changes are not sufficiently plentiful or prominent for a reliable diagnosis, the preparation(s) should be sent to a veterinary clinical pathologist/cytologist for interpretation, or an alternative diagnostic procedure should be employed. Occasionally, clinical and/or cytologic evidence of specific organism involvement is sufficient to merit a prolonged search for the organism suspected. For example, if a patient has clinical signs of coccidioidomycosis, and macrophages and inflammatory giant cells are found in the cytologic preparation, a prolonged search for *Coccidioides immitis* might be rewarding. However, even in these cases, you should not spend so much time searching for the organism that you become frustrated. Instead, send the cytologic preparation(s) to a veterinary clinical pathologist/cytologist or use an alternative procedure, such as biopsy or serologic testing.

Probably the most important judgment to be made when interpreting a cytologic sample is whether the lesion is inflammatory or neoplastic in nature. If the lesion is strictly inflammatory, it can be treated with antiinflammatories, antibiotics or other medical therapy. If the lesion is neoplastic in nature, however, it may need to be resected and/or treated by chemotherapy. Often, the decision of whether the lesion is inflammatory or neoplastic is simple. Samples containing only inflammatory cells or inflammatory cells and a few nondysplastic tissue cells indicate an inflammatory lesion, whereas samples containing only tissue cells indicate a neoplastic or hyperplastic process. An admixture of inflammatory cells and tissue cells suggests either neoplasia with secondary inflammation, or inflammation with secondary tissue cell dysplasia.

If there is confusion concerning whether the lesion is inflammatory or neoplastic, 2 approaches can be taken. First, the lesion can be treated with appropriate antibiotic therapy. If the lesion regresses, it was inflammatory. If the lesion does not regress, another aspirate can be taken to see if the inflammatory component has resolved, making the lesion recognizable as neoplastic. If the lesion does not regress and the decision of inflammation or neoplasia still cannot be made cytologically, the lesion can be removed or biopsied and submitted for histopathologic evaluation. Alternatively, without attempting treatment, the lesion can be removed and submitted for histopathologic examination.

Lesions determined to be inflammatory in nature can be classified into different categories of inflammation. Often, neoplastic lesions can be recognized as malignant or benign and as epithelial, mesenchymal (spindle-cell) or discrete round-cell tumors. Chart 1 presents an algorithm to aid in general evaluation of cytologic preparations.

Inflammation

To determine the type of inflammatory lesion, the abundance and proportions of different inflammatory cells are evaluated. Types of inflammatory cells include neutrophils, eosinophils, tissue macrophages, epithelioid macrophages and inflammatory giant cells. Also, a few mast cells may be present during some inflammatory responses, *eg*, allergic inflammation.

Inflammation can be classified using terminology implying duration (acute, subacute, chronic-active, chronic) or by the type of inflammatory process (purulent, suppurative, granulomatous, eosinophilic hypersensitivity reaction). The qualifiers mild, moderate and marked can be used to classify the severity of the inflammatory reaction.

The inflammatory process can be classified as acute when >70% of the inflammatory cells are neutrophils, as subacute or chronic-active when 50-70% of the inflammatory cells are neutrophils and 30-50% of the inflammatory cells are macrophages, and chronic when >50% of the inflammatory cells are macrophages.[9,10] The inflammatory response can be classified as purulent or suppurative if >85% of the inflammatory cells are neutrophils, granulomatous if inflammatory giant cells and/or numerous epithelioid macrophages are present, and eosinophilic or allergic if eosinophils are numerous. The classifications of purulent/suppurative, granulomatous and eosinophilic/allergic are not mutually exclusive. For example, purulent and granulomatous inflammation is termed pyogranulomatous inflammation.

Neoplasia

When the cellular components of the sample indicate the process is neoplastic, the neoplasm often can be recognized as an epithelial, mesenchymal (spindle-cell) or discrete round-cell tumor, and/or as benign or malignant.

Introduction

Chart 1. An algorithm to aid evaluation of cytologic preparations.

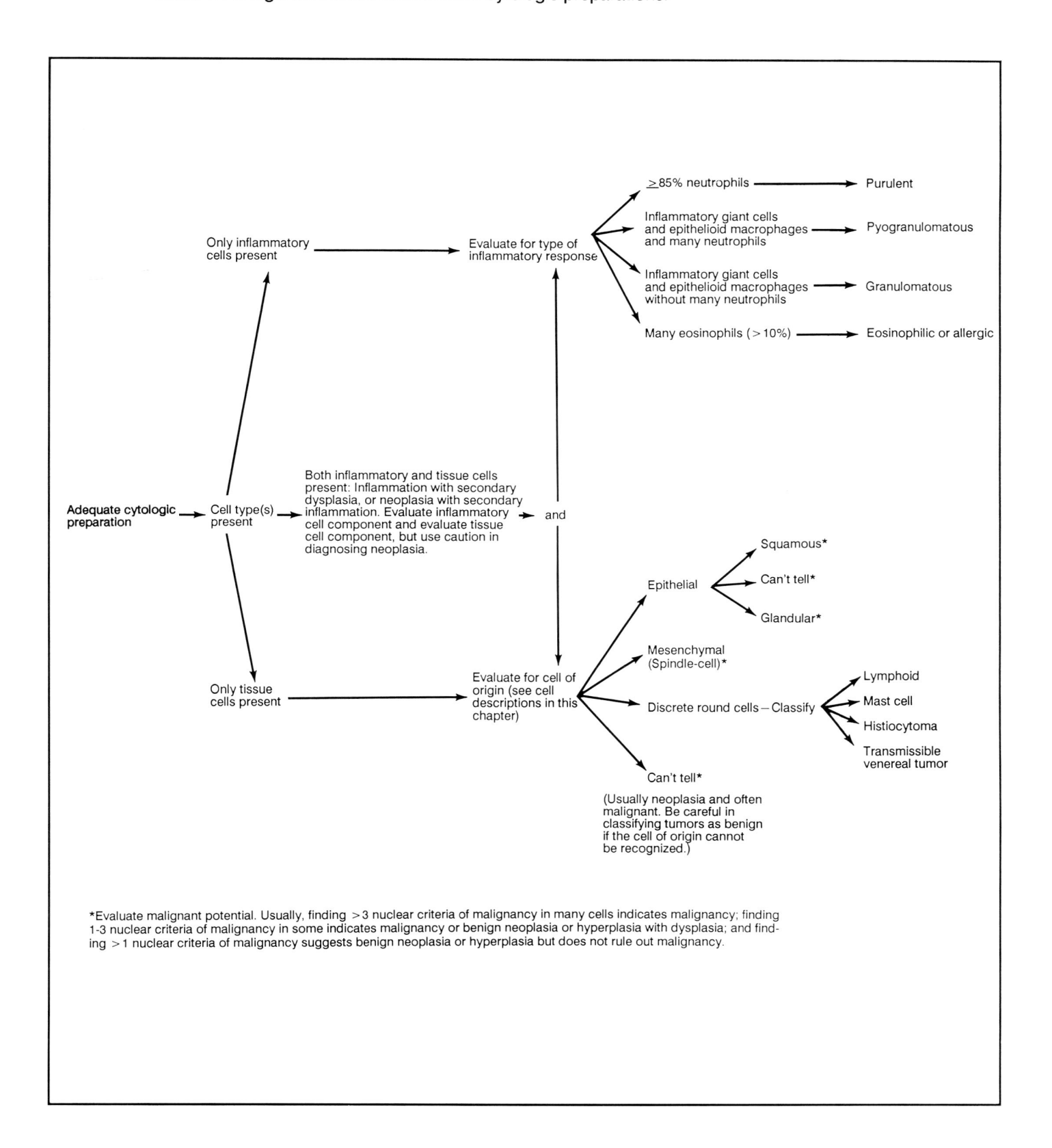

```
Adequate cytologic preparation → Cell type(s) present
```

- **Only inflammatory cells present** → Evaluate for type of inflammatory response
  - ≥85% neutrophils → Purulent
  - Inflammatory giant cells and epithelioid macrophages and many neutrophils → Pyogranulomatous
  - Inflammatory giant cells and epithelioid macrophages without many neutrophils → Granulomatous
  - Many eosinophils (>10%) → Eosinophilic or allergic

- **Both inflammatory and tissue cells present:** Inflammation with secondary dysplasia, or neoplasia with secondary inflammation. Evaluate inflammatory cell component and evaluate tissue cell component, but use caution in diagnosing neoplasia. → *and*

- **Only tissue cells present** → Evaluate for cell of origin (see cell descriptions in this chapter)
  - Epithelial
    - Squamous*
    - Can't tell*
    - Glandular*
  - Mesenchymal (Spindle-cell)*
  - Discrete round cells — Classify
    - Lymphoid
    - Mast cell
    - Histiocytoma
    - Transmissible venereal tumor
  - Can't tell*
    (Usually neoplasia and often malignant. Be careful in classifying tumors as benign if the cell of origin cannot be recognized.)

*Evaluate malignant potential. Usually, finding >3 nuclear criteria of malignancy in many cells indicates malignancy; finding 1-3 nuclear criteria of malignancy in some indicates malignancy or benign neoplasia or hyperplasia with dysplasia; and finding >1 nuclear criteria of malignancy suggests benign neoplasia or hyperplasia but does not rule out malignancy.

Table 3. General appearance of the 3 basic tumor categories.

Tumor Type	General Cell Size	General Cell Shape	Schematic Representation	Cellularity of Aspirates	Clumps or Clusters Common
Epithelial	Large	Round to caudate		Usually high	Yes
Mesenchymal (spindle cell)	Small to medium	Spindle to stellate		Usually low	No
Discrete round cell	Small to medium	Round	Mast cell; Lymphosarcoma; Transmissible venereal tumor; Histiocytoma	Usually high except histiocytoma	No

Evaluation of Tumor Cell Types: Tumors are classified as epithelial, mesenchymal (spindle-cell) or discrete round-cell tumors, based on size, shape and exfoliation characteristics (tendency to exfoliate individual cells or groups of cells and tendency to exfoliate numerous cells or only a few cells) (Table 3). Some tumors do not demonstrate sufficient characteristics to be classified by cell types. Often, these tumors can be recognized as malignant. However, if not, extreme caution should be used in classifying them as benign, since some types of malignant tumors show few cytologic criteria of malignancy. General characteristics of the different tumor cell types are described below.

Epithelial neoplasms tend to exfoliate cells in sheets or clumps, though some individual cells usually are seen. Acinar or ductal arrangements may be identified with adenomas and adenocarcinomas. Cells from epithelial-cell tumors tend to be large to very large, with moderate to abundant cytoplasm and a round nucleus. The nucleus generally has a smooth to slightly coarse chromatin pattern that becomes more coarse and ropy as the tumor's malignant potential increases. The nucleus usually contains one or more prominent nucleoli that become larger and often irregular in shape as the tumor's malignant potential increases. Malignant epithelial-cell tumors often show marked variation in cellular, nuclear and nucleolar size and shape. These variations are most significant when they occur within the same cell or same group of cells. Malignant epithelial-cell tumors also often show a markedly increased nucleus:cytoplasm ratio and may show nuclear molding.

Benign epithelial-cell tumors not undergoing dysplasia subsequent to local inflammation or other irritation usually exfoliate cells indistinguishable from normal cells of the tissue of origin or cells that may be slightly more active than normal cells from the tissue of origin. The nucleolus may be a bit more prominent but still round and of reasonable size, the cytoplasm may be slightly more basophilic, and the nucleus:cytoplasm ratio may be mildly increased.

Local inflammation or other irritation can cause epithelial cells to become dysplastic. Epithelial cells undergoing dysplasia may show mild to moderate variation in cell, nuclear and nucleolar size and shape, increased nucleus:cytoplasm ratio, and coarse chromatin in a few cells. Dysplasia usually does not cause bizarre nuclear and nucleolar morphology. Again, when there is concern that the abnormal tissue cell morphology observed in a cytologic sample is caused by dysplasia, a biopsy from the lesion should be submitted for histopathologic evaluation, or the cause of dysplasia should be treated and the lesion re-evaluated cytologically.

Mesenchymal tumors are commonly referred to as spindle-cell tumors. These tumors tend to yield individual cells instead of groups, clumps or sheets of cells, but a few groups of cells usually can be found. The term spindle cell arises from the fusiform or spindle shape of a few or many of the cells (depending on the specific cell of origin and malignant potential of the tumor). Spindle cells have a fusiform shape, with cytoplasmic tails trailing away from the nucleus in 1 or 2 directions. They usually are small to medium sized and have a moderate amount of light to medium-blue cytoplasm. Nuclei are round to oval, stain with medium intensity and have a smooth or fine lacy chromatin pattern. Nucleoli usually are not visible in nonneoplastic spindle cells. As malignant potential increases, nucleoli become prominent and the chromatin pattern becomes coarser. Also, the spindle shape of the cells becomes less prominent. Cytoplasmic basophilia and nucleus:cytoplasm ratio increase, and cell, nuclear and nucleolar size and shape vary markedly.

Spindle-cell tumors are often difficult or impossible to name cytologically. Also, granulation tissue produces plump, young fibroblasts that may have prominent criteria of malignancy. As a result, granulation tissue can be very difficult to differentiate from a spindle-cell neoplasm. In some cases, histopathologic examination may be necessary to definitively diagnose spindle-cell tumors.

Local inflammation or other irritation can cause mesenchymal cells to become dysplastic. Cellular morphologic changes caused by dysplasia are very similar to the changes caused by neoplasia, but are usually only mildly to moderately severe. Nuclear and nucleolar changes are less sensitive to dysplasia than cytoplasmic changes. If there is concern that the cellular morphology is altered due to dysplasia instead of neoplasia, a biopsy of the lesion should be submitted for histopathologic evaluation or, if possible, the stimulus for dysplasia (inflammation or other irritation) can be treated and the lesion reevaluated cytologically.

Table 4. Easily recognized general and nuclear criteria of malignancy.

Criteria	Description	Schematic Representation
General Criteria		
Anisocytosis and macrocytosis	Variation in cell size, with some cells ≥ 1.5 times larger than normal.	
Hypercellularity	Increased cell exfoliation due to decreased cell adherence.	Not depicted
Pleomorphism (except in lymphoid tissue)	Variable size and shape in cells of the same type.	
Nuclear Criteria		
Macrokaryosis	Increased nuclear size. Cells with nuclei larger than 10 μ in diameter suggest malignancy.	RBC
Increased nucleus: cytoplasm ratio (N:C)	Normal nonlymphoid cells usually have a N:C of 1:3 to 1:8, depending on the tissue. Ratios ≥ 1:2 suggest malignancy.	See "macrokaryosis"
Anisokaryosis	Variation in nuclear size. This is especially important if the nuclei of multinucleated cells vary in size.	
Multinucleation	Multiple nucleation in a cell. This is especially important if the nuclei vary in size.	
Increased mitotic figures	Mitosis is rare in normal tissue.	normal abnormal
Abnormal mitosis	Improper alignment of chromosomes.	See "increased mitotic figures"
Coarse chromatin pattern	The chromatin pattern is coarser than normal. It may appear ropy or cord-like.	
Nuclear molding	Deformation of nuclei by other nuclei within the same cell or adjacent cells.	
Macronucleoli	Nucleoli are increased in size. Nucleoli ≥ 5μ strongly suggest malignancy. For reference, RBC are 5-6μ.	RBC
Angular nucleoli	Nucleoli are fusiform or have other angular shapes, instead of their normal round to slightly oval shape.	
Anisonucleoliosis	Variation in nucleolar shape or size (especially important if the variation is within the same nucleus.	See "angular nucleoli"

Discrete round-cell tumors are also called cutaneous round-cell tumors and cutaneous discrete-cell tumors. These tumors tend to exfoliate small to medium-sized, single, round cells. The discrete round-cell tumors are mast-cell tumors, lymphosarcomas, histiocytomas and transmissible venereal tumors. Occasionally, malignant melanomas and basal-cell tumors also yield discrete round cells in cytologic smears.

Evaluation of Malignant Potential: The malignant potential of tumors is estimated by evaluating tumor cells for indications of anaplasia and asynchronous development (criteria of malignancy) (Table 4). Nuclear criteria of malignancy are more reliable than cytoplasmic criteria for estimating malignant potential. Cytoplasmic criteria of malignancy are more sensitive to cellular physiologic alterations caused by nonneoplastic processes, such as inflammation, than are nuclear criteria. As a result, cytoplasmic criteria of malignancy are encountered due to hyperplasia and/or dysplasia more commonly than nuclear criteria. Recognition of more than 3 nuclear criteria of malignancy in a high percentage of tumor cells is strong evidence that the tumor is malignant. When 1-3 criteria of malignancy are recognized in some tumor cells, the tumor may be malignant or benign and histopathologic examination may be needed for definitive determination.

If malignant criteria are not recognized, the tumor is most likely benign. However, some tumors, such as canine thyroid tumors, may be malignant but show few, if any, criteria of malignancy. Therefore, if the cell type of a tumor cannot be recognized or if the evaluator is not aware of which malignant tumor types are less likely to show criteria of malignancy, caution must be exercised in classifying the tumor as benign. Instead, the cytologic preparation can be sent to a veterinary clinical pathologist/cytologist for interpretation, or a biopsy can be submitted for histopathologic examination.

Submission of Cytologic Preparations and Samples for Interpretation

When in-house evaluation of a cytologic preparation does not furnish sufficient reliable information for managing a case, the preparation can be submitted to a veterinary clinical pathologist/cytologist for interpretation, or an alternative procedure, such as biopsy and histopathologic evaluation, can be performed. If possible, the person to whom the cytologic preparation is sent should be contacted, and specifics concerning sample handling should be discussed, such as the number of smears to send, whether to fix or stain the smears before mailing, etc. The following discussion gives some general guidelines for submitting cytologic preparations for interpretation.

When possible, 2-3 air-dried unfixed smears, and 2-3 air-dried Romanowsky-stained smears should be submitted. The air-dried unfixed smears can be stained by the pathologist with the Romanowsky-type or new methylene blue stains of his or her choice. The Romanowsky-stained smears are a safety factor. Some tissues stain poorly when they are air dried but not stained for several days. Also, slides occasionally are shattered during transport and cannot be stained upon receipt. Sometimes, microscopic examination of shards from the broken pre-stained smears allows diagnosis. If only a couple of smears can be prepared from the sample, one should be submitted air dried and unfixed, and the other submitted air dried and stained. Smears should be well labeled with pencil, alcohol-resistant ink or another permanent labeling method.

If a Papanicolaou-type stain is to be used, several wet-fixed smears should be submitted.

Fluid samples should have smears prepared from them immediately. Both direct smears and concentrated smears should be submitted. Also, an EDTA (lavender top) and sterile serum tube (red top) fluid sample should be submitted. A total nucleated cell count and total protein concentration can be performed on the EDTA tube sample and, if necessary, chemical analyses can be performed on the serum tube sample.

Slides must be well protected when mailed. Simple cardboard mailers do not provide sufficient protection to prevent slide breakage if they are mailed in unpadded envelopes. Marking the envelope with such phrases as "Fragile," "Glass," "Breakable" and "Please Hand Cancel" have little success. Usually, placing a pad of bubble-paper or styrofoam on each side of the slide holder prevents slide breakage. Also, slides can be mailed in plastic slide holders or innovative holders, such as small pill bottles.

Slides should not be mailed with formalin-containing samples and should be protected against moisture. Formalin fumes alter the staining characteristics of smears and water causes cell lysis.

Submission of Samples for Culture

Culture results are strongly influenced by sample collection, preparation and transport. The following procedures are suggested to optimize success in culturing lesions and fluids:

- Call the laboratory before collecting the sample.
- Collect the sample as aseptically as possible.
- Submit fresh samples for culture.
- Use proper equipment for collection and transport of the sample.
- Use a timely transportation service.

Call the Lab Before Collecting the Sample

Techniques, media, days when cultures are read or subcultures are performed, etc, often vary from laboratory to laboratory. By contacting the laboratory to which the sample will be submitted, such things as optimum sample type, transport medium, day of the week to submit the sample, etc, can be discussed. Also, some laboratories furnish culture supplies. Expensive and/or quickly outdated supplies, such as blood culture tubes, may be ordered from the laboratory as needed. Early communication with the laboratory also allows the laboratory to prepare for the sample and ensure that any special media required are available.

Collect Samples as Aseptically as Possible

All samples should be collected as aseptically as possible. Even samples collected from lesions that naturally are exposed to secondary contamination, such as cutaneous ulcers, should be protected from further contamination. When samples are collected from more than one lesion, care should be taken not to cross-contaminate the samples. Finding the same organism in several different lesions is strong evidence that the organism is involved in development of the lesions. Therefore, cross-contamination of samples from different lesions can lead to misinterpretation of culture results. When fluids are collected, anticoagulant and serum tubes should not be assumed to be sterile.[8,21] Also, EDTA, through its effect on bacterial cell walls, can be bacteriostatic or bactericidal.

Submit Fresh Samples

Samples should be submitted as soon after collection as possible. Fluid aspiration, resection of lesions to be cultured, exploratory surgeries during which culture is anticipated, and other procedures that may produce samples to be cultured should be scheduled to allow immediate transporation of samples to the laboratory. During transport, samples should be kept cool but not frozen.

Tissue and fluid samples usually are more rewarding than swab samples for isolation of a causative agent. Individual tissue samples submitted for culture should be about 4 cm square or larger. Whirl-Pak (Nasco, Ft Atkinson, WI), Ziploc or heat-sealed plastic bags are excellent for submitting tissue samples for culture. Such samples as abscesses and skin, known to contain bacteria, must be packaged separately from other tissues. Culturette-type transport systems should be used to prevent small biopsies from drying during transport. Avoid shipping biopsies in sterile saline, as this may cause negative culture results.

Fluid samples (urine, milk, joint fluid, thoracic fluid, abdominal fluid, abscess aspirates) can be submitted in sterile Vacu-Tainer tubes, small Whirl-Pak bags or sterile disposable syringes. Fluids for anaerobic cultures should be collected in syringes, with air excluded, and then capped and transported immediately to the laboratory for culture. However, for optimal results or if a time delay is anticipated, the fluid should be placed in a transport system that supports both aerobic and anaerobic bacteria. These systems often can be obtained from the laboratory performing the culture. Transport culture tubes, such as Port-A-Cul Tubes (BBL Microbiology Systems, Cockeysville, MD) are commercially available for samples obtained on swabs. Containers, such as Port-A-Cul Vials (BBL) are commercially available for fluid samples. These systems usually support a wide variety of anaerobic and aerobic organisms for up to 72 hours at 20-25 C.

If separate aerobic and anaerobic transport systems are used, a culturette-like transport system, such as Culture Collection and Transport Tube (Curtin Matheson Scientific, Burbank, CA) containing Amies medium with charcoal, is suggested for aerobic cultures. These seem to be excellent transport and holding media for fastidious bacteria. Anaerobic transport systems, such as B-D Vacu-Tainer Anaerobic Specimen Collector (Becton-Dickinson, Rutherford, NJ), can be used to transport fluid, small tissue specimens or swabs. However, they are large and cumbersome for mailing, and must be packaged well to prevent the glass vial from breaking. Anaerobic transport systems, such as the Marion Scientific Anaerobic Culturette (Kansas City, MO), have prereduced Cary-Blair transport medium to prevent the swab from drying. These small plastic units are sturdy and easy to handle and mail. However, they can only be used for swabs.

When biopsies or aspirates are not obtainable or warranted, swabs are useful for sample collection, especially of mucosal surfaces and deep within soft tissue lesions. Culturette-type transport swabs are preferred; those containing Amies medium with charcoal are superior for fastidious organisms. Anaerobic systems, such as mentioned above, are necessary for transport of swabs for anaerobic culture. Swabs without medium can dry out in transport, resulting in false-negative results, whereas swabs submitted in broth medium often are overgrown by contaminants. Separate swabs should be submitted if additional cultures for fungi and/or viruses are desired.

In general, samples submitted for fungal culture should be collected and transported in the same manner as samples for bacterial culture. Again, tissues and body fluids are preferred to swabs. Swab samples should never be submitted for dermatophyte cultures. Communication with the laboratory chosen to perform the cultures is especially important before samples for fungal culture are collected.

References

1. Allen and Prasse: Cytologic diagnosis of neoplasia and perioperative implementation. *Comp Cont Ed Pract Vet* 8:72-80, 1986.
2. Barton: Cytologic diagnosis of neoplastic diseases: an algorithm. *Texas Vet Med J* 45:11-13, 1983.
3. Boon *et al*: A cytologic comparison of Romanowsky stains and Papanicolaou-type stains. I. Introduction, methodology and cytology of normal tissues. *Vet Clin Pathol* 11:22-30, 1982.
4. DeNicola: Diagnositic cytology, collection techniques and sample handling. *Proc 4th Ann Mtg ACVIM*, 1987. pp 15-25.
5. Griffith and Lumsden: Fine needle aspiration cytology and histologic correlation in canine tumors. *Vet Clin Pathol* 13:13-17, 1984.
6. Meyers and Feldman: Diagnostic cytology in veterinary medicine. *Southwestern Vet* 25:277-282, 1972.
7. Meyers and Franks: Clinical cytology, management of tissue specimens. *Mod Vet Pract* 67:255-259, 1986.
8. O'Rourke: Cytology technics. *Mod Vet Pract* 64:185-189, 1983.
9. Rebar: Diagnostic cytology in veterinary practice. *Proc 54th Ann Mtg AAHA*, 1987. pp 498-504.
10. Rebar, in Kirk: *Current Veterinary Therapy VII*. Saunders, Philadelphia, 1980. pp 16-27.
11. Seybold *et al*: Exfoliative cytology. *VM/SAC* 77:1029-1033, 1982.
12. Bottles *et al*: Fine needle aspiration biopsy. *Am J Med* 81:525-529, 1986.
13. Cochland-Priolett *et al*: Comparison of cytologic examination of smears and histologic examination of tissue cores obtained by fine needle aspiration biopsy of the liver. *Acta Cytol* 31:476-480, 1987.
14. Kline and Neal: Needle aspiration biopsy: A critical appraisal. *JAMA* 239:36-39, 1978.
15. Kline *et al*: Needle aspiration biopsy: Diagnosis of subcutaneous nodules and lymph nodes. *JAMA* 235:2848-2850, 1976.
16. Ljung *et al*: Fine needle aspiration biopsy of the prostate gland: A study of 103 cases with histological follow-up. *J Urol* 135:955-958, 1986.
17. Lundquist: Fine needle aspiration biopsy of the liver. *Acta Med Scand* (suppl) 520:1-28, 1971.
18. Mills and Griffiths: The accuracy of clinical diagnoses by fine-needle aspiration cytology. *Aust Vet J* 61:269-271, 1984.
19. Livraghi *et al*: Risk in fine needle abdominal biopsy. *J Clin Ultrasound* 11:77-81, 1983.
20. Zajicek: Aspiration biopsy cytology: 1. Cytology of supradiaphragmatic organs. *Monogr Clin Cytol* 4:1-211, 1974.
21. Meyer: The management of cytology specimens. *Comp Cont Ed Pract Vet* 9:10-16, 1987.

2

Cutaneous & Subcutaneous Lesions:
Masses, Cysts, Ulcers and Fistulous Tracts

R.D. Tyler, R.L. Cowell and J.H. Meinkoth

Cytologic examination can be very useful when a cutaneous or subcutaneous lesion is not easily diagnosed by simple clinical evaluation. Certainly, when lesions are not responsive to therapy, cytologic evaluation can be very helpful. Cutaneous and subcutaneous lesions are easily accessible and there are no significant contraindications to collecting samples from them. Tranquilization and/or anesthesia is seldom needed for sample collection. Often the cytologic preparation can be collected, prepared, stained and microscopically evaluated in minutes, providing a diagnosis, prognosis, indication of appropriate therapy, and/or guidance for the next diagnostic procedure.

Collection Techniques

Lesions may be swabbed, imprinted, scraped and/or aspirated, depending on the character of the lesion and tractability of the patient. Ulcerated lesions should be imprinted, then cleaned, dried and reimprinted. After the imprints are made, scrapings should be obtained. Aspirates are then collected from deep within the lesion or mass. Obviously, lesions without an eroded or ulcerated surface must be aspirated.

Swabs

Generally, cytologic swab smears are made only when imprints, scrapings and aspirates cannot be collected. Sterile cotton swabs moistened with sterile isotonic fluid, such as 0.9% NaCl, are used. Moistening the swab helps minimize cell damage during sample collection and smear preparation but is unnecessary if the lesion itself is very moist. After sample collection, the swab is gently rolled along the flat surface of a clean glass slide. Do not rub the swab across the slide surface, as this causes excessive cell damage. If a Romanowsky-type stain is used, the smears are air dried before staining (Chapter 1).

Imprints

Imprints are made by removing any scab covering the lesion and then touching the dry surface of a clean glass slide to the surface of the lesion. If *Dermatophilus congolensis* infection is suspected, the underside of the scab is imprinted also. The lesion is then cleaned with a nonirritating antiseptic, wiped dry with a sterile gauze sponge or other clean absorbent material, and reimprinted.

Scrapings

Scrapings of cutaneous lesions are made by rubbing the edge of a blunt instrument, such as a glass slide or the back of a scalpel blade, across the lesion. The accumulated cells along the edge of the blunt instrument are then spread onto a clean, dry glass slide by one of the techniques described in Chapter 1.

Aspirates of Solid Masses

Aspirates are obtained by using a 21- to 25-ga needle attached to a 3- to 20-ml syringe. If microbiologic examination is to be performed on a portion of the sample, the area of aspiration should be surgically prepared. Otherwise, skin preparation is essentially that required for vaccination or venipuncture. An alcohol swab can be used to clean the area.

The mass to be aspirated is held firmly to aid penetration and control the direction of the needle. The needle, attached to a syringe, is introduced into the center of the mass and strong negative pressure is applied by withdrawing the plunger about one-half to three-fourths the volume of the syringe (Fig 1, Chapter 1). Several areas of the mass must be sampled, but aspiration of the sample into the barrel of the syringe and contamination of the sample by aspiration of tissue surrounding the mass must be avoided. To accomplish this, when the mass is large enough to allow the needle to be redirected and moved to several areas in the mass without danger of the needle's leaving the mass, negative pressure is maintained during redirection and movement of the needle. However, when the mass is not large enough for the needle to be redirected and moved without danger of the needle's leaving the mass, the negative pressure is relieved during redirection and movement of the needle. In this situation, negative pressure is applied only when the needle is static.

Often, high-quality collections do not have the sample showing in the syringe and sometimes not even in the hub of the needle. Negative pressure is then released from the syringe. If negative pressure is not released before the needle is removed from the tissue being aspirated, aspiration of cells and blood from the subcutaneous tissues and skin into the sample may interfere with interpretation of the aspirate. If negative pressure remains on the syringe when the needle exits the skin, the portion of the sample in the barrel and hub of the needle will be aspirated into the syringe.

Frequently, when only a small amount of sample has been collected and it is aspirated into the syringe, the sample cannot be recovered from the syringe and another sample must be collected. Once the negative pressure has been fully released, the needle is removed from the mass and skin. The needle is then removed from the syringe and air is aspirated into the syringe. Next, the needle is replaced onto the syringe and some of the tissue in the barrel and hub of the needle is expelled onto the middle of a glass slide by rapidly depressing the plunger.

Aspirate Smear Preparation

A combination of slide preparation techniques should be used to spread aspirates of solid masses (Figs 2-5, Chapter 1). One combination procedure (Fig 2, Chapter 1) is to first spray the aspirate onto the middle of a slide (prep slide). Next, keeping the prep slide on a flat, solid, horizontal surface, pull another slide (spreader slide) backward at a 45° angle to the first slide until it contacts about one-third of the aspirate. The spreader slide is then slid forward smoothly and rapidly as if making a blood smear. Next, the spreader slide is placed horizontally over the back one-third of the aspirate at a right angle to the prep slide. Allow the weight of the top slide to spread the material, resisting the temptation to compress the slides manually. Keeping the top slide flat and horizontal, quickly and smoothly slide it across the prep slide. This makes a squash prep of the back third of the aspirates. The middle third of the aspirate is left untouched. This procedure leaves the front third of the aspirate gently spread. If the aspirate is of fragile tissue, this area should contain sufficient unruptured cells to interpret. The back third of the aspirate has been spread with the shear forces of a squash prep. If the aspirate contains clumps of cells that are difficult to spread, there should be some clumps sufficiently spread in the back one-third of the preparation. If the aspirate is of very low cellularity, the middle third remains more concentrated and is the most efficient area to study.

The squash preparation (Fig 3, Chapter 1) is a commonly used sample-spreading technique. In expert hands this procedure can yield excellent cytologic smears; however, in less experienced hands it often yields smears that cannot be evaluated because too many cells are ruptured or the sample is not sufficiently spread. A squash prep is made by expelling the aspirate onto the middle of a microscope slide (prep slide). A second slide (spreader slide) is placed over the aspirate at right angles to the first slide. Keeping the spreader slide horizontal to the prep slide, the spreader slide is then rapidly and smoothly slid across the prep slide. A modification of the squash preparation that has less tendency to rupture cells is to lay the second slide over the aspirate, rotate the second slide 45° and lift it upward (Fig 4, Chapter 1).

Another technique for spreading aspirates (Fig 5, Chapter 1) is to drag the aspirate peripherally in several directions with the point of a needle, producing a starfish shape of the aspirate. This technique tends not to damage fragile cells, but leaves a thick layer of tissue fluid around the cells. Sometimes the thick layer of fluid prevents the cells from spreading well and interferes with evaluation of cell detail. Usually, some acceptable areas are present.

Aspirates of Fluid-Filled Masses and Cysts

Aspirates can be collected from fluid-filled masses and cysts with a 21- to 25-ga needle attached to a 3-ml syringe. When possible, enough fluid should be aspirated to prepare several cytologic smears, perform a nucleated cell count and total protein analysis, and obtain a sample for culture. Usually 1-3 ml is sufficient.

The lesion is prepared as described above for solid masses. Smears can be prepared directly from the aspirated fluids or from the sediment of centrifuged fluids using the blood smear, line smear and/or squash prep techniques as described in Chapter 1.

When lesions contain solid areas and fluid areas, separate aspirates of each type area should be collected.

General Appearance of the Lesion

The general physical appearance of the lesion is helpful in interpreting the cytologic findings.

Fistulous Tracts

Fistulous tracts are usually caused by infectious agents or foreign bodies. They should be probed for foreign bodies, and culture and swab samples should be collected from deep within the tracts. Cytologic preparations should be carefully perused for filamentous rods staining light blue, with intermittent pink to purple areas, with Romanowsky-type stains (Plate 3). This morphology is characteristic of *Nocardia* spp and *Actinomyces* spp, which often cause fistulous tracts, but occasionally occurs with some anaerobic bacteria also, such as *Fusobacterium* spp.

Ulcerated Lesions

Ulcerated lesions may be areas of skin that have been injured and/or infected, and become ulcerated and indurated due to the subsequent inflammatory reaction, or may be areas of ulcerated skin overlying a cutaneous or subcutaneous mass. Generally, examination of the lesion indicates whether there is an underlying mass. Ulcerated lesions can result from infectious, foreign body, allergic, parasitic or neoplastic causes.

Nonulcerated Masses

Nonulcerated masses may be solid or fluid filled. Nonulcerated solid masses usually are neoplastic in origin. However, inflammatory conditions occasionally produce solid nonulcerated masses. Fluid-filled nonulcerated masses usually are nonneoplastic in origin but occasionally represent cystic neoplasia.

General Evaluation of Cytologic Smears

The first step in cytologic evaluation of a smear is to determine if sufficient intact cells are present, and if the sample is spread and stained adequately to allow evaluation of cell morphology. If repeated collection attempts fail to yield sufficient numbers of cells for cytologic evaluation, an alternative procedure, such as biopsy or culture (depending on the character of the lesion), may be necessary.

Once a suitable cytologic preparation is achieved, smears are evaluated for evidence of inflammation and/or neoplasia (Chart 1). If all the cells from a solid mass are tissue cells (*ie*, no inflammatory cells are present), the lesion was missed or is due to either neoplasia or hyperplasia. If all the cells are inflammatory cells, an inflammatory process is most likely the cause of the lesion, but an inflamed neoplasm cannot be ruled out. An admixture of inflammatory cells and dysplastic tissue cells can be caused by inflammation with secondary tissue cell dysplasia, or neoplasia with secondary inflammation. Therefore, caution must be used in making the diagnosis of malignancy if evidence of inflammation is detected.

Evaluation of an Inflammatory Cell Population

Chart 2 provides an algorithm to aid in evaluation of the inflammatory cell component of cutaneous and subcutaneous lesions. Table 1 gives some general considerations for some inflammatory responses. If most of the inflammatory cells are neutrophils (Plates 1 and 3), especially if degenerate neutrophils are present, but no bacteria are found, a covert infection may be present or the neutrophilic inflammatory response may be due to one of the conditions listed under "Marked predominance of neutrophils" in Table 1. The lesion can be cultured to identify a covert infection. If culture results reveal an infectious agent, appropriate therapy can be instituted. If culture results do not reveal an infectious agent or if therapy for the infectious agent identified

Chapter 2

Chart 1. An algorithm to aid in classifying cellular components of cytologic preparations from solid lesions.

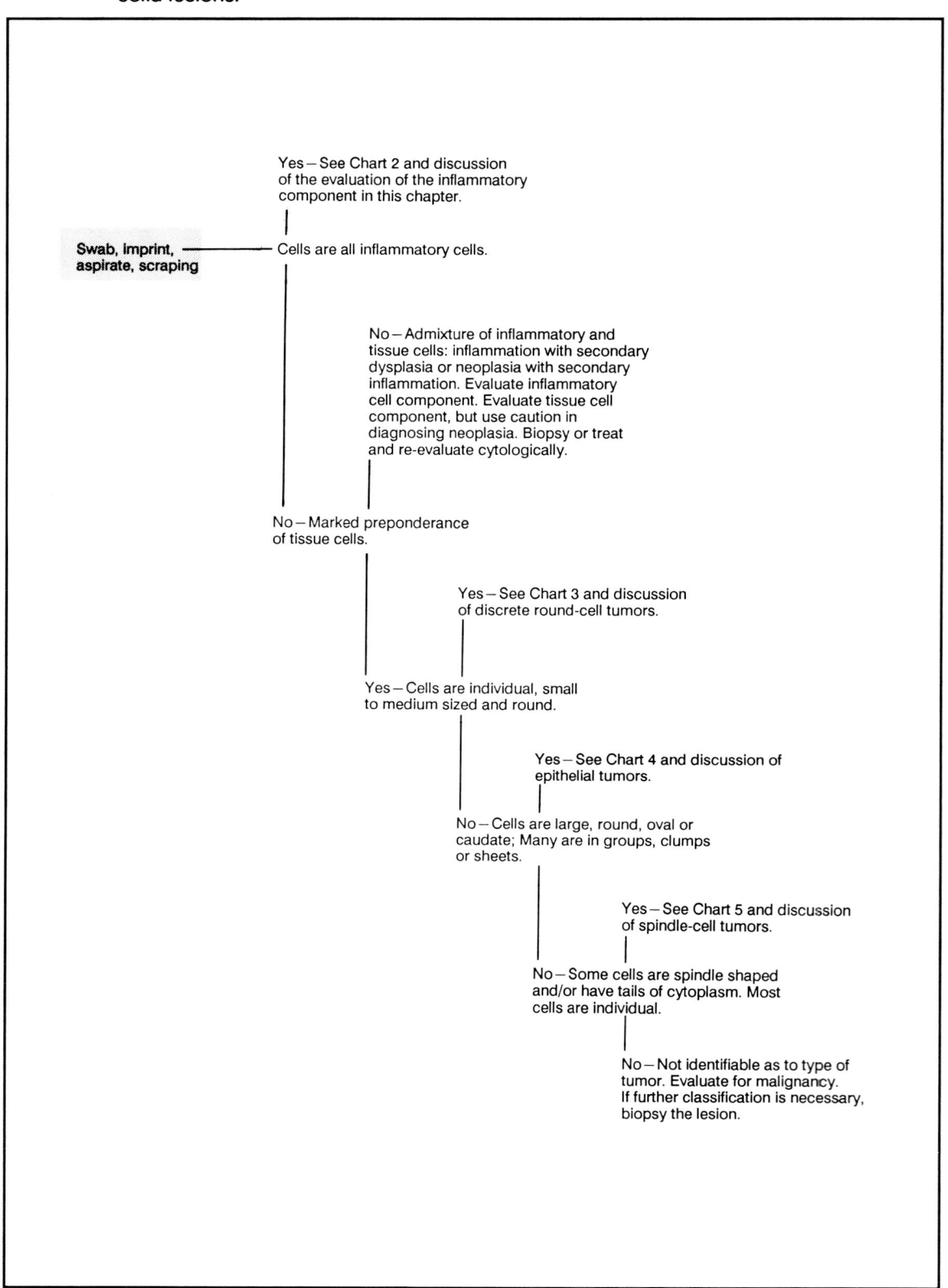

Swab, imprint, aspirate, scraping — Cells are all inflammatory cells.

- Yes — See Chart 2 and discussion of the evaluation of the inflammatory component in this chapter.

- No — Admixture of inflammatory and tissue cells: inflammation with secondary dysplasia or neoplasia with secondary inflammation. Evaluate inflammatory cell component. Evaluate tissue cell component, but use caution in diagnosing neoplasia. Biopsy or treat and re-evaluate cytologically.

No — Marked preponderance of tissue cells.

Yes — Cells are individual, small to medium sized and round.

- Yes — See Chart 3 and discussion of discrete round-cell tumors.

No — Cells are large, round, oval or caudate; Many are in groups, clumps or sheets.

- Yes — See Chart 4 and discussion of epithelial tumors.

No — Some cells are spindle shaped and/or have tails of cytoplasm. Most cells are individual.

- Yes — See Chart 5 and discussion of spindle-cell tumors.

No — Not identifiable as to type of tumor. Evaluate for malignancy. If further classification is necessary, biopsy the lesion.

Table 1. Some conditions suggested by certain proportions of inflammatory cells.

Inflammatory Cell Population	First Considerations	Second Considerations
Marked predominance (85%) of neutrophils:		
Many neutrophils are degenerate	Gram-negative bacteria Gram-positive bacteria	Abscess secondary to neoplasia, foreign bodies, etc
A few neutrophils are degenerate	Gram-positive bacteria Gram-negative bacteria Higher bacteria (*Nocardia*, *Actinomyces*, etc)	Fungi Protozoa Foreign body Immune mediated Chemical or traumatic injury Abscess secondary to neoplasia
No neutrophils are degenerate	Gram-positive bacteria Higher bacteria (*Nocardia*, *Actinomyces*, etc) Chemical or traumatic injury Panniculitis	Gram-negative bacteria Fungi Foreign body Abscess secondary to neoplasia
Admixture of inflammatory cells:		
15-40% macrophages	Higher bacteria (*Nocardia*, *Actinomyces*, etc) Fungi Protozoa Neoplasia Foreign body Panniculitis Any resolving inflammatory lesions	Nonfilamentous Gram-positive bacteria Parasites, chronic allergic inflammation and eosinophilic granuloma if eosinophil numbers are increased
>40% macrophages	Fungi Foreign body Protozoa Neoplasia Panniculitis Any resolving inflammatory lesions	Parasites, chronic allergic inflammation and eosinophilic granuloma if eosinophil numbers are increased
Giant inflammatory cells present	Fungi Foreign body Protozoa Collagen necrosis Panniculitis Parasites (if eosinophils are present)	
>10% eosinophils	Allergic inflammation Parasites Eosinophilic granuloma Collagen necrosis Mast-cell tumor	Neoplasia Foreign body Hyphating fungi

by culture is not effective, cytologic examination can be repeated or a biopsy can be submitted for histopathologic evaluation.

When >15% of the inflammatory cells present are macrophages (Plates 2 and 3) and/or giant inflammatory cells are present (Plate 3), fungal infection or foreign body granuloma should be considered. The slide should be carefully perused for organisms or signs of a foreign body, such as refractile debris (Fig 1). Also, historical information concerning possible introduction of foreign material should be sought. If no organisms are found and there is no historical information indicating introduction of a foreign substance into the area, the tissue can be cultured or a biopsy can be submitted for histopathologic examination.

If the proportion of eosinophils exceeds 10% (Plate 3), an allergic, parasitic, foreign body reaction or eosinophilic granuloma complex lesion should be considered. Again, the slide should be carefully searched for organisms or signs of foreign material. If none is found, the lesion can be cultured (including fungal cultures) or a biopsy can be submitted for histopathologic evaluation. If the lesion is cultured but not biopsied, and the culture fails to yield an organism, the lesion may be treated as an eosinophilic granuloma if the historical and clinical evidence indicates an eosinophilic granuloma complex lesion. In this situation, the lesion should be watched carefully. If the response to therapy is not appropriate, a biopsy of the lesion should be submitted for histopathologic evaluation.

Figure 1. Fine-needle aspirate from a foreign body reaction in a dog. Refractile foreign material is scattered throughout the photomicrograph. A large clump of cell debris and refractile foreign body material is in the center. (Wright's stain, original magnification 100X)

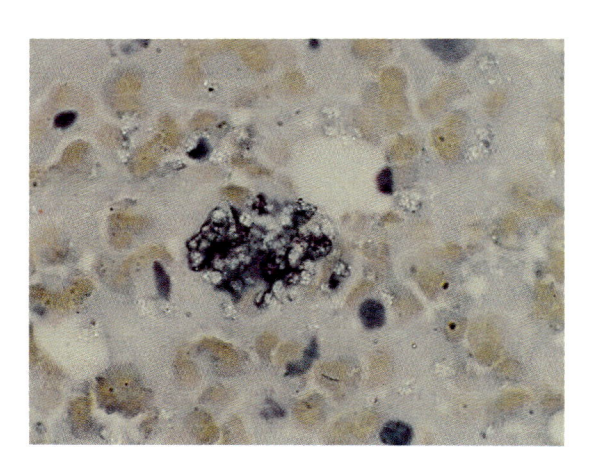

Figure 2. Aspirate from a dog with a nasal polyp caused by *Rhinosporidium seeberi*. Note the dysplastic epithelial cells (mild anisocytosis, anisokaryosis, prominent nucleoli, coarse chromatin, cytoplasmic basophilia) and the numerous neutrophils. *Rhinosporidium* organisms were found in other areas of the smear. (see Chap 3, Fig 5) (Wright's stain, original magnification 100X)

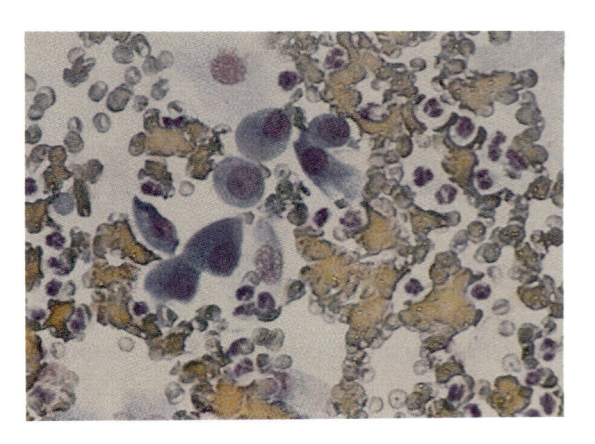

When tissue cells showing criteria of malignancy are accompanied by inflammatory cells (Fig 2), the sample should be interpreted cautiously. Dysplasia in tissue adjacent to inflammatory reactions can alter tissue cell morphology. As a result, cells undergoing dysplasia in response to a local inflammatory process can be erroneously classified as neoplastic cells. As the intensity of the inflammatory reaction increases, the assurance with which a diagnosis of neoplasia can be made decreases.

Selected Infectious Agents

Infectious agents invariably cause lesions characterized by the presence of inflammatory cells. Bacterial agents usually produce lesions characterized by >85% neutrophils (Plates 1 and 3) (many of which may be degenerate), a few macrophages, and a few lymphocytes and plasma cells. On the other hand, mycotic agents produce lesions that tend to have more macrophages than in bacterial lesions, but neutrophils often predominate and occasionally eosinophils are plentiful with hyphating fungi. Mycotic lesions often contain lymphocytes, plasma cells and fibroblasts also. The infectious agent, location of the lesion, chronicity of the lesion, and immune status of the animal influence the character of the lesion.

Cocci: Pathogenic bacterial cocci are usually Gram positive and of the genus *Staphylococcus*, *Streptococcus*, *Streptopeptococcus* or *Peptococcus* (Plate 3). Staphylococci usually occur in clusters of 4-12 bacteria, while streptococci,

Chart 2. An algorithm to aid in evaluating aspirates containing a preponderance of inflammatory cells.

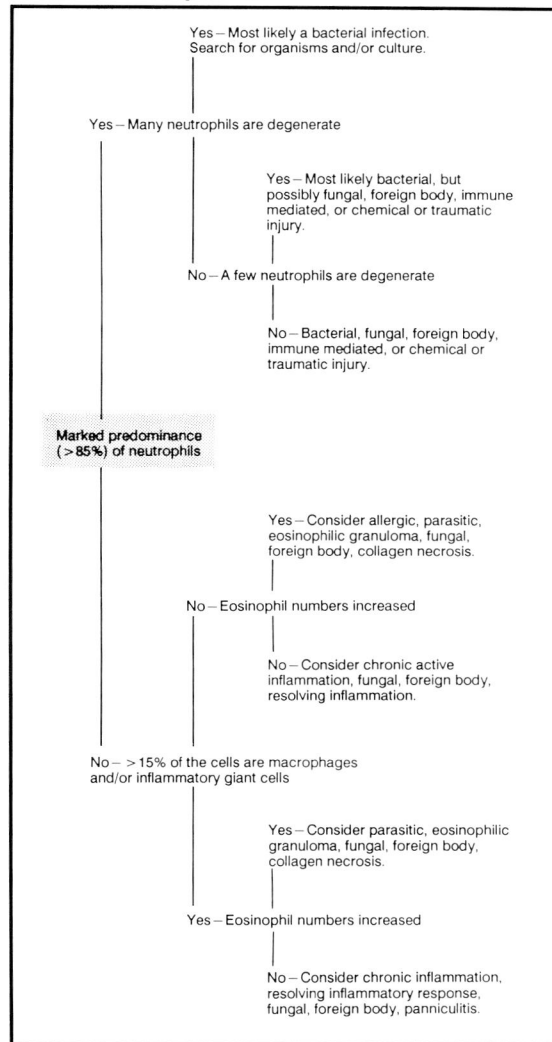

```
                    Yes — Most likely a bacterial infection.
                          Search for organisms and/or culture.
                    |
        Yes — Many neutrophils are degenerate
                    |
                    Yes — Most likely bacterial, but
                          possibly fungal, foreign body, immune
                          mediated, or chemical or traumatic
                          injury.
                    |
        No — A few neutrophils are degenerate
                    |
                    No — Bacterial, fungal, foreign body,
                         immune mediated, or chemical or
                         traumatic injury.

Marked predominance
( >85%) of neutrophils
                    Yes — Consider allergic, parasitic,
                          eosinophilic granuloma, fungal,
                          foreign body, collagen necrosis.
                    |
        No — Eosinophil numbers increased
                    |
                    No — Consider chronic active
                         inflammation, fungal, foreign body,
                         resolving inflammation.

No — >15% of the cells are macrophages
and/or inflammatory giant cells
                    |
                    Yes — Consider parasitic, eosinophilic
                          granuloma, fungal, foreign body,
                          collagen necrosis.
                    |
        Yes — Eosinophil numbers increased
                    |
                    No — Consider chronic inflammation,
                         resolving inflammatory response,
                         fungal, foreign body, panniculitis.
```

streptopeptococci and peptococci tend to occur in short or long chains of organisms. Staphylococci and streptococci are aerobic, while streptopeptococci and peptococci are anaerobic. When cocci are identified in cytologic preparations, aerobic and anaerobic cultures and sensitivity tests should be performed to identify the organism and the optimum antibacterial. Because most cocci are Gram positive, antibacterial therapy effective against Gram-positive organisms should be used when it is necessary to start therapy before culture and sensitivity results are received.

Small Bacilli: Most small bacilli are Gram negative. Some can be recognized as bipolar rods (Plate 3). All pathogenic bipolar bacilli are Gram negative. Bacillary infections are usually associated with a marked neutrophilic inflammatory response. When small bacilli are recognized in cytologic preparations, the lesion should be cultured to identify the organism and sensitivity tests performed to determine the optimum antibacterial therapy. If it is necessary to institute antibacterial therapy before culture and sensitivity results are received, the therapy employed should be effective against Gram-negative organisms, since most pathogenic small bacilli are Gram negative.

Filamentous Rods: Pathogenic filamentous rods that cause cutaneous or subcutaneous lesions are usually *Nocardia* spp or *Actinomyces* spp (Plate 3). Rarely, *Mycobacterium* spp and some anaerobes, such as *Fusobacterium*, may be filamentous. *Nocardia* and *Actinomyces* generally have a distinctive morphology in cytologic preparations stained with Romanowsky-type stains. They are characterized by long, slender (filamentous) strands that stain pale blue and have intermittent, small, pink to purple areas. This morphology is characteristic of both *Nocardia* and *Actinomyces* spp, and the filamentous form of *Fusobacterium* spp. When these features are recognized cytologically, cultures should be performed specifically for *Nocardia*, *Actinomyces* and anaerobes.

Mycobacterium spp, on the other hand, often do not stain with Romanowsky-type stains. As a result, negative images (Plate 4) may be observed in the cytoplasm of macrophages and/or inflammatory giant cells. When epithelioid macrophages and/or inflammatory giant cells are encountered in cytologic preparations not containing any obvious organisms, a careful search for negative images of *Mycobacterium* spp should be made. *Mycobacterium* spp stain with acid-fast stains. Therefore, when negative images are encountered or when the character of the lesion suggests *Mycobacterium* spp, an acid-fast stain can be performed to demonstrate the organism, and/or cultures for *Mycobacterium* spp can be performed to identify the organism.

Because *Nocardia* spp, *Actinomyces* spp, anaerobes and *Mycobacterium* spp are often refractory to common antimicrobial therapy and reliable culture of these organisms has special requirements, cytologic examination is very useful in indicating that special cultures are needed.

Large Bacilli: Large bacilli found in cytologic preparations usually are not pathogenic. Large bacilli that are pathogenic and sometimes infect cutaneous and subcutaneous tissues include *Clostridium* spp and, infrequently, *Bacillus* spp. When large bacilli are thought to be pathogenic, both aerobic and anaerobic cultures should be performed. Also, the smears should be inspected for large bacilli containing spores (Plate 3). If spore forms are found, clostridia are most likely.

Sporothrix schenckii: *Sporothrix schenckii* infection (sporothricosis) can cause raised proliferative, often ulcerated, lesions in the skin of dogs and cats. In cats, many organisms are produced and cytologic evaluation leads to easy diagnosis. In dogs, however, organisms are scarce and cytologic preparations must be perused carefully. If organisms are not found, the lesion should be cultured or a biopsy of the lesion should be submitted for histopathologic evaluation.

In cytologic preparations stained with Romanowsky-type stains, *Sporothrix schenckii* organisms are round to oval or fusiform (cigar shaped). They are about 3-9 μ long and 1-3 μ wide, and stain pale to medium blue with a slightly eccentric pink to purple nucleus (Plate 4). They may be confused with *Histoplasma capsulatum* if only a few organisms are found and the classic fusiform (cigar shape) is not seen.

Histoplasma capsulatum: Though *Histoplasma capsulatum* usually infects the lungs and/or other internal organs, it can infect the skin, with or without concurrent involvement of internal organs. Cutaneous histoplasmosis lesions are raised and proliferative, and may ulcerate. They usually yield many organisms within macrophages and some extracellular organisms. A few organisms may be found in neutrophils. In cytologic preparations stained with Romanowsky-type stains, *Histoplasma capsulatum* organisms are round to slightly oval, but are not fusiform or cigar shaped. They are 2-4 μ in diameter (one-fourth to one-half the size of a RBC), stain pale to medium blue, and contain an eccentric pink- to purple-staining nucleus (Plate 4). There is usually a clear halo around the yeast.

Blastomyces dermatitidis: *Blastomyces dermatitidis* infection (blastomycosis) can involve the skin, eyes and internal organs. Cutaneous lesions of blastomycosis usually are raised and proliferative, and often ulcerate. Cutaneous lesions should be sought when any form of blastomycosis is suspected. Imprints of these lesions usually have a cell composition characteristic of pyogranulomatous inflammation (Plate 3), and a few to many organisms. In cytologic preparations stained with Romanowsky-type stains, the organisms are blue, spherical, 8-10 μ in diameter, and thick walled (Plate 4). Most organisms are single, but occasionally organisms showing broad-based budding are found.

Cryptococcus neoformans: *Cryptococcus neoformans* infection (cryptococcosis) can involve subcutaneous tissues, causing subcutaneous swellings, but more commonly involves the upper respiratory and central nervous systems. Cryptococcosis usually evokes a granulomatous response (Plate 3) of epithelioid macrophages and/or inflammatory giant cells. In some cytologic preparations, *Cryptococcus* organisms may outnumber inflammatory and tissue cells. The organism is spherical and usually has a thick mucoid capsule, but occasionally, unencapsulated (rough) forms are found. The organism is 4-8 μ in diameter without its capsule and 8-40 μ in diameter with its capsule. In cytologic preparations stained with Romanowsky-type stains, the organism stains deep pink to bluish purple and may be slightly granular (Plate 4). The capsule usually is clear and homogeneous, but it may stain light to medium pink.

Coccidioides immitis: *Coccidioides immitis* infections (coccidioidomycosis) generally involve the lungs and bones of dogs. However, cutaneous lesions (masses) and draining tracts from bony lesions develop in some cases. Cytologic preparations usually have a cell composition characteristic of pyogranulomatous or granulomatous inflammation (Plate 3). *Coccidioides* organisms usually are scarce.

Figure 3. Scraping from a dog with ringworm. Several degenerating neutrophils are present, along with RBCs and a row of dermatophyte organisms attached to a hair shaft. (Wright's stain, original magnification 330X)

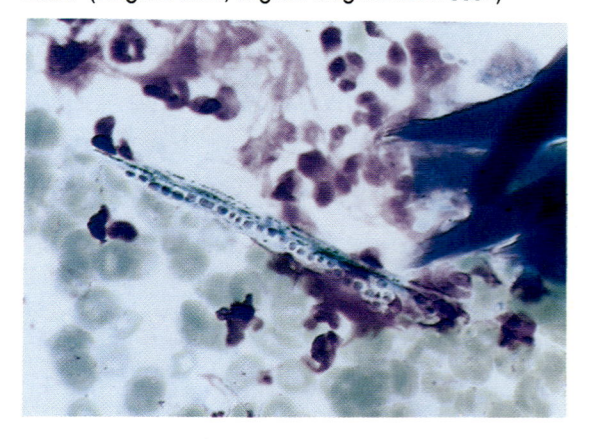

Therefore, cytologic preparations from suspected coccidioidomycosis lesions should be examined carefully. In cytologic preparations stained with Romanowsky-type stains, the organism is a large (10-100 μ in diameter), double-contoured, blue to blue-green sphere, with finely granular protoplasm (Plate 5). Round endospores 2-5 μ in diameter may be seen in some of the larger organisms. The tremendous variation in size, presence of endospores, and green tint to the organism differentiate *Coccidioides immitis* from nonbudding *Blastomyces dermatitidis*.

Prototheca zopfii, P wickerhami: *Prototheca* spp are colorless algae that are ubiquitous in the southern regions of America, but only rarely cause disease (protothecosis). In dogs, the disease is often disseminated, but in cats only cutaneous protothecosis has been reported.[1-4] Cytologic preparations reveal an inflammatory response characteristic of pyogranulomatous or granulomatous inflammation (Plate 3), and a few to numerous organisms. The organisms are round to oval and 1-14 μ wide and 1-16 μ long. When stained with Romanowsky-type stains, they have granular basophilic cytoplasm and a clear cell wall about 0.5 μ thick (Plate 5). The organisms, except small immature organisms, contain a small nucleus staining pink to deep purple. A single organism may consist of 2, 4 or more endospores. Most organisms are extracellular, but small forms may be found in macrophages and neutrophils.

Dermatophytes: The dermatophytes *Microsporum* spp and *Trichophyton* spp commonly cause ringworm in dogs and cats. Scrapings from the edge of the lesion are the best cytologic sample for finding dermatophytes. They can be identified in cytologic preparations using the standard 10% potassium hydroxide stain for hair, in wet-mount preparations stained with new methylene blue, or air-dried preparations stained with Romanowsky-type stains. Cytologically, fungal mycelia and spores are found within hair shafts (*Trichophyton* spp) or on the hair shaft surface (*Microsporum* spp). With Romanowsky-type stains, the mycelia and spores stain medium to dark blue with a thin clear halo (Fig 3). An inflammatory reaction composed of an admixture of neutrophils, macrophages, lymphocytes and plasma cells may be seen in cytologic preparations from skin scrapings.

Fungi That Form Hyphae in Cutaneous and Subcutaneous Tissues: Many fungi can form hyphae in cutaneous and subcutaneous tissue. They usually cause small to very large, raised proliferative lesions that often ulcerate. These fungi induce a granulomatous inflammatory response characterized by epithelioid macrophages and inflammatory giant cells (Plate 3). Neutrophil, lymphocyte, plasma cell and eosinophil numbers are variable (Plate 5). Phaeohyphomycosis refers to infections by pigmented fungi. Some fungi, such as *Phycomycetes*, do not stain and are recognized as negative images (Plate 5). Fungal culture or histopathologic examination with special immunohistochemical stains may be used to definitively classify the fungus.

Leishmania: *Leishmania donovani* can infect skin and subcutaneous tissues of dogs, producing small to very large, thickened, ulcerated areas. Imprints, scrapings and aspirates yield numerous admixed neutrophils, macrophages, lymphocytes and plasma cells. Either neutrophils or macrophages may predominate. Usually, numerous organisms are found within macrophages and free in the preparation (Plate 5).

Dermatophilus congolensis: *Dermatophilus congolensis* infects the superficial epidermis, causing crusty lesions. Cytologic preparations from the undersurface of scabs from these crusty lesions are most rewarding in demonstrating organisms. The preparations usually contain mature epithelial cells, keratin bars, debris and organisms (Fig 4). A few neutrophils may also be found. *Dermatophilus congolensis* replicates by transverse

Figure 4. Imprint from the underside of a scab caused by *Dermatophilus congolensis*. There is a background of squamous debris and 2 chains of bacterial doublets. (Wright's stain, original magnification 250X)

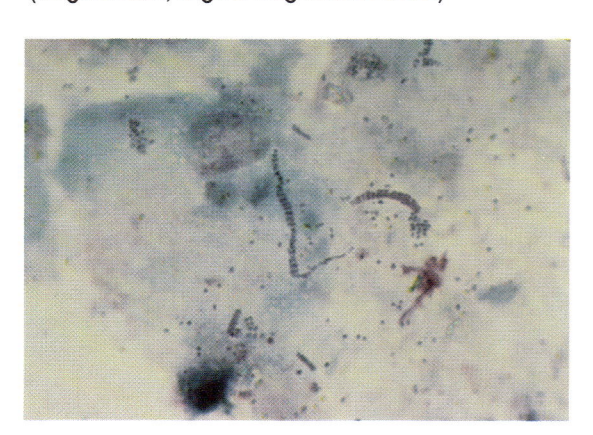

Figure 5. Aspirate from an eosinophilic granuloma. Several eosinophils are present, along with a neutrophil and a fibroblast. (Wright's stain, original magnification 250X)

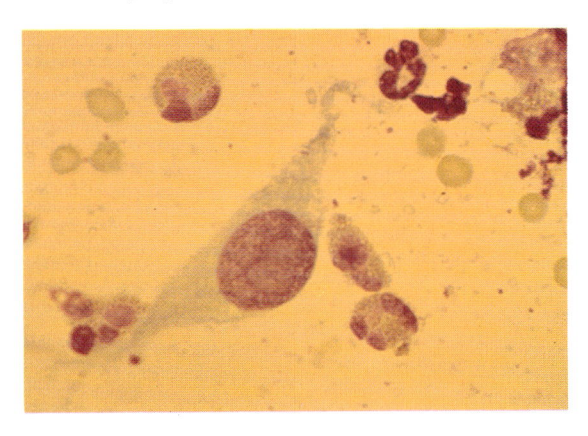

and longitudinal division, producing long chains of coccoid bacterial doublets. These chains resemble small, blue railroad tracks.

Noninfectious Inflammatory Lesions

Some inflammatory lesions are not caused by infectious agents. Such conditions as immune-mediated diseases, allergic reactions and sterile foreign body reactions elicit inflammatory lesions. Cytologic evaluation along with clinical evaluation may be helpful in diagnosing these lesions.

Linear Eosinophilic Granulomas, Eosinophilic Plaques: Linear granulomas and eosinophilic plaques occur most commonly in cats, but also may occur in dogs. Cytologically, these lesions are characterized by a predominance of eosinophils in association with a few neutrophils and macrophages (Fig 5). A few lymphocytes, plasma cells and fibroblasts may be present also. Some of the fibroblasts may have anaplastic characteristics, including cytomegaly, basophilic cytoplasm, large nuclei and large prominent nucleoli (Fig 5). Occasionally, aspirates from eosinophilic granulomas fail to yield eosinophils. Biopsies from these lesions may be submitted for histopathologic evaluation to confirm clinical suspicion of linear eosinophilic granuloma or eosinophilic plaque.

Cytologically, linear eosinophilic granulomas and eosinophilic plaques cannot always be differentiated from allergic and parasite-induced inflammatory reactions. If clinical evidence in conjunction with cytologic findings is not sufficient to establish the diagnosis, a biopsy of the lesion can be submitted for histopathologic evaluation.

Allergic Inflammatory Reactions: Cytologically, allergic inflammatory reactions are characterized by numerous eosinophils (Plate 3). Neutrophil and mast cell numbers are variable. Lymphocytes, plasma cells and macrophages may also be present if the condition is chronic.

Parasite-Induced Inflammatory Reactions: Parasite-induced inflammatory reactions are characterized by numerous eosinophils and a few to many neutrophils. Macrophages may be present in large numbers also. Variable numbers of lymphocytes and plasma cells may be present. Occasionally, the parasitic organism is found.

Immune-Mediated Skin Lesions: Cytologic preparations from immune-mediated skin lesions, such as pemphigus, usually contain neutrophils and necrotic debris. Occasionally, a few lymphocytes and plasma cells may also be present. The lesion may be secondarily infected. Histopathologic evaluation of a properly collected and prepared biopsy is necessary for diagnosis of immune-mediated skin lesions.

Virus-Induced Skin Lesions: Cytologic preparations from virus-induced skin lesions generally contain necrotic material and a few to many neutrophils. A few lymphocytes may also be present. The lesion may be secondarily infected. Histopathologic evaluation of biopsies from the lesions may be helpful in achieving a diagnosis.

Traumatic Skin Lesions: Traumatic skin lesions may be caused by trauma or caustic injury. Cytologic preparations from traumatic skin lesions usually contain numerous neutrophils and may contain abundant necrotic material and/or bacteria from secondary infection. The history and physical examination usually help establish the suspicion of either physical or caustic injury.

Sterile Foreign Body-Induced Inflammation: Cytologic preparations from inflammatory lesions induced by sterile foreign bodies usually contain an admixture of neutrophils and macrophages. Many of the macrophages present in foreign body reactions may be epithelioid macrophages; inflammatory giant cells may be present also. Occasionally, eosinophils are present. Lymphocytes and plasma cells may be present in variable numbers. Sometimes, refractile material can be found

Figure 6. Cytologic preparation from an area of fat necrosis in a dog. Note the dysplastic cells with small to large vacuoles in their cytoplasm. Cell borders are indistinct. (Wright's stain, original magnification 250X). (Courtesy of the University of Georgia, College of Veterinary Medicine)

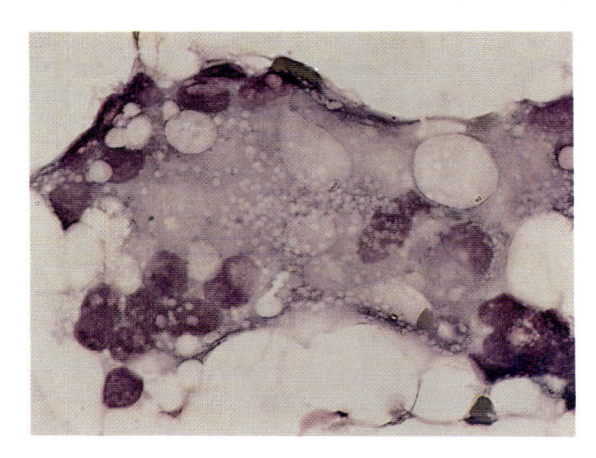

(Fig 1). When a sterile foreign body is suspected, the smear can be viewed under polarized light. Some foreign material refracts polarized light, whereas endogenous debris, such as hemosiderin, that might be mistaken as particulate foreign body material does not refract polarized light (Fig 1).

Fat Necrosis/Steatitis/Panniculitis: Necrosis and inflammation of adipose tissue (steatitis/panniculitis) can occur in dogs or cats. In cats, vitamin E deficiency is a common cause of fat necrosis/steatitis/panniculitis and should be investigated when steatitis/panniculitis is recognized. Cytologic preparations from areas of fat necrosis/steatitis/panniculitis usually contain variable numbers of neutrophils, macrophages, inflammatory giant cells and reactive spindle cells (Fig 6). The reactive spindle cells may contain clear vacuoles, indicating fat-cell origin. Often, the spindle cells are dysplastic and, if caution is not used, can be misclassified as neoplastic.

Collagen Necrosis: Collagen necrosis elicits an inflammatory response characterized by marked infiltration of eosinophils and monocytes, with development of epithelioid macrophages and inflammatory giant cells. As a result, cytologic preparations from areas of collagen necrosis contain numerous eosinophils and variable numbers of macrophages, epithelioid macrophages and inflammatory giant cells. Lymphocytes and plasma cells are scarce. Histopathologic evaluation of a biopsy from the lesion usually is necessary for definitive diagnosis.

Insect Bites: Cytologic preparations from welts caused by acute allergic reactions, such as bee stings, usually contain only a few local tissue cells and a few neutrophils and/or eosinophils. Older lesions caused by insect bites may contain a few neutrophils, eosinophils, macrophages, lymphocytes and plasma cells, along with a few local tissue cells.

Snake Bites: Cytologic preparations from recent snake bites tend to be of low cellularity. The cells present are local tissue cells and a few neutrophils. Neutrophil infiltration of the bitten area is very rapid. Within a few hours of the bite, neutrophil numbers begin to increase markedly. Neutrophil numbers in cytologic preparations from older snake bites increase accordingly. Within a couple of days they contain necrotic debris, numerous neutrophils and variable numbers of macrophages.

Evaluation of Tumor Cells

Tissue cells found on cytologic smears may arise from normal tissue, hyperplastic and/or dysplastic tissue, or neoplastic tissue. The skin is the most common site for neoplasms in dogs and cats.[5,6] In one survey, neoplasms of cutaneous and subcutaneous tissues accounted for 67.5% of all canine tumors.[5] Cutaneous and subcutaneous neoplasms may be of epithelial or mesenchymal (spindle-cell tumors) origin, or may be discrete round-cell tumors. Cytologic examination often indicates the cell of origin and/or malignant potential of the tumor. In general, epithelial tumors yield

Figure 7. Aspirate from a histiocytoma showing 2 histiocytoma cells, a neutrophil and several RBCs. (Wright's stain, original magnification 330X)

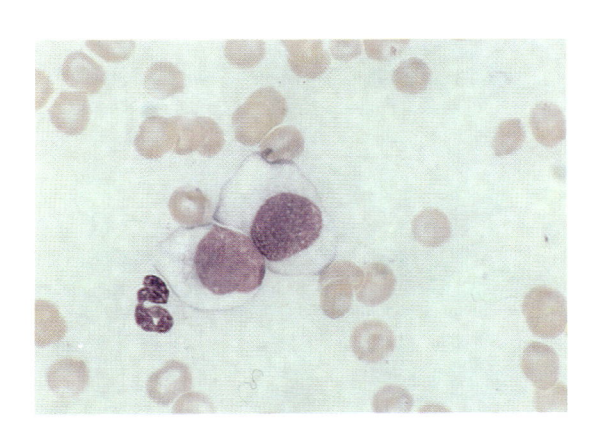

medium to large, round to caudate cells, with many clumps, groups or sheets of cells. Mesenchymal tumors yield a few to many cells, some of which are fusiform or stellate in shape. Most of the cells exfoliate individually, but a few cell groups may be found. Discrete round-cell tumors yield small to medium, round, individual cells.

The cellular morphology should be evaluated for criteria of malignancy (Table 4, Chapter 1). When no inflammatory cells are present, criteria of malignancy are more meaningful than when inflammatory cells are present. If many of the cells show 3 or more nuclear criteria of malignancy and no inflammatory cells are present, the lesion is most likely a malignant neoplasm. If less significant criteria of malignancy are present or only a few cells are affected, the cytologic preparation should be referred for interpretation or a biopsy of the lesion should be submitted for histopathologic examination. Sometimes tumors cannot be classified as spindle-cell tumors, epithelial-cell tumors or discrete round-cell tumors cytologically. However, these tumors often demonstrate sufficient criteria of malignancy for classification as malignant.

Charts 3-5 provide algorithms to aid in evaluating cytologic smears containing discrete round cells, epithelial cells and spindle cells, respectively. The typical cytologic characteristics of selected tumors are discussed below.

Discrete Round-Cell Tumors

Discrete round-cell tumors (Fig 7; Plate 7) yield cytologic preparations containing individual, small to medium-sized, round cells. Lymphosarcoma, mast-cell tumor, histiocytoma and transmissible venereal tumor (TVT) are the most common discrete round-cell tumors.[7-10] Occasionally, melanomas and basal-cell tumors exfoliate as discrete round cells. Discrete round-cell tumors are discussed below. Chart 3 provides an algorithm to aid in evaluating aspirates containing discrete round cells.

Lymphosarcomas: Several forms of lymphoid neoplasia can occur in the skin of dogs and cats. They usually produce multiple plaque-like lesions, but occasionally produce solitary nodules.[9,11,12] Aspirates of these lesions usually yield highly cellular cytologic preparations (Plate 7).

Preparations from *lymphoblastic lymphosarcoma* (the most common cutaneous lymphoid neoplasm) contain numerous lymphoblasts. Lymphoblasts are larger than neutrophils and have a small to moderate amount of light to medium blue-staining cytoplasm that is usually displaced to one side of the nucleus and not as abundant as in the other discrete round-cell tumors. They have indented to irregular nuclei, with smudged to stippled chromatin patterns and often several prominent nucleoli.

Preparations from *lymphocytic lymphosarcoma* are composed of small lymphocytes that cannot be readily differentiated from normal lymphocytes. These tumors require histopathologic examination for definitive diagnosis.

Preparations from *histiocytic lymphosarcoma* (reticulum-cell sarcomas) contain cells with morphology similar to histiocytoma cells (described below). Some multinucleated cells may be found, and cells containing pleomorphic indented nuclei, similar to monocyte nuclei, occasionally are found. Histiocytic lymphosarcomas tend to occur as multiple rapidly growing plaque-like lesions in middle-aged or older dogs. In contrast, histiocytomas tend to occur as solitary nodular lesions on the head and extremities of young dogs.

Mast-Cell Tumors: Mast-cell tumors yield a few to many cells with a moderate amount of cytoplasm, usually containing small, red-purple granules. Most mast-cell tumors yield cells that contain many granules; however, some yield cells containing only a few granules. The cells usually have round nuclei that often stain palely because of the intense staining of the highly granulated cytoplasm (Plate 7). Occasionally, anaplastic mast-cell tumors contain only rare granules and have convoluted nuclei. Sometimes, Diff-Quik fails to stain mast-cell granules.

Histiocytomas: Histiocytomas usually yield only a few cells. These cells have a moderate amount of pale blue cytoplasm that often has ill-defined boundaries and may contain a few small vacuoles (Fig 7). Their nuclei have finely etched, lacy to finely stippled chromatin patterns, and contain multiple indistinct nucleoli.

Transmissible Venereal Tumors: Transmissible venereal tumors exfoliate many cells on scrapings, aspirates and imprints. The cells have a moderate amount of light smoky blue to medium blue cytoplasm with distinct boundaries and usually many distinct vacuoles. Their nuclei tend to be round, with coarse, cord-like chromatin patterns and 1-2 large, very prominent nucleoli (Plate 7).

Epithelial Tumors

Epithelial cells tend to form cell-to-cell bridges. As a result, epithelial-cell tumors tend to exfoliate clumps of cells, but usually some individual cells are present also. Acinar or ductal arrangements may be identified with adenomas and adenocarcinomas. Cells from epithelial-cell tumors tend to be large to very large, with moderate to abundant cytoplasm and round nuclei. The nuclei generally have smooth to slightly coarse chromatin patterns that become more coarse and ropy as malignant potential increases. The nuclei usually contain one or more prominent nucleoli that become larger and irregular in shape as malignant potential increases. Malignant epithelial-

Figure 8. Aspirate from a basal-cell tumor in a dog. A. Many of the basal cells have morphology similar to that of histiocytoma cells. The 2 cells containing numerous cytoplasmic vacuoles probably are sebaceous cells. (Wright's stain, original magnification 250X). B. These basal cells show row formation sometimes seen in cytologic preparations from basal-cell tumors. (Wright's stain, original magnification 400X)

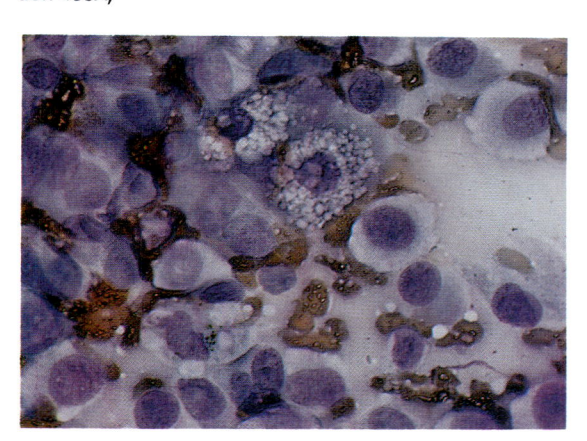

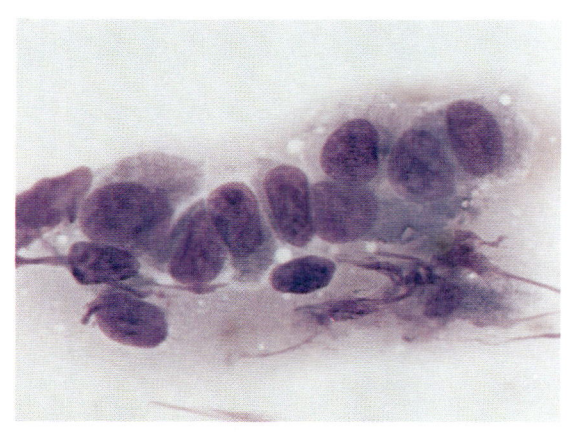

Figure 9. Aspirate from a perianal adenoma in a dog. A. A cluster of perianal adenoma cells. (Wright's stain, original magnification 100X). B. Three perianal adenoma cells. (Wright's stain, original magnification 250X)

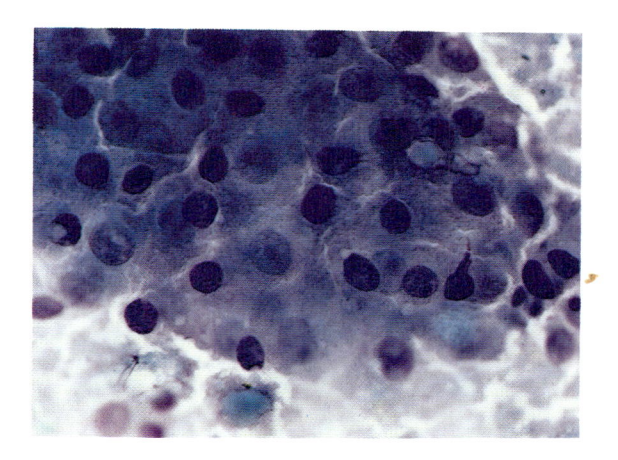

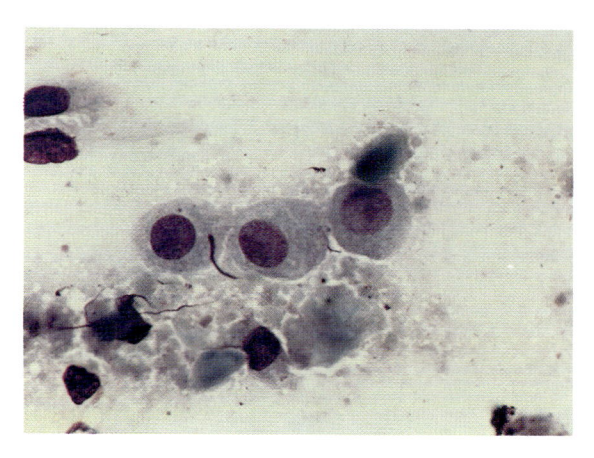

cell tumors often show marked variation in cellular, nuclear and nucleolar size and shape. These variations are most significant when they occur within the same cell or same group of cells. Malignant epithelial-cell tumors also often show a markedly increased nucleus:cytoplasm ratio and may show nuclear molding.

Local inflammation or other irritation can cause epithelial cells to become dysplastic. Epithelial cells undergoing dysplasia may show mild to moderate variation in cell, nuclear and nucleolar size and shape, increased nucleus:cytoplasm ratio, and coarse chromatin in a few cells. Dysplasia usually does not cause bizarre nuclear and nucleolar morphology. When there is concern that the abnormal cell morphology observed in a cytologic sample is caused by dysplasia instead of neoplasia, a biopsy from the lesion should be submitted for

Chapter 2

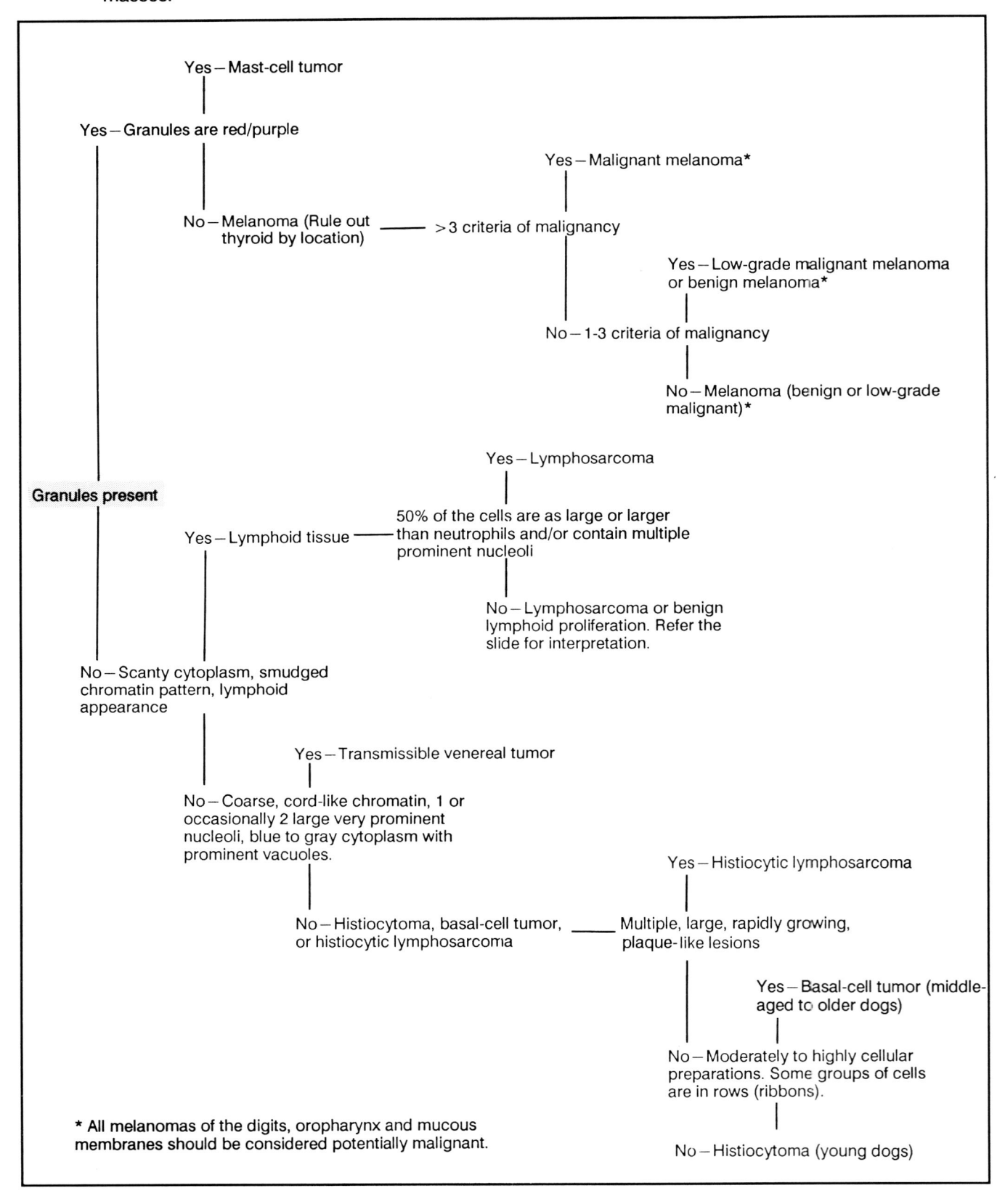

Chart 3. An algorithm to aid in evaluating aspirates containing discrete round cells from solid masses.

```
                          Yes — Mast-cell tumor
                          |
        Yes — Granules are red/purple
        |                                           Yes — Malignant melanoma*
        |                                           |
                No — Melanoma (Rule out ——— >3 criteria of malignancy
                      thyroid by location)          |
                                                    |         Yes — Low-grade malignant melanoma
                                                    |               or benign melanoma*
                                                    |         |
                                                    No — 1-3 criteria of malignancy
                                                              |
                                                              No — Melanoma (benign or low-grade
                                                                    malignant)*

                                          Yes — Lymphosarcoma
                                          |
                          50% of the cells are as large or larger
              Yes — Lymphoid tissue ——— than neutrophils and/or contain multiple
                                          prominent nucleoli
Granules present                          |
                                          No — Lymphosarcoma or benign
                                                lymphoid proliferation. Refer the
                                                slide for interpretation.

        No — Scanty cytoplasm, smudged
              chromatin pattern, lymphoid
              appearance

                                          Yes — Transmissible venereal tumor
                                          |
                No — Coarse, cord-like chromatin, 1 or
                      occasionally 2 large very prominent
                      nucleoli, blue to gray cytoplasm with
                      prominent vacuoles.
                                                              Yes — Histiocytic lymphosarcoma
                                                              |
                      No — Histiocytoma, basal-cell tumor, ——— Multiple, large, rapidly growing,
                            or histiocytic lymphosarcoma       plaque-like lesions
                                                                        |
                                                                        Yes — Basal-cell tumor (middle-
                                                                              aged to older dogs)
                                                                        |
                                                                        No — Moderately to highly cellular
                                                                              preparations. Some groups of cells
                                                                              are in rows (ribbons).
                                                                                    |
* All melanomas of the digits, oropharynx and mucous                                No — Histiocytoma (young dogs)
  membranes should be considered potentially malignant.
```

Cutaneous and Subcutaneous Lesions

Chart 4. An algorithm to aid in evaluating cytologic smears containing epithelial cells (large, round to caudate cells with many cell clumps) from cutaneous or subcutaneous tissues.

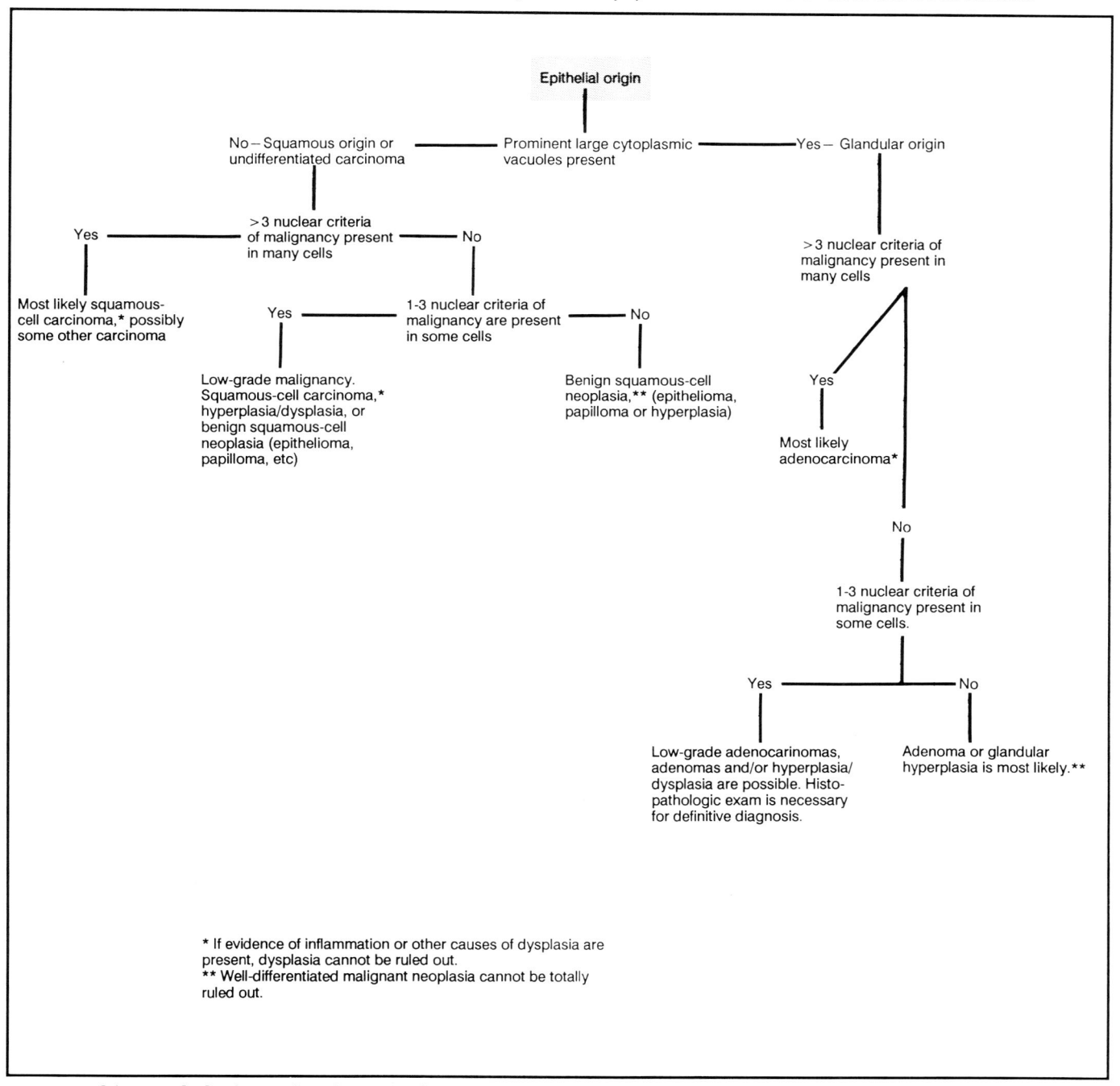

```
                                    Epithelial origin
                                          |
        No—Squamous origin or ——— Prominent large cytoplasmic ——— Yes— Glandular origin
        undifferentiated carcinoma        vacuoles present                |
                  |                                                        |
  Yes ——— >3 nuclear criteria                                    >3 nuclear criteria of
          of malignancy present ——— No                           malignancy present in
          in many cells              |                           many cells
   |              |                  |                                    |
 Most likely     Yes ——— 1-3 nuclear criteria of ——— No                  Yes
 squamous-                malignancy are present      |                   |
 cell carcinoma,*         in some cells               |                 Most likely
 possibly         |                                   |                 adenocarcinoma*
 some other    Low-grade malignancy.           Benign squamous-cell      |
 carcinoma     Squamous-cell carcinoma,*       neoplasia,** (epithelioma, No
               hyperplasia/dysplasia, or       papilloma or hyperplasia)  |
               benign squamous-cell                                      1-3 nuclear criteria of
               neoplasia (epithelioma,                                   malignancy present in
               papilloma, etc)                                           some cells.
                                                                Yes ——————————— No
                                                                 |               |
                                                        Low-grade adenocarinomas,  Adenoma or glandular
                                                        adenomas and/or hyperplasia/ hyperplasia is most likely.**
                                                        dysplasia are possible. Histo-
                                                        pathologic exam is necessary
                                                        for definitive diagnosis.
```

* If evidence of inflammation or other causes of dysplasia are present, dysplasia cannot be ruled out.
** Well-differentiated malignant neoplasia cannot be totally ruled out.

histopathologic evaluation, or the cause of dysplasia should be treated and the lesion reevaluated cytologically.

Neoplasms of epithelial origin are often ulcerated and may have a superficial secondary infection. Imprints of ulcerated areas on epithelial-cell tumors often yield only inflammatory cells with or without bacteria. When cells are collected by imprintation of ulcerated areas, the changes in cellular morphology caused by neoplasia are difficult to distinguish from dysplastic changes caused by inflammation. It is more rewarding, therefore, to collect cytologic samples from ulcerated lesions by deep aspiration or deep scraping of the lesion

Chapter 2

Chart 5. An algorithm to aid in evaluating aspirates containing spindle cells.

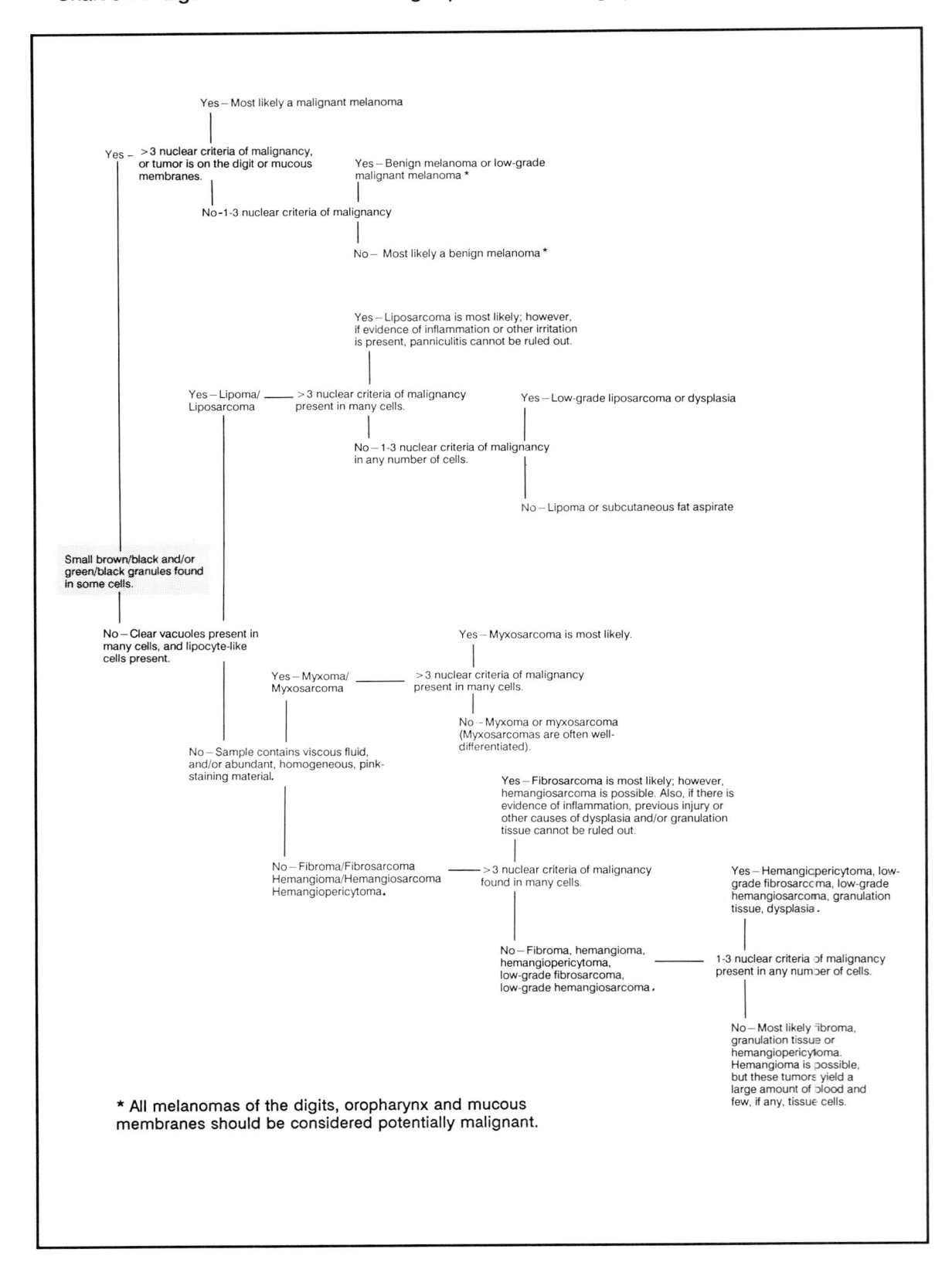

```
                                              Yes — Most likely a malignant melanoma
                                              │
         Yes — >3 nuclear criteria of malignancy,
               or tumor is on the digit or mucous
               membranes.                     Yes — Benign melanoma or low-grade
               │                                    malignant melanoma *
               │                              │
               No — 1-3 nuclear criteria of malignancy
                                              │
                                              No — Most likely a benign melanoma *


                                                      Yes — Liposarcoma is most likely; however,
                                                            if evidence of inflammation or other irritation
                                                            is present, panniculitis cannot be ruled out.
                                                      │
         Yes — Lipoma/ ——— >3 nuclear criteria of malignancy        Yes — Low-grade liposarcoma or dysplasia
               Liposarcoma    present in many cells.                │
                              │                                     │
                              No — 1-3 nuclear criteria of malignancy
                                   in any number of cells.
                                   │
                                   No — Lipoma or subcutaneous fat aspirate

Small brown/black and/or
green/black granules found
in some cells.
│
No — Clear vacuoles present in              Yes — Myxosarcoma is most likely.
     many cells, and lipocyte-like          │
     cells present.                         │
     │                    Yes — Myxoma/ ——— >3 nuclear criteria of malignancy
     │                          Myxosarcoma  present in many cells.
     │                          │            No — Myxoma or myxosarcoma
     │                          │                 (Myxosarcomas are often well-
     │                          │                 differentiated).
     │                          │
     │                                            Yes — Fibrosarcoma is most likely; however,
     │                                                  hemangiosarcoma is possible. Also, if there is
     │                                                  evidence of inflammation, previous injury or
     │                                                  other causes of dysplasia and/or granulation
     │                                                  tissue cannot be ruled out.
     │                          No — Sample contains viscous fluid,
     │                               and/or abundant, homogeneous, pink-
     │                               staining material.
     │                               │
     │                               │                                                    Yes — Hemangiopericytoma, low-
     │                               No — Fibroma/Fibrosarcoma  ——— >3 nuclear criteria of malignancy    grade fibrosarcoma, low-grade
     │                                    Hemangioma/Hemangiosarcoma  found in many cells.               hemangiosarcoma, granulation
     │                                    Hemangiopericytoma.         │                                  tissue, dysplasia.
     │                                                                │
     │                                                                No — Fibroma, hemangioma,
     │                                                                     hemangiopericytoma,      ——— 1-3 nuclear criteria of malignancy
     │                                                                     low-grade fibrosarcoma,       present in any number of cells.
     │                                                                     low-grade hemangiosarcoma.
     │                                                                                                   No — Most likely fibroma,
     │                                                                                                        granulation tissue or
     │                                                                                                        hemangiopericytoma.
     │                                                                                                        Hemangioma is possible,
     │                                                                                                        but these tumors yield a
     │                                                                                                        large amount of blood and
                                                                                                              few, if any, tissue cells.
```

* All melanomas of the digits, oropharynx and mucous
  membranes should be considered potentially malignant.

after it has been cleaned and debrided. Scrapings have the advantage of collecting many tissue cells. A disadvantage is that the sample is collected from an area undergoing an inflammatory response that may have caused sufficient cellular dysplasia to impair cytologic interpretation. Aspirations from deep within the lesion have the advantage of being collected farther from the site of possible inflammation. A disadvantage is that they usually yield fewer cells for evaluation.

Chart 4 provides an algorithm to aid identification of epithelial tumors. Some epithelial tumors are discussed below:

Normal Squamous Epithelium: Normal superficial squamous epithelial cells (Plate 6) are very large, appear flattened, have abundant light blue to blue-green-staining cytoplasm, and are anucleate or have a small, contracted, dark-staining nucleus without a discernible nucleolus. Normal squamous epithelial cells from the basal layer (Plate 6) tend to be round, with a moderate amount of light to medium blue cytoplasm. They have a single medium to dark purple-staining nucleus with a smooth to slightly coarse chromatin pattern. Their nuclei may contain a single small, round, indistinct nucleolus. As maturation progresses, the morphology of squamous epithelial cells changes from that of basal squamous epithelial cells to that of mature superficial squamous epithelial cells. As a result, cells with morphology varying from that of normal basal epithelial cells to that of normal mature squamous epithelial cells may be collected

Figure 10. Aspirate from a liposarcoma. Note the vacuolated cytoplasm with indistinct borders, large nucleus, ropy chromatin pattern, and multiple prominent nucleoli. (Wright's stain, original magnification 400X). (Courtesy of the University of Georgia, College of Veterinary Medicine)

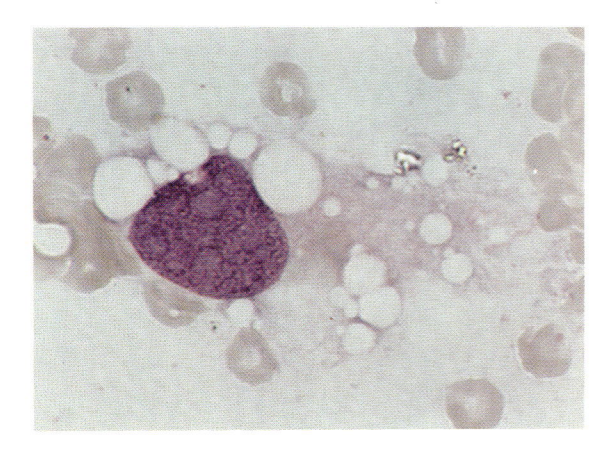

Figure 11. Aspirate from a hemangiopericytoma in a dog. Note the spindle shape of most of the cells and the prominent nucleoli. One cell has a somewhat caudate shape and a tail of cytoplasm trailing away from it. (Wright's stain, original magnification 250X)

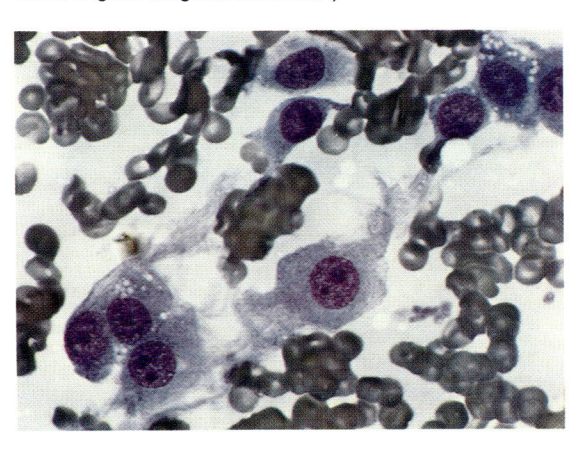

from cutaneous lesions, depending upon the manner of collection and the erosiveness of the lesion.

Benign Tumors of Squamous Epithelium: Benign epithelial-cell tumors not undergoing dysplasia subsequent to local inflammation or other irritation usually exfoliate cells either indistinguishable from normal cells of the tissue of origin or slightly more active. Nucleoli may be a bit more prominent, but still round and of reasonable size. The cytoplasm may be slightly more basophilic, and the nucleus:cytoplasm ratio may be mildly increased.

Benign tumors of squamous epithelium, such as epitheliomas and papillomas, yield cytologic samples predominantly composed of mature squamous epithelial cells (Plate 6). A few basal and intermediate stages of squamous maturation may also be present. If there is any concern that the lesion might be a well-differentiated squamous-cell carcinoma, a biopsy of the lesion should be submitted for histopathologic evaluation.

Epidermal Cysts: Epidermal cysts are discussed below under "Cysts."

Basal-Cell Tumors: Basal-cell tumors usually are benign but can be malignant. Their malignant potential is difficult to predict by cytologic or histopathologic examination.[9] Basal-cell tumors yield some cells in groups and some as individuals. Sometimes a row or ribbon of several cells is found (Fig 8). This pattern is caused by the tendency of basal cells to line up along basement membranes within the tumor. This gives the characteristic ribbon-like histologic pattern of the basal-cell tumor.

Individual cells of basal-cell tumors have morphology similar to normal basal cells (Plate 6). Cytologically, they may appear similar to histiocytoma cells; however, basal-cell tumors usually exfoliate more cells that histiocytomas. Identification of rows or ribbons of cells helps differentiate them from histiocytomas. Since aspirates from basal-cell tumors do not always contain rows or ribbons of cells, their absence does not totally rule out basal-cell tumors.

Squamous-Cell Carcinomas: Squamous-cell carcinomas may occur anywhere in the skin of dogs and cats. They are often ulcerated with a secondary superficial bacterial infection. Imprints of ulcerated areas may yield only bacteria and inflammatory cells (Plate 6). Scrapings of cleaned and debrided ulcerated areas may yield numerous tissue cells, but interpretation often is impaired by secondary inflammation. Deep aspirates from squamous-cell carcinomas usually do not yield as many cells as scrapings but usually are very helpful in diagnosis, since interpretation usually is not impaired by local inflammation.

Squamous-cell carcinomas tend to yield groups of cells and a few individual cells. Many of the groups may be too thick to evaluate, but thinner groups and individual cells can be evaluated to determine the cell of origin and malignant potential. Often, there is marked variation in cell, nuclear and nucleolar size, nucleolar number and shape, nucleus: cytoplasm ratio, and cytoplasmic basophilia. Some cells may contain small clear vacuoles. Occasionally, the vacuoles may aggregate around the nucleus (perinuclear vacuolation) and appear to coalesce, forming a clear ring around the nucleus. These cells strongly suggest carcinoma. The cytoplasm of some cells may stain homogeneous blue-green. Occasionally, an individual cell has the cytoplasm displaced to one side and a blunted cytoplasmic tail. These "tadpole cells" are considered suggestive of squamous-cell carcinoma. Individual cellular morphology varies from normal large, mature squamous cells to small or medium-sized round cells, with a small amount of very basophilic cytoplasm and large, round nuclei that may have a very coarse, ropy chromatin pattern and contain multiple, prominent, irregularly shaped and sized nucleoli.

Sebaceous-Cell Adenomas: Sebaceous-cell adenomas are most common in older dogs and usually appear as wart-like growths. They generally exfoliate cells in groups; however, a few individual cells may be present. Occasionally, the cells of a group may be arranged in an acinar pattern. The morphology of sebaceous adenoma cells is very similar to that of normal sebaceous cells. They are large cells, with foamy cytoplasm and a small, central to slightly eccentric nucleus. The nucleus usually stains darkly and has a slightly coarse chromatin pattern. Usually, the nucleolus is indistinct or indiscernible. In preparations from sebaceous-cell adenomas, some cells may have a slightly larger nucleus that stains with less intensity, has a slightly coarse chromatin pattern, and has a small to medium-sized, round, discernible nucleolus.

Figure 12. Aspirate from a myxosarcoma in a dog. A. Low magnification shows numerous rows of cells embedded in a pink substance. (Wright's stain, original magnification 50X). B. A higher magnification shows many cells with a plasmacytoid appearance and a background of pink material. A few cells are spindle shaped. (Wright's stain, original magnification 100X)

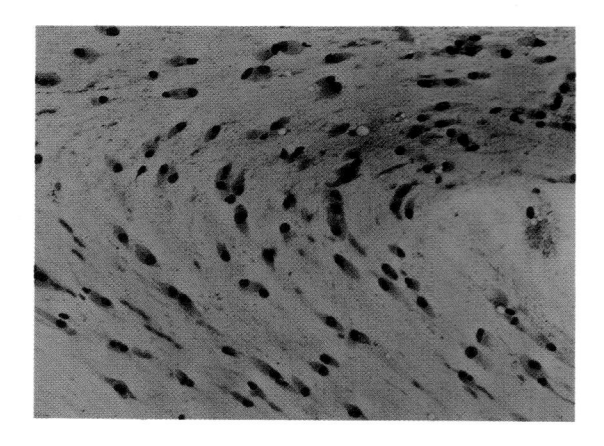

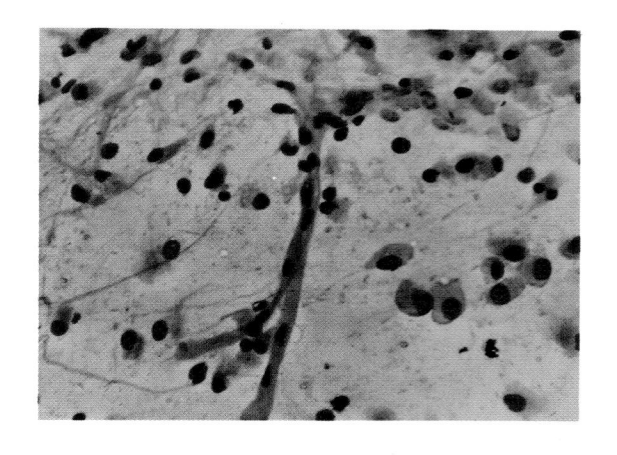

Figure 13. Aspirate from a malignant fibrous histiocytoma (giant-cell tumor) in a dog showing several multinucleated cells. One cell has a tail of cytoplasm trailing away from it. A few histiocytic cells are also present. (Wright's stain, original magnification 200X)

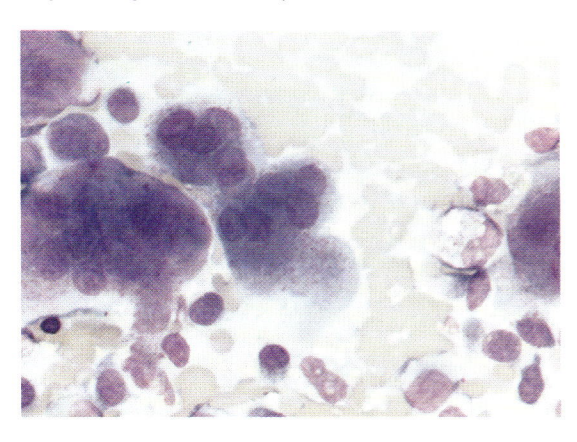

Basilar reserve cells may be found also. These cells are immature and contain little or no secretory material. They have basophilic cytoplasm and a nucleus:cytoplasm ratio of about 1:2. As a result, they may be misinterpreted as malignant. Sebaceous cysts are described below under "Cysts."

Sebaceous-Cell Adenocarcinomas: Sebaceous-cell adenocarcinomas are much less common than sebaceous-cell adenomas. The cytologic characteristics are similar to those of other adenocarcinomas (Plate 6). Cytologic preparations usually consist of groups of extremely basophilic reserve cells showing numerous criteria of malignancy. Cells containing secretory material are scarce; however, signet-ring cells (cells containing large secretory vacuoles that press the nucleus against the cell membrane) occasionally may be found.

Sweat-Gland Adenomas/Adenocarcinomas: In cats, sweat-gland tumors are most often located at the base of the ear, dorsum of the head and neck, and base of the tail.[6] They are usually 1-2 cm in diameter and attached to the skin, and sometimes are cystic. In cats, they frequently ulcerate and may resemble a chronic inflammatory process.

Sweat-gland adenomas usually yield cytologic preparations that are moderately cellular. Most cells are in clumps. The cells are of medium size and round to oval, and have a slightly eccentric nucleus. They may contain one or more large droplets of secretory material.

Sweat-gland adenocarcinomas yield groups of basophilic round cells similar to those found with other adenocarcinomas (Plate 6). These cells often show numerous criteria of malignancy (Table 4, Chapter 1). Sweat-gland adenocarcinomas metastasize to regional lymph nodes and the lungs.[6]

Perianal-Gland Adenomas/Adenocarcinomas: The perianal glands encircle the anus of dogs. A few perianal-gland cells are also located in the skin of the tail, prepuce, thigh and dorsum. Perianal adenomas and adenocarcinomas can occur at any of these locations. They often ulcerate and may become secondarily infected. Cytologically and histopathologically perianal-gland hyperplasia is difficult to differentiate from benign neoplasia.[9]

Cytologic preparations from perianal gland adenomas/hyperplasia usually are very cellular. Most cells are in clumps, but a few individual cells usually are present (Fig 9). They are medium sized and have a moderate to large amount of gray to tan cytoplasm, and uniform round nuclei that may contain 1-2 small round nucleoli. At high magnification, the cytoplasm may appear granular. Because these cells resemble hepatocytes, perianal-gland neoplasms are sometimes referred to as hepatoid tumors. A few flattened reserve cells may be present also. The cytoplasm of the reserve cells is more basophilic, and the nucleus:cytoplasm ratio is between 1:1 and 1:2.

Perianal-gland adenocarcinomas may show numerous criteria of malignancy or may be well differentiated and difficult to differentiate from perianal-gland adenomas. Varia-

Figure 14. Aspirate from an epidermal cyst in a dog showing numerous squamous cells and abundant blue amorphous debris. (Wright's stain, original magnification 25X)

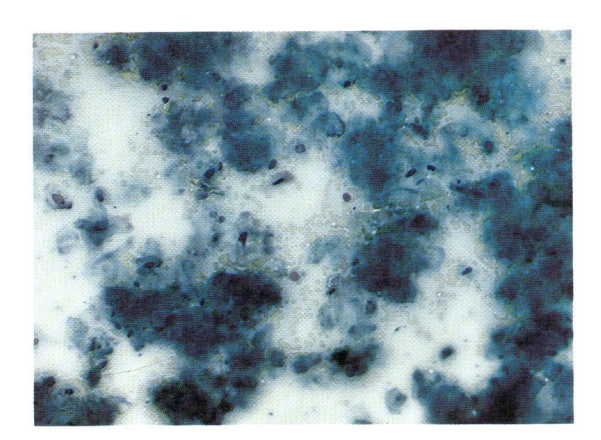

tion in nuclear size, nucleolar size and nucleolar number per cell are the most common malignant features of perianal-gland adenocarcinomas.[9]

Tumors of the Subcutaneous Glandular Tissues: These tumors (salivary, mammary, thyroid, etc) are discussed in Chapter 7.

Undifferentiated Carcinomas: Undifferentiated carcinomas are malignant tumors that morphologically appear of epithelial origin, but the specific cell of origin (squamous epithelial cell or glandular epithelial cell) cannot be determined. Obviously, these tumors may vary greatly in cellular morphology. To classify them as carcinomas, characteristics of epithelial cells must be present without characteristics of spindle cells. Because of their undifferentiated (anaplastic) nature, numerous criteria of malignancy usually are present and they are easily recognized as malignant.

Tumors of Mesenchymal Origin (Spindle-Cell Tumors)

Tumors of mesenchymal origin are commonly referred to as spindle-cell tumors. These tumors tend to yield individual cells instead of groups, clumps or sheets of cells, but a few groups of cells usually can be found. The term spindle cell arises from the fusiform or spindle appearance that a few to many (depending on the specific cell of origin and malignant potential of the tumor) cells may show. Spindle cells have a fusiform shape with cytoplasmic tails trailing away from the nucleus in 1-2 directions. They usually are small to medium sized and have a moderate amount of light to medium blue cytoplasm, and a round to oval nucleus that stains with medium intensity and has a smooth to fine lacy chromatin pattern. Nucleoli usually are not visible in nonneoplastic spindle cells. As the malignant potential of spindle-cell tumors increases, nucleoli become prominent. The spindle shape becomes less prominent, and cell, nuclear and nucleolar size and shape vary markedly. The chromatin pattern becomes coarser, and cytoplasmic basophilia and the nucleus:cytoplasm ratio increase.

Spindle-cell tumors are often difficult or impossible to name cytologically. Also, granulation tissue produces plump, young fibroblasts that may have prominent criteria of malignancy. As a result, granulation tissue can be very difficult to differentiate from a spindle-cell neoplasm. In some cases, histopathologic examination is necessary to definitively diagnose spindle-cell tumors.

Local inflammation or other irritation can cause mesenchymal cells to become dysplastic. Cellular morphologic changes caused by dysplasia are very similar to the changes caused by neoplasia, but usually are mildly to moderately severe. Nuclear and nucleolar changes are less sensitive to dysplasia than cytoplasmic changes. If there is concern that cellular morphology is altered due to dysplasia instead of neoplasia, a biopsy of the lesion should be submitted for histopathologic evaluation. Alternatively, the stimulus for dysplasia (inflammation or other irritation) can be treated and the lesion re-evaluated cytologically.

Chart 5 provides an algorithm to aid identification of spindle-cell tumors. Some spindle-cell tumors are discussed below.

Fibromas: Fibromas can occur in the dermis or subcutaneous tissue. They seldom ulcerate. Aspirates and imprints yield very few cells. Scrapings from excised fibromas yield more cells, but even scrapings do not yield many cells. The cells collected usually are individuals, but an occasional group of 2 to several cells may be found.

Cells from fibromas are uniform in size and shape (Plate 7). They tend to have very elongated spindle shapes, with a moderate amount of light blue cytoplasm streaming away from the nucleus in 2 opposing directions. Their nuclei are round to oval and stain with medium to marked intensity, have a smooth to lacy chromatin pattern, and may contain 1-2 small, round, indistinct nucleoli.

Fibrosarcomas: Fibrosarcomas can arise from cutaneous or subcutaneous tissues. They may ulcerate and become secondarily infected. Aspirates, imprints and scrapings from fibrosarcomas tend to collect more cells than from fibromas.

Cells from fibrosarcomas are less spindle shaped than cells from fibromas (Plate 7). Many cells may be plump and/or oval shaped. Others may be stellate or have only a single, indistinct tail of cytoplasm. Occasionally, multinucleated fibroblasts may be found. Mild to marked variation in cell, nuclear and nucleolar size and shape, cytoplasmic basophilia, increased nucleus:cytoplasm ratio, and enlarged and/or angular nucleoli develop as malignant potential increases.

Granulation Tissue: Granulation tissue is composed of proliferating fibroblasts and small vessels. Since fibroblasts are young plump spindle cells with anaplastic characteristics, granulation tissue cannot be reliably differentiated from fibrous tissue neoplasia cytologically. If granulation tissue is suspected, a biopsy of the lesion should be submitted for histopathologic evaluation to definitively differentiate granulation tissue from fibrous tissue neoplasia.

Lipomas: Lipomas most frequently occur in the subcutaneous tissue of the shoulders, thighs and trunk. They seldom ulcerate. Aspirates of lipomas usually yield abundant free fat and a few lipocytes. As a result, cytologic smears have an oily appearance and do not dry. Fat does not stain with Romanowsky-type stains and is dissolved by alcohol in alcohol-containing stains. Therefore, microscopic evaluation of the smear reveals clear areas and a variable number of lipocytes. Lipocytes have pyknotic nuclei that are pressed against the side of the cell membrane by huge fat globules (Plate 8). Fat stains, such as Sudan IV and oil red O, may be used on fresh smears before alcohol fixation to establish the presence of lipids. Though lipomas are benign tumors, occasionally they infiltrate between muscle masses.[13] These infiltrative lipomas are difficult or impossible to remove and can lead to the patient's demise.

Lipomas usually do not become secondarily infected. Therefore, when inflammatory cells are found concurrently with lipid and lipocytes, inflammation of fat tissue (fat necrosis/steatitis/panniculitis) should be suspected.

Liposarcomas: Liposarcomas occur most frequently in the subcutaneous tissue of the shoulders, thighs and trunk. Aspirates, imprints and scrapings from liposarcomas may contain free fat, some mature lipocytes and lipoblasts, and appear greasy. Or they may contain very little free fat and few mature lipocytes, along with many lipoblasts, and not appear greasy.

Cells from liposarcomas often have very light cytoplasm with indistinct cell borders (Fig 10). Within the same tumor, cells may vary in morphology from that of lipocytes to that of bizarre blastic cells similar to those found in fibrosarcomas. Large to small lipid globules may be found in any of the cells. However, in general, the more immature and anaplastic cells have fewer and smaller fat globules. Smears that have not been exposed to alcohol or other lipid solvents can be stained with fat stains, such as Sudan IV and oil red O, to establish the presence of lipid.

Inflammation can cause fat cells to become dysplastic. The cellular morphology of fat cells

Figure 15. Aspirate from an epidermal cyst in a dog. Several cholesterol crystals are located in the center. (Wright's stain, original magnification 25X)

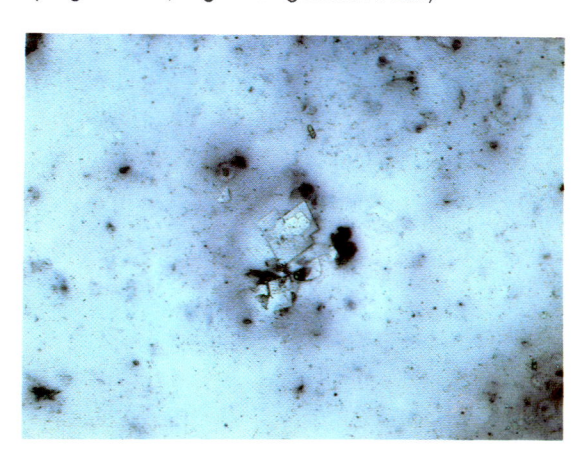

undergoing dysplasia can be similar to that of cells from liposarcomas. Since liposarcomas do not usually become secondarily infected or inflamed, evidence of inflammation concurrent with cellular changes suggestive of dysplasia or neoplasia suggests inflammation or necrosis of fat tissue (fat necrosis/steatitis/panniculitis) (Fig 6), but secondary inflammation of neoplastic fat tissue cannot be totally ruled out. To definitively differentiate neoplasia from dysplasia, a biopsy of the lesion can be submitted for histopathologic evaluation.

Hemangiopericytomas: Hemangiopericytomas most frequently occur in the subcutaneous tissues of the distal limbs of dogs. They seldom ulcerate. Aspirates, imprints and scrapings usually yield a moderate number of individual cells and a few small groups of cells. Cell morphology varies from very spindled with cytoplasmic tails trailing away from a round or oval nucleus in 2 opposing directions, to caudate with a moderate amount of cytoplasm without a distinct tail (Fig 11). The cytoplasm of hemangiopericytoma cells stains light to medium blue, and is usually devoid of any granules or vacuoles. Nuclei have a lacy to moderately coarse chromatin pattern and contain 1-2 round, indistinct to prominent nucleoli. Because of the vascular association of the neoplasm, a large amount of blood usually is present.

Hemangiomas: Hemangiomas may occur in the skin or subcutaneous tissue at any location in dogs and cats. They usually do not ulcerate. Hemangiomas are benign tumors of blood vessel endothelium and are contiguous with the blood vascular system. Aspirates of hemangiomas usually yield a large amount of blood that may contain a few endothelial cells. Because of the tendency for neutrophils to marginate, neutrophil numbers may be higher in blood aspirated from hemangiomas and hemangiosarcomas than in peripheral blood. Even when a few tumor cells are collected, they are difficult to differentiate from nonneoplastic endothelial cells. They tend to be oval, spindle or stellate in shape, have moderate to abundant amounts of light to medium blue cytoplasm, and contain a medium-sized round to slightly oval nucleus (Plate 7). The nucleus usually has a smooth to fine lacy chromatin pattern and may have 1-2 small, round, indistinct nucleoli. Because hemangiosarcomas may be well differentiated, tumors thought to be hemangiomas or hemangiosarcomas that do not yield sufficient cytologic evidence for classification as hemangiosarcomas should not be classified as hemangiomas by cytologic examination alone. Instead, they should be excised and submitted for histopathologic evaluation.

Cytologic examination can be used to differentiate hemangiomas and hemangiosarcomas from hematomas. Blood collected from hemangiomas and hemangiosarcomas contains platelets, whereas aspirates collected from hematomas do not unless blood has hemorrhaged into the hematoma within a few hours of sample collection or blood contamination has occurred during sample collection. Also, aspirates from hematomas usually contain macrophages with phagocytized RBCs (Plate 2) and/or RBC-breakdown products, whereas blood from hemangiomas and hemangiosarcomas does not.

Hemangiosarcomas: Hemangiosarcomas may occur in the skin and subcutaneous tissue at any location in dogs and cats. They seldom ulcerate. Hemangiosarcomas are malignant tumors of the vascular endothelium and are contiguous with the vascular system. Aspirates from hemangiosarcomas usually yield abundant blood, with a few endothelial cells. Occasionally, a moderate number of endothelial cells may be collected. Because of the tendency of neutrophils to marginate, neutrophil numbers in blood collected from hemangiosarcomas may exceed neutrophil numbers in peripheral blood. Neoplastic endothelial cells collected from hemangiosarcomas range in morphology from apparently normal endothelial cells to medium or large cells with marked variation in cell, nuclear and nucleolar size, and increased nucleus:cytoplasm ratio, nucleolar prominence, nucleolar angularity and cytoplasmic basophilia (Fig 8, Chapter 17).

When 3 or more nuclear criteria of malignancy (Table 4, Chapter 1) are prominent in many of the cells collected and there is no evidence of inflammation, the tumor can be classified as malignant. However, often sufficient numbers of cells are not collected or the criteria of malignancy are not sufficiently prominent to allow the tumor to be classified as malignant. Tumors thought to be hemangiomas or hemangiosarcomas should not be classified as hemangiomas based on cytologic examination alone. Instead, they should be excised and submitted for histopathologic evaluation.

Melanomas (Benign/Malignant): Melanomas are very common in dogs but rare in cats. In dogs, most cutaneous melanomas are benign, but melanomas of the lips, oral cavity and digits frequently are malignant.

Cytologic preparations from melanomas usually are moderately cellular and contain a small to moderate amount of blood, but occasionally they are of low cellularity and contain a large amount of blood. Most of the cells are found as individual cells, but a few small groups of cells may be found. The cells may be round, oval, stellate or spindle shaped. Melanomas composed predominantly of round to oval cells may be confused with round-cell tumors. Generally, however, a few spindle-shaped cells can be found. The cells have a moderate to abundant amount of cytoplasm. Even cells from malignant melanomas often contain a large amount of cytoplasm and, therefore, have a low nucleus:cytoplasm ratio. The cytoplasm usually contains granules of brown-black to green-black pigment (Plate 8). These granules may be densely packed and obscure the nucleus in some cells or may be absent from other cells. Amelanotic melanomas, which are usually malignant, contain only a small amount of pigment that is often not discernible by histopathologic examination. However, a careful search of cytologic preparations invariably identifies a few cells containing a few small pigment granules interspersed throughout their cytoplasm. Some malignant melanomas demonstrate numerous cytologic criteria of malignancy, but others are well differentiated and do not demonstrate significant criteria of malignancy. Therefore, caution should be used in classifying melanomas as benign by cytologic evaluation alone.

Melanocytes must be differentiated from melanophages (macrophages containing phagocytized melanin), hemosiderophages (macrophages containing hemosiderin) and mast cells. Melanophages (Plate 8) usually contain a few clear vacuoles, along with a few to many large phagocytic vacuoles packed with melanin pigment. These melanin-packed vacuoles are much larger than the small granules in melanocytes and melanoblasts. Hemosiderophages have a few to many phagocytic vacuoles stuffed with hemosiderin. The hemosiderin-laden vacuoles are blue-black to brown-black, and usually are much larger than the small granules of melanocytes and melanoblasts. Mast cells (Plate 2) are round to oval and contain a few to many red-purple granules. Usually, these granules are larger than the small green-black to brown-black granules of melanocytes and melanoblasts, but are smaller than the melanin-laden phagocytic vacuoles of melanophages and the hemosiderin-laden phagocytic vacuoles of hemosiderophages.

Myxomas/Myxosarcomas: Myxomas and myxosarcomas are rare tumors of subcutaneous tissues. On aspiration, a small to large amount of viscid material usually is obtained. Cytologic preparations of myxomas and myxosarcomas contain a few to many individual cells in a background of pink homogeneous material. The cells vary in morphology from oval to stellate or spindle shaped, and have a small to abundant amount of cytoplasm that sometimes contains small vacuoles of pink secretory material (Fig 12). The oval cells often have eccentric nuclei and medium to dark blue cytoplasm, giving them an appearance similar to plasma cells. Myxosarcomas exhibit variable degrees of criteria of malignancy.

Neurofibromas/Neurofibrosarcomas: These are tumors of the nerve-cell sheath. They can occur in subcutaneous tissue but are rare. Cytologically, they cannot be reliably differentiated from other spindle-cell tumors, such as fibromas and fibrosarcomas. Histologic demonstration of tumor involvement with a nerve sheath is necessary for definitive diagnosis.

Malignant Fibrous Histiocytomas (Giant-Cell Tumors of Soft Parts): These tumors occur more commonly in cats than in dogs but are not common in either species. When located in subcutaneous tissues, they are infiltrative and aggressive but rarely metastasize.[9]

Cytologic preparations are best collected by scrapings, but aspiration often yields sufficient cells for diagnosis. The preparations generally consist of multinucleated giant cells (Fig 13), fibroblastic cells (see description of fibrosarcoma above), and smaller round cells that resemble histiocytes (see description of "Histiocytomas" in this chapter).

Undifferentiated Sarcomas: Undifferentiated sarcomas are malignant tumors that morphologically appear to be of mesenchymal origin, but the specific cell of origin (fibroblasts, endothelial cell, etc) cannot be determined. Obviously, these tumors may vary greatly in cellular morphology. To classify them as sarcomas, some spindling must be recognized. Because of their undifferentiated and anaplastic nature, they usually are easily recognized as malignant. Their cellular characteristics are those described above in the general description of spindle-cell tumors.

Carcinosarcomas: Carcinosarcomas are malignant tumors that do not show sufficient cellular differentiation to be classified as carcinomas or sarcomas. Because of the anaplastic nature of these tumors, they usually are easily classified as malignant. Their cellular characteristics are a variable admixture of the characteristics for carcinomas and sarcomas.

Evaluation of Fluid-Filled Lesions

Fluid-filled lesions may be neoplastic or nonneoplastic in origin. Neoplastic fluid-filled lesions of the cutaneous and subcutaneous tissues include hemangiomas/hemangiosarcomas, adenomas/adenocarcinomas, neurofibromas/neurofibrosarcomas, myxomas/myxosarcomas and epidermal cysts. Nonneoplastic fluid-filled lesions of the cutaneous and subcutaneous tissues include hematomas, seromas, hygromas and abscesses. Cytologic evaluation of fluid from these lesions can be very helpful in their differentiation. Chart 6 provides an algorithm to aid in evaluation of fluid-filled lesions. Some common fluid-filled lesions are discussed below.

Epidermal Cysts

Epidermal cysts can arise from tumors of sebaceous- or squamous-cell differentiation. Fluid from epidermal cysts is usually creamy white, to brown or gray. With previous hemorrhage or peripheral blood contamination during collection, the fluid may appear pink to red.

Chapter 2

Chart 6. An algorithm to aid in evaluating cytologic preparations from fluid-filled lesions.

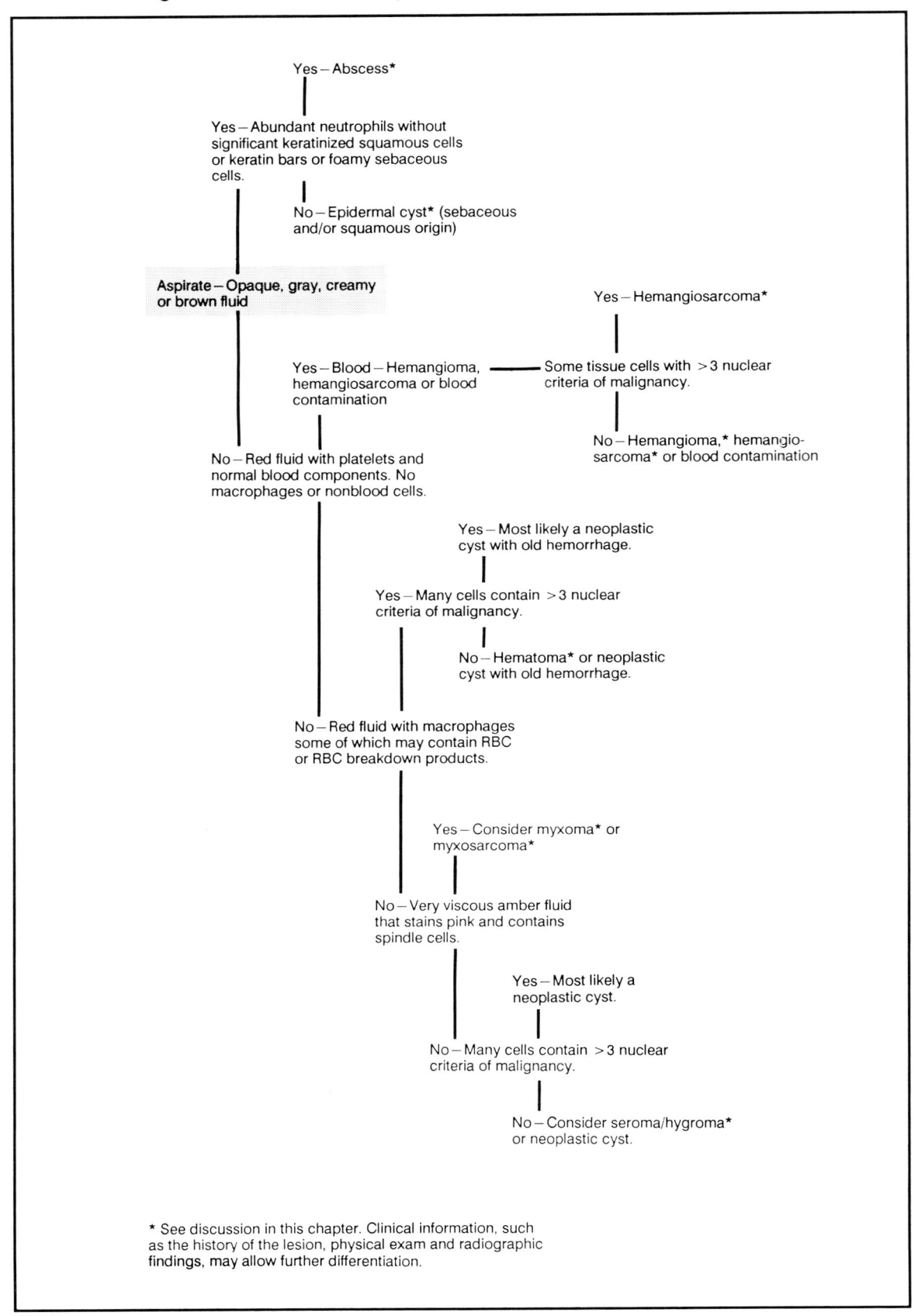

```
                            Yes — Abscess*
                              |
              Yes — Abundant neutrophils without
              significant keratinized squamous cells
              or keratin bars or foamy sebaceous
              cells.
                |
                   No — Epidermal cyst* (sebaceous
                        and/or squamous origin)

  Aspirate — Opaque, gray, creamy             Yes — Hemangiosarcoma*
  or brown fluid                                |
                |                                |
                   Yes — Blood — Hemangioma, ——— Some tissue cells with >3 nuclear
                   hemangiosarcoma or blood      criteria of malignancy.
                   contamination                  |
                |                                    No — Hemangioma,* hemangio-
  No — Red fluid with platelets and                       sarcoma* or blood contamination
  normal blood components. No
  macrophages or nonblood cells.
                |
                                Yes — Most likely a neoplastic
                                cyst with old hemorrhage.
                                  |
                   Yes — Many cells contain >3 nuclear
                   criteria of malignancy.
                                    |
                                    No — Hematoma* or neoplastic
                                    cyst with old hemorrhage.
                |
  No — Red fluid with macrophages
  some of which may contain RBC
  or RBC breakdown products.
                |
                     Yes — Consider myxoma* or
                     myxosarcoma*
                       |
                   No — Very viscous amber fluid
                   that stains pink and contains
                   spindle cells.
                         |
                             Yes — Most likely a
                             neoplastic cyst.
                               |
                         No — Many cells contain >3 nuclear
                         criteria of malignancy.
                               |
                               No — Consider seroma/hygroma*
                               or neoplastic cyst.
```

* See discussion in this chapter. Clinical information, such as the history of the lesion, physical exam and radiographic findings, may allow further differentiation.

Smears prepared from these cysts contain abundant amorphous blue to gray-staining material, and a few to many squamous epithelial cells and/or sebaceous cells (Fig 14). Neutrophils and macrophages may be present if the cyst has ruptured. Blood components (RBCs, neutrophils, etc) are present if hemorrhage or blood contamination has occurred. Sometimes, cholesterol clefts and/or cholesterol crystals are seen (Fig 15). Cholesterol crystals develop from cholesterol that accumulates from degradation of cells exfoliating into the cyst. Cholesterol clefts are the negative images left after cholesterol crystals have been dissolved by the alcohol in Romanowsky-type stains. When cholesterol crystals are abundant, some may remain undissolved in Romanowsky-stained smears. Cholesterol clefts and/or crystals commonly occur in epidermal cysts.

Hematomas

Fluid from hematomas is red to red-brown. Supernatant from centrifuged samples usually has a total protein content between 2.5 g/dl and that of peripheral blood. Cytologically, the fluid contains nondegenerate neutrophils, macrophages and numerous RBCs. A few lymphocytes may be present also. Usually, the macrophages are activated and often contain intact RBCs (Plate 2), hematoidin (Plate 2) and other RBC-breakdown products. Platelets are not found in fluid from hematomas unless there has been hemorrhage into the hematoma within a few hours of sample collection, or the sample is contaminated with peripheral blood. Differentiation of hematomas from hemangiomas and hemangiosarcomas is discussed in the "Hemangiomas" section of this chapter.

Seromas/Hygromas

Fluid from seromas/hygromas is typically clear to amber, and usually has a total protein concentration >2.5 g/dl. The fluid usually is of low cellularity. The cell population is composed predominantly of mononuclear cells with characteristics of macrophages or cyst lining cells. These cells are medium to large and round, and have moderate to abundant cytoplasm that is often highly vacuolated. Their nuclei may be centrally located but are often eccentric. Usually, the nucleus is round, has a smooth to fine lacy chromatin pattern, and may contain 1-2 indistinct nucleoli. A few nondegenerate neutrophils may also be found. A few cyst lining cells may be spindloid. Occasionally, some cells may be very dysplastic and exhibit criteria of malignancy.

With hemorrhage into the seroma/hygroma or if the sample is contaminated with peripheral blood, a combination of the cytologic characteristics of hematomas and/or peripheral blood and the cytologic characteristics of seromas/hygromas is found.

Abscesses

Fluid from abscesses usually is creamy, yellow, pink or brown. The total protein concentration usually cannot be determined because of the turbidity of the fluid. Even the supernatant of centrifuged samples often is too turbid for accurate total protein measurement. When the total protein concentration can be determined, it usually is >4 g/dl.

Smears prepared from abscesses are highly cellular. The cell composition usually is >90% neutrophils, with a few macrophages. Scattered lymphocytes and plasma cells may be present also. Abscesses caused by Gram-negative bacteria usually contain numerous degenerate neutrophils (Plate 1). Abscesses caused by Gram-positive bacteria often contain a few to many degenerate neutrophils. Other abscesses usually contain only a few or no degenerate neutrophils. Occasionally, macrophages may compose >50% of the nucleated cells, especially with sterile abscesses. Sterile foreign body abscesses, such as those caused by oil-based injections, may contain refractile material as well as inflammatory cells (Fig 1).

References

1. Coloe and Allison: Protothecosis in a cat. *JAVMA* 180:78-79, 1982.

2. Kaplan, *et al*: Protothecosis in a cat: First recorded case. *Sabouraudia* 14:281-286, 1976.

3. Finnie and Coloe: Cutaneous protothecosis in a cat. *Aust Vet J* 57:307-308, 1981.

4. Lorenz, in Ettinger: *Textbook of Veterinary Internal Medicine.* Saunders, Philadelphia, 1983. pp 1346-1372.

5. Dorn *et al*: Survey of animal neoplasms in Alameda and Contra Costa counties, California. II. Cancer morbidity in dogs and cats from Alameda County. *J Natl Cancer Inst* 40:307-318, 1968.

6. Susaneck: Feline skin tumors. *Comp Cont Ed Pract Vet* 5:251-257, 1983.

7. Duncan and Prasse: Cytologic examination of the skin and subcutis. *Vet Clin No Am* 6:637-645, 1976.

8. Duncan and Prasse: Cytology of canine cutaneous round cell tumors. *Vet Pathol* 16:673-679, 1979.

9. Barton: Cytologic diagnosis of cutaneous neoplasia: An algorithmic approach. *Comp Cont Ed Pract Vet* 9:20-33, 1987.

10. Rebar: *Handbook of Veterinary Cytology.* Ralston Purina, St. Louis, 1979.

11. Brown *et al*: Cutaneous lymphosarcoma in the dog: A disease with variable clinical and histologic manifestations. *JAAHA* 16:565-572, 1980.

12. McKeever *et al*: Canine cutaneous lymphoma. *JAVMA* 180:531-536, 1982.

13. Kramek *et al*: Infiltrative lipoma in three dogs. *JAVMA* 186:81-82, 1985.

3

Nasal Exudates and Masses

C.B. Andreasen, P.M. Rakich and K.S. Latimer

Indications

Pathologic conditions in the nasal cavity are often characterized by sneezing, nasal discharge, epistaxis, ocular discharge, pawing at the nose or facial deformity. Epistaxis may also result from primary coagulopathies, secondary coagulopathies (*eg*, canine ehrlichiosis) and hyperviscosity syndromes. Cytologic findings are interpreted in light of historical, physical, rhinoscopic, radiographic and clinical laboratory findings to arrive at a diagnosis. Rhinoscopy and cytologic evaluation are simple noninvasive procedures that may yield a definitive diagnosis. Cytologic evaluation is a method of screening the nasal cavity for the underlying etiology; however, negative or nonspecific findings do not exclude a fungal infection, neoplasm or foreign body if only superficial inflammatory cells are obtained. In some cases, surgical exploration of the nasal cavity and biopsy/cytologic evaluation may be necessary for definitive diagnosis.

Detailed examination of the nasal cavity and most sample collections are optimally performed while the animal is under general anesthesia, with an endotracheal tube in place and the cuff inflated. Radiographs and rhinoscopy should be performed before biopsy or flushing techniques so radiographic detail and visualization are not altered by resulting hemorrhage and manipulation of the nasal tissues.[1]

The nasal cavity may be examined with equipment that varies from simple to sophisticated (Fig 1). In some animals, an otoscope may be used to examine the rostral nares; however, a flexible 4-mm fiberoptic endoscope should be used to view the ventral nasal meatus or nasopharynx.[2] The oronasal cavity can be examined by retracting the soft palate with forceps and using a dental mirror or flexible endoscope (Fig 1). These procedures can aid visualization of abnormal tissues but copious exudates or hemorrhage may preclude adequate examination.

Sampling Techniques

Cytologic specimens from the nasal cavity may be obtained by flushing or aspiration techniques. These methods are safe if care is taken not to penetrate the cribriform plate with the

Figure 1. Schematic diagram indicating major landmarks and communication of the airways and food passages 1. nasal cavity, 2. nasopharynx, 3. palate, 4. oropharynx, 5. epiglottis, and 6. esophagus. The nasal cavity (1) may be sampled rostrad through the nares or caudad through the nasopharynx (2) as the soft palate (3) is retracted.

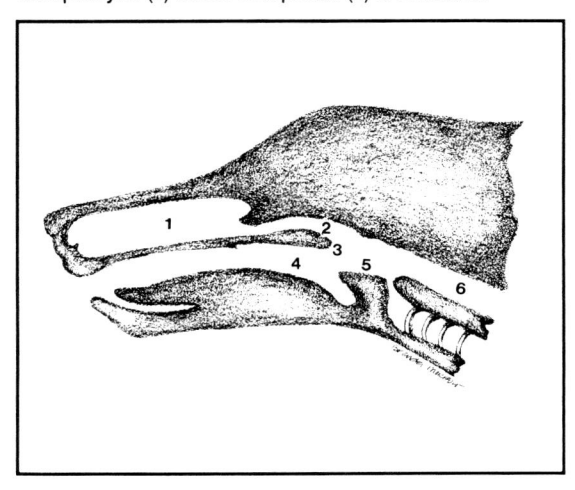

instruments used for obtaining samples and if precautions are taken to prevent inhalation of blood and fluids during sampling. Some hemorrhage may occur during manipulation of the nasal cavity, but this should not be a complicating factor unless a coagulopathy is present.

For the nasal flushing technique, the depth of the nasal cavity is estimated and a soft rubber catheter is passed caudad through the external nares or retrograde from caudal to the nasopharynx. A syringe containing about 10 ml of nonbacteriostatic sterile saline is attached to the catheter and multiple flushes are performed using intermittent positive and negative pressure.[1,2] Dislodged particulate matter can be caught in a gauze sponge placed caudal to the soft palate or rostral to the nares, depending on the direction of the flushing procedure. Aqueous cytologic material can be collected within the syringe barrel by aspiration.

Aspiration, the second means of obtaining samples from the nasal cavity, is useful when a mass is localized radiographically or visually. This technique involves use of a large-gauge polypropylene urinary catheter, a Sovereign plastic needle guard (Monoject), or a tomcat catheter cut at a 45-degree angle to form a sharp cutting edge.[3] Proper catheter length is determined by measuring the distance from the external nares to the medial canthus of the eye. Catheter length is important to prevent penetration of the cribriform plate during the procedure. The catheter is attached to a syringe and advanced into the nasal cavity until moderate resistance is felt. Suction is applied while several advances are made into the mass. Gentle negative pressure is maintained as the catheter is removed from the mass and nasal cavity to retain solid tissue fragments.

Alternatively, a biopsy needle (Tru-Cut: Travenol Labs) may be passed through the nares to the mass and a biopsy obtained. Samples may also be obtained with a biopsy forceps attachment during endoscopic examination. Needle and endoscopic biopsies are large enough for cytologic touch imprint preparations and, if necessary, histopathologic examination.

Nasal swabs often do not yield satisfactory diagnostic material because they cannot be inserted far enough into the nasal cavity and are not abrasive enough to obtain representative samples of deep mucosal lesions. A diagnosis may be obtained using nasal swabs if a causative agent, such as *Cryptococcus neoformans*, is present in the nasal exudate or rostral nares.

Cytologic preparations are made from touch imprints or squash preparations of tissue fragments, smears of flush samples and swabs, and smears of centrifuged nasal flush sediments. These preparations are air-dried, stained and examined by routine methods. (See Chapter 1 for further discussion concerning specimen preparation and staining.) A portion of the samples can be reserved for microbiologic culture and sensitivity testing if an infectious agent is suspected or found on stained cytologic preparations. After imprinting for cytologic evaluation, tissue fragments can be preserved in 10% neutral buffered formalin for histopathologic evaluation, if necessary.

Normal Cytologic Findings

It is important to distinguish normal from pathologic cell and bacterial populations in cytologic preparations. In nasal flush specimens, oropharyngeal organisms of variable morphology and epithelial cells may be obtained from healthy animals. *Simonsiella* spp are large, stacked, rod-shaped bacteria that are inhabitants of the oral cavity of dogs and cats and are seen commonly in smears contaminated by oral secretions (Plate 3).[4] Epithelial cell morphology varies with the site and depth of the specimen. Nonkeratinized squamous epithelial cells, often with adherent bacteria, are obtained from the external nares and oropharynx. Ciliated pseudostratified columnar epithelial cells and associated mucus originate from the nasal turbinates (Fig 2). Basal epithelial cells are smaller and rounded and have darker blue cytoplasm (Plate 6). Hemorrhage during sampling results in the presence of RBC and WBC in similar proportions to peripheral blood (about 1 WBC for every 500-1000 RBC).

Infectious Agents

Neutrophils usually predominate in exudates associated with bacterial, viral and some fungal infections. In addition to neutrophils, variable numbers of macrophages, lymphocytes and plasma cells may be present with any inflammatory condition (Plates 1 and 2). Pathogenic bacterial infection should be suspected when bacterial organisms (Plate 3) are seen within neutrophils as compared to normal bacterial flora that colonize squamous epithelial cells in the absence of neutrophils (Fig 3). Since bacteria from the oral cavity are usually a pleomorphic population, a monomorphic bacterial population suggests infection.[5]

Figure 2. A row of normal ciliated columnar respiratory epithelial cells (630X).

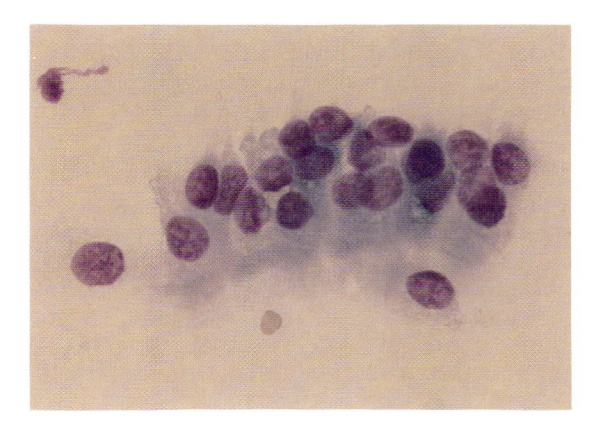

Classification of bacteria on the basis of a Gram-stained exudate is often unreliable; however, with routine hematologic stains, homogeneous populations of cocci usually represent Gram-positive organisms, such as *Staphylococcus* or *Streptococcus* spp, while homogeneous populations of bipolar rods often indicate Gram-negative organisms. Samples should be submitted for microbiologic culture, identification and sensitivity testing.

Bacterial infections are usually secondary to mucosal injury from trauma or foreign bodies, but also may be associated with viral infection, fungal infection and neoplasia. Oronasal fistulas can result in chronic bacterial rhinitis. These fistulas most commonly involve canine, premolar and molar teeth.[6]

Figure 3. Septic purulent exudate with a monomorphic population of intracellular and extracellular paired cocci (400X).

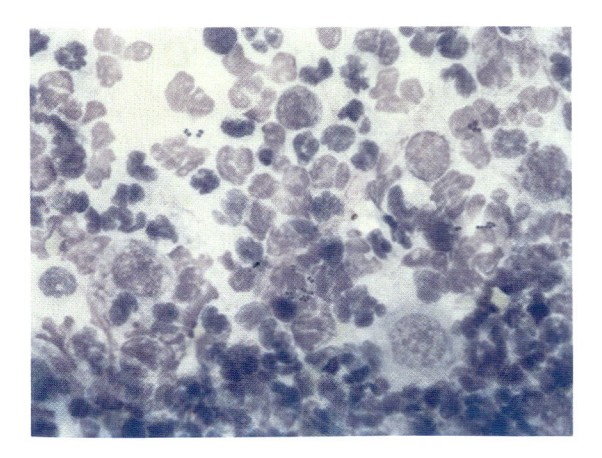

Viral inclusions are infrequently seen in nasal cytology specimens. Herpesvirus infection in cats may produce intranuclear inclusions within epithelial cells.[7] Since inclusions are rarely found in Wright's-stained cytologic preparations, definitive diagnosis of viral inclusions is best accomplished by fluorescent antibody examination.

Fungal infections, foreign bodies and neoplasia of the nasal cavity should be suspected when sinusitis is unresponsive to antibacterial therapy. In the case of mycotic rhinitis, fungal hyphae frequently are present within dense accumulations of cells and debris (Plate 5). Hyphae may be difficult to discern because they may not stain well with Romanowsky and new methylene blue stains and appear as clear filamentous structures (Plate 5). If a fungal infection is suspected but no fungal elements are identified on cytologic preparations, slides can be submitted to a laboratory for examination with special stains, such as periodic acid-Schiff (PAS) or Gomori's methenamine silver (GMS), to enhance visualization of fungal organisms. Additionally, fungal cultures are more reliable in identifying a fungal species than are morphologic characteristics.

Aspergillus spp and/or *Penicillium* spp reportedly produce nasal cavity and sinus infections in dogs and cats. These agents are associated with serosanguineous to mucopurulent nasal exudates, nasal mucosal necrosis, and turbinate destruction.[8-10] Both *Aspergillus* spp and *Penicillium* spp appear as 2- to 4.5-μ-wide septate, branching hyphae on cytologic preparations (Plate 5); therefore, specific identification requires fungal culture.[10]

Cryptococcus neoformans is a saprophytic yeast that causes rhinitis and sinusitis and occurs most commonly in cats.[11,12] The organism may sometimes be found in touch imprints or aspirates of nasal lesions without nasal flushing or biopsy techniques. This basophilic yeast is round to oval, 3.5-7.0 μ in diameter, surrounded by a thick polysaccharide capsule (1-30 μ) that stains poorly with Wright's or Diff-Quik (Dade Diagnostics) stains (Fig 4 and Plate 4). Though India ink is often proposed as an aid in identifying *Cryptococcus neoformans*, air bubbles and fat globules can be mistaken for organisms, particularly by inexperienced microscopists.

Rhinosporidiosis in dogs is characterized by polypoid nasal growths and caused by *Rhinosporidium seeberi*, a fungal organism of uncertain taxonomy and incompletely defined life cycle.[13,14] Diagnosis is based upon finding

Figure 4. Numerous variably sized, spherical yeasts with thick unstained capsules are typical of *Cryptococcus neoformans* (400X).

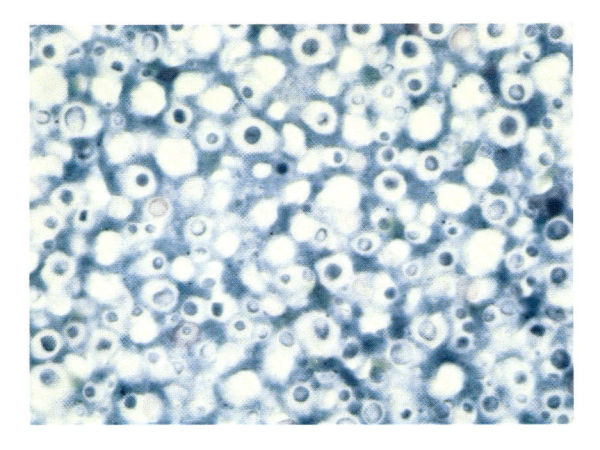

round to oval, 7-μ-diameter spores in nasal exudates or tissue imprints. The spores stain bright pink, have internal eosinophilic globules and are surrounded by thin bilamellar cell walls (Fig 5). Finding large sporangia containing numerous endospores supports the diagnosis; however, these structures are infrequently seen.[15]

Though parasitic diseases of the nasal cavity and sinuses are infrequent causes of clinical signs in small animals, infections with the arthropods *Pneumonyssus caninum* and *Linguatula serrata* have been reported in dogs.[6,16] Adult or larval forms of the nasal mite *P caninum* may be found on the nasal mucosa. The mites may be an incidental finding or may be associated with mucosal irritation and sneezing. *Linguatula serrata* is a pentastome that attaches to the nasal mucosa and may induce sneezing, coughing and epistaxis. Adult parasites may be visualized endoscopically or larvated eggs may be found in nasal exudates. Exudates associated with these parasites often contain increased numbers of eosinophils.

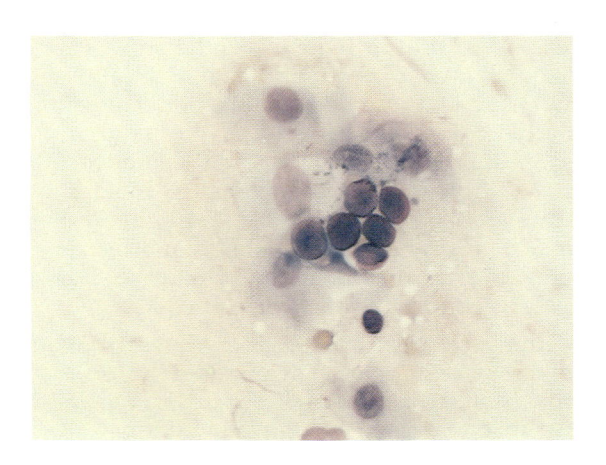

The helminth parasite *Capillaria aerophila* usually is found in the distal respiratory tract but may be found within the nasal sinuses.[6,17] Inflammatory exudates may contain characteristic barrel-shaped eggs with bipolar end plugs, neutrophils and eosinophils (Fig 6). Sedimentation of nasal flush samples may be helpful in obtaining ova.

Figure 6. Barrel-shaped egg with bipolar end plugs characteristic of *Capillaria* spp (1000X).

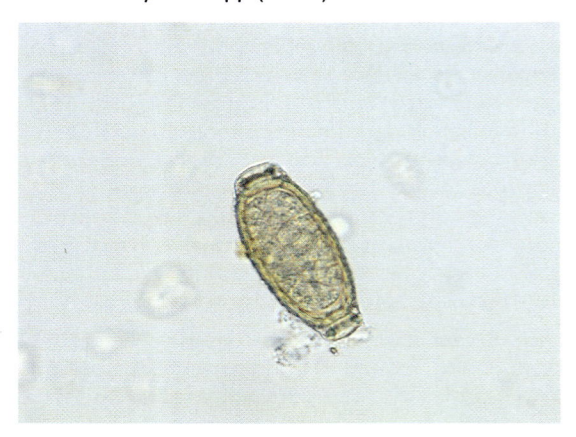

Figure 5. Round, eosinophilic, bilamellar-walled spores of *Rhinosporidium seeberi* (400X).

Noninfectious Conditions

Nasal foreign bodies most frequently consist of inhaled plant material, such as grass awns or foxtails. Cytologic preparations should be examined closely for foreign material consisting of variably sized and shaped particles with distinct cell walls, fibers and various degrees of pigmentation. A common sequel to this problem is chronic rhinitis due to persistence of foreign material, with damage to the nasal mucosa.

Exudates with a predominance of eosinophils may result from environmental inhalant allergens (Plate 3). Since eosinophils may be present in response to parasites, fungi, bacteria and neoplasms, these conditions should be ruled out cytologically and/or radiographically before allergic inhalant rhinitis is diagnosed.

Neoplastic Disorders

Neoplasia involving nasal passages and sinuses generally occurs in older animals, with a mean age of 8-10 years.[6,18,19] Nasal tumors are malignant in 80-90% of reported cases, but metastasis is uncommon.[18] Tumors can arise from epithelial or mesenchymal tissues of the nasal cavity, extend from the oral cavity into the nasal passages, or be transplanted into the nasal cavity, *eg*, transmissible venereal tumor.

Clinical presentation, history and radiographic lesions may lead to presumptive diagnosis of neoplasia; however, cytologic or histologic examination is needed to confirm the diagnosis. Cytologic specimens of any tumor type may contain RBC, inflammatory cells, bacteria and necrotic debris. Neoplastic cells may or may not be present. Fine-needle aspiration or catheter biopsy of a tumor is more likely to yield identifiable neoplastic cells than a nasal flush. Usually, only normal superficial nasal epithelial cells or inflammatory cells are obtained from a nasal flush.

Most nasal tumors are of epithelial-cell origin. Adenocarcinomas are most common, followed by squamous-cell carcinomas and undifferentiated carcinomas.[18,20] Carcinomas usually consist of clusters of round to oval cells, with variable nucleus:cytoplasm ratios (Plate 6). These characteristics of malignancy are less pronounced in well-differentiated carcinomas, which may be difficult to distinguish from hyperplastic epithelial cells. Adenocarcinomas may be associated with production of mucus, apparent as amorphous to fibrillar deeply pink-staining material. Squamous-cell carcinomas generally consist of various developmental stages ranging from small hyperchromatic cells to large round or angular cells with pale basophilic cytoplasm and large nuclei (Fig 7). Perinuclear clearing, if present, strongly suggests squamous-cell origin.

Figure 7. Cells from a squamous-cell carcinoma with characteristic pale basophilic cytoplasm, large nuclei and perinuclear clearing (400X).

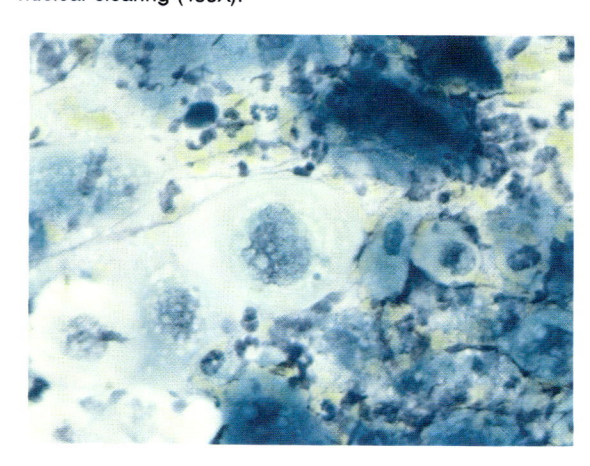

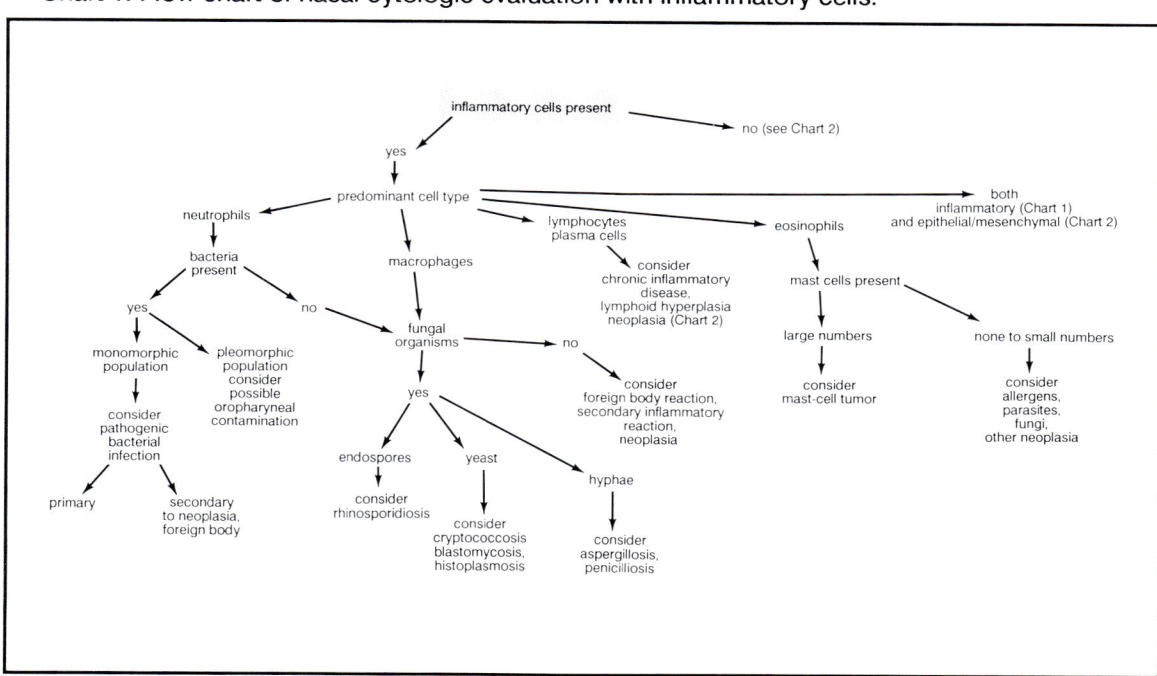

Chart 1. Flow chart of nasal cytologic evaluation with inflammatory cells.

Chapter 3

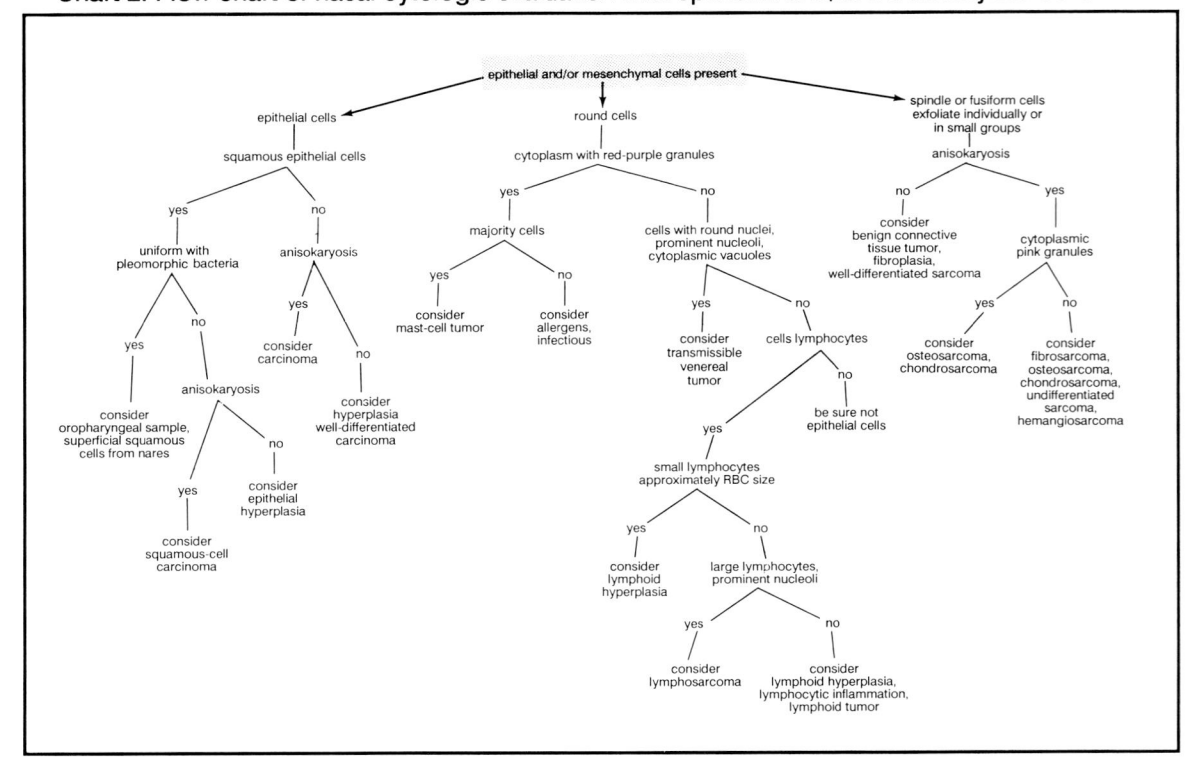

Chart 2. Flow chart of nasal cytologic evaluation with epithelial and/or mesenchymal cells.

Mesenchymal tumors of the nasal cavity primarily include fibrosarcomas, chondrosarcomas, osteosarcomas, hemangiosarcomas and undifferentiated sarcomas.[20] As with sarcomas in any location, these tumors do not exfoliate readily. Aspirates or catheter biopsy imprints tend to produce a more cellular sample for evaluation than do nasal flushes. Sarcoma cells range from plump oval to fusiform or spindle shaped, with cytoplasm streaming away from the nucleus. These cells also tend to exfoliate individually or in small clumps, as compared to carcinomas, which often exfoliate in large sheets (Plate 7). In osteosarcomas and chondrosarcomas, cells may have abundant basophilic cytoplasm and pink granules (Chapter 11, Fig 5). Reactive fibroplasia and fibrosarcoma may be difficult or impossible to differentiate cytologically. Definitive identification of the type of sarcoma usually requires histologic examination.

Round-cell tumors of the nasal cavity include transmissible venereal tumors, lymphosarcomas and mast-cell tumors (Plate 7). Generally these tumors exfoliate as a homogenous population of individual round cells with distinct cell margins. Lymphosarcoma usually is characterized by a monomorphic population of large immature lymphocytes (Plate 7). In contrast, small mature lymphocytes predominate in nonneoplastic conditions with submucosal lymphoid hyperplasia. (See Chapter 8 on lymph node cytology for further discussion on differentiating lymphoid hyperplasia from lymphosarcoma.)

Mast-cell neoplasia is characterized by bloody aspirates containing numerous mast cells with fewer eosinophils (Plate 7). In contrast, allergic rhinitis is characterized by few mast cells and many eosinophils. Other cell types present may include plasma cells and lymphocytes.

Transmissible venereal tumors are more commonly associated with genital neoplasms but may be transplanted to the nasal mucosa due to the social habits of dogs, especially males.[21] The tumor cells have round nuclei, variable chromatin pattern, and a single prominent nucleolus. Cytoplasm is lightly basophilic and moderate in amount, and usually contains clear vacuoles (Plate 7). Mitoses may be numerous and inflammatory cells of mixed type may be present.

References

1. Meyer: The management of cytology specimens. *Comp Cont Ed Pract Vet* 9:10-16, 1987.

2. Rudd and Richardson: A diagnostic and therapeutic approach to nasal disease in dogs. *Comp Cont Ed Pract Vet* 7:103-112, 1985.

3. Withrow et al: Aspiration and punch biopsy techniques for nasal tumors. *JAAHA* 21:551-554, 1985.

4. Nyby et al: Incidence of *Simonsiella* in the oral cavity of dogs. *J Clin Microbiol* 6:87-88, 1977.

5. French: The use of cytology in the diagnosis of chronic nasal disorders. *Comp Cont Ed Pract Vet* 9:115-120, 1987.

6. O'Brien and Harvey, in Ettinger: *Textbook of Veterinary Internal Medicine*. 2nd ed. Saunders, Philadelphia, 1983. pp 692-722.

7. Perman et al: *Cytology of the Dog and Cat*. American Animal Hospital Association, Denver, CO, 1979. pp 142-143.

8. Harvey et al: Nasal penicilliosis in six dogs. *JAVMA* 178:1084-1087, 1981.

9. Goring et al: A contrast rhinographic diagnosis of nasal and sinusoidal aspergillosis in the dog: a case report. *JAAHA* 19:920-924, 1983.

10. Barsanti, in Greene: *Clinical Microbiology and Infectious Diseases of the Dog and Cat*. Saunders, Philadelphia, 1984. pp 728-737.

11. Barsanti, in Greene: *Clinical Microbiology and Infectious Diseases of the Dog and Cat*. Saunders, Philadelphia, 1984. pp 700-709.

12. Macy and Small, in Ettinger: *Textbook of Veterinary Internal Medicine*. 2nd ed. Saunders, Philadelphia, 1983. pp 237-269.

13. Barsanti, in Greene: *Clinical Microbiology and Infectious Diseases of the Dog and Cat*. Saunders, Philadelphia, 1984. pp 738-746.

14. Mosier and Creed: Rhinosporidiosis in a dog. *JAVMA* 185:1009-1010, 1984.

15. Easley et al. Nasal rhinosporidiosis in the dog. *Vet Pathol* 23:50-56, 1986.

16. Barsanti and Prestwood, in Kirk: *Current Veterinary Therapy VIII*. Saunders, Philadelphia, 1983. pp 241-246.

17. Evinger et al: Ivermectin for treatment of nasal capillariasis in a dog. *JAVMA* 186:174-175, 1985.

18. Legendre et al: Canine nasal and paranasal sinus tumors. *JAAHA* 19:115-123, 1983.

19. Madewell et al: Neoplasms of the nasal passages and paranasal sinuses in domesticated animals as reported by 13 veterinary colleges. *Am J Vet Res* 37:851-856, 1976.

20. Norris: Intranasal neoplasms in the dog. *JAAHA* 15:231-236, 1979.

21. Moulton, in Moulton: *Tumors in Domestic Animals*. 2nd ed. Univ California Press, Berkeley, 1978. pp 307-345.

4

The Oropharynx and Tonsils

R.D. Tyler, R.L. Cowell and J.H. Meinkoth

Indications

Foul breath, dysphagia, loose teeth, drooling, pain and/or persistent hemorrhage from the mouth warrant a thorough examination of the oropharynx, including palpation of the gums, teeth, cheeks and jaws. Visual examination of the oropharynx, especially the pharyngeal area, is occasionally impaired by pain caused by manipulation of the jaws. Occasionally, enlargements in the facial, intermandibular or cranial cervical areas suggest a lesion involving the oropharynx. When nasal structures are involved, upper respiratory signs (epistaxis, sneezing, etc) may be present.

Cytologic examination is often useful in evaluating lesions of the oropharynx and tonsils. These lesions may be ulcers, masses, draining tracts, plaques or enlarged tonsils. Such lesions as ulcers may initially be treated with antibiotics or other therapies, and cytologic examination may be employed only after they fail to respond to treatment. However, masses are often cytologically evaluated before therapy is instituted. Ulcers, draining tracts and plaques are often cultured at the same time they are cytologically evaluated.

Techniques

Cytologic samples may be obtained from *in-situ* lesions or from excised tissue. Lesions may be aspirated, scraped or imprinted *in situ* to obtain cytologic samples. When collecting cytologic samples from the oral cavity, the disinfectant used to clean the lesion must be nontoxic. Otherwise, the procedures for collection of cytologic samples detailed in Chapter 1 are followed. Cytologic preparations from excised tissue are obtained by the procedures detailed in Chapter 1.

Sometimes, cytologic samples can be collected from the oral cavity without anesthesia. Depending on the type of sample being collected, the painfulness of the lesion, and the stoicism of the animal, the level of chemical restraint required ranges from none, to tranquilization, to surgical-plane anesthesia. The level of restraint, whether manual or chemical, is the minimal level required for safe collection of an adequate sample. On the other hand, collection of cytologic samples from the pharyngeal region usually requires tranquilization and/or anesthesia. Positioning of the animal is dependent on the location of the lesion. The animal should be placed in the position allowing the collector to most comfortably approach the lesion and collect the sample.

Imprints may be diagnostically rewarding in the evaluation of ulcers, whereas aspirates are usually more diagnostic when evaluating masses. Scrapings are usually rewarding in evaluating ulcers and plaques, and are often rewarding in evaluating ulcerated masses. However, scrapings and imprints often contain sufficient numbers of inflammatory cells to prevent definitive diagnosis of neoplasia. Also, squamous cells collected by imprinting or scraping may impair determination of the type of neoplasia present. Therefore, aspirates of masses are usually more rewarding in establishing the presence of neoplasia and determining the neoplastic cell type.

Interpretation

Cytologic samples from the oropharynx and tonsils may contain normal tissue cells, inflammatory cells and/or cells from primary or metastatic neoplasms. Cells that may be collected from the normal tissues of the oropharynx and tonsils include squamous epithelial cells, fibrocytes/fibroblasts, cuboidal or columnar epithelial cells from salivary glands and ducts of the oropharynx, and lymphoid cells from the tonsils. Also, bacilli, cocci and spirochetes may be collected from the normal oropharynx, or may be primary or secondary pathogens. One bacterium in particular, *Simonsiella* (Plate 3), is a normal inhabitant of the oropharynx and should not be considered a pathogen.

Squamous Epithelial Cells

Squamous epithelial cells (Plate 6) may be collected from the normal epithelium lining the oral cavity and pharynx, and covering the tonsils. These cells are large, flat and angular. They may be anuclear or contain a very small, dark-staining, centrally located nucleus without a visible nucleolus. They are usually collected on imprints and scrapings regardless of the cause of the lesion. Deep aspirates of oropharyngeal or tonsillar lesions usually do not contain many squamous epithelial cells unless the lesion is neoplastic, such as squamous-cell carcinoma (Plate 6), or the operator continues aspirating as the needle is withdrawn.

Fibrocytes/Fibroblasts

Fibrocytes and/or fibroblasts (Plate 7) may be collected on imprints of ulcerated lesions, scrapings or aspirates. These cells are derived from connective tissue underlying the squamous epithelium lining the oropharynx. Fibrocytes and fibroblasts are spindle cells. Fibrocytes are very fusiform, with a moderate amount of light blue cytoplasm that pulls away from the nucleus in 1-2 directions. They have a single, dark-staining nucleus with a smooth chromatin pattern, and indistinct or unrecognizable nucleoli. Fibroblasts are more plump spindle cells, with a moderate amount of cytoplasm that pulls away from the nucleus in 1-2 directions. Their nuclei are moderately dark staining, but not as dark staining as fibrocyte nuclei, have a smooth or fine chromatin pattern, and contain indistinct to prominent nucleoli. Fibroblasts may be found as a result of fibroplasia stimulated by an inflammatory or neoplastic lesion in the area or as a result of fibrous neoplasia, fibroma or fibrosarcoma (Plate 7). Differentiation of fibrous neoplasia from fibroplasia is difficult to impossible cytologically. Therefore, histopathologic examination may be necessary for definitive diagnosis of fibroma or fibrosarcoma.

Cuboidal and Columnar Epithelial Cells

Occasionally, epithelial cells (Fig 5, Chapter 7) may be collected from the salivary glands and ducts of the oral cavity. These cells are medium sized and round, with a moderate amount of medium to dark blue cytoplasm. They contain a single nucleus that is dark to moderately dark staining, have a coarse chromatin pattern, and contain a single indistinct, round nucleolus. Occasionally, ranulas develop in the salivary ducts of the oral cavity. These are easily identified cytologically by the presence of large foamy epithelial cells and/or macrophages (Fig 6, Chapter 7). Rarely, adenocarcinomas (Plate 6) develop within the oral cavity. See Chapter 7 for further discussion of salivary cysts, neoplasia and inflammation.

Lymphoid Cells

The tonsils are a lymphoid organ covered by squamous epithelium. Lymphoid cells and sometimes squamous epithelial cells are collected on imprints, scrapings or aspirates of the tonsils. Lymphoid aggregates or follicles may form in other areas of the pharynx and the caudal portion of the tongue. Typically, >80% of the lymphoid cells collected from a normal tonsil or lymphoid aggregate are small lymphocytes (Plate 1). The remainder of the lymphoid cells are medium-sized lymphocytes (prolymphocytes) (Plate 1) and large lymphocytes (lymphoblasts), (Plates 1 and 7). In normal samples, medium-sized lymphocytes markedly outnumber large lymphocytes.

Small lymphocytes (Plate 1) are smaller than neutrophils and have indented round nuclei about the same size as a canine RBC and about 1.25-1.5 times the size of a feline RBC. The nuclei have densely aggregated chromatin that prevents visualization of the nucleoli. The chromatin pattern often appears smudged. The cytoplasm is scant and pale blue, and often can be visualized only on one side of the nucleus (area of the Golgi apparatus).

Medium lymphocytes (Plate 1) are about the same size as neutrophils, have a small amount (slightly more than small lymphocytes) of light to medium blue cytoplasm, and contain nuclei that are moderately dark staining (but less dark staining than the nuclei of small lymphocytes), with a smudged, moderately aggregated chromatin pattern and indistinct multiple nucleoli.

Large lymphocytes (Plates 1 and 7) are recognizably larger than neutrophils and have a small to moderate amount of medium to dark blue cytoplasm. Their nuclei stain less darkly than medium lymphocyte nuclei, and have a smudged, stippled chromatin pattern, and multiple nucleoli.

Lymphoid cells may be collected on imprints, scrapings or aspirates of normal lymphoid tissue such as the tonsil, areas of inflammation in which the inflammatory response contains a lymphoid component, or lymphoid tumors. Collections from lymphoid neoplasia (Plate 7) usually yield >50% large lymphocytes (lymphoblasts), while collections from inflamed lymphoid tissue (Fig 8, Chapter 8), inflamed tissue in which lymphoid cells are a portion of the inflammatory component, or normal or hyperplastic lymphoid tissue (Figs 1-5, Chapter 8) usually yield <20% of the lymphoid cells as large lymphocytes (lymphoblasts). Evaluation of lymphoid tissue is further discussed in Chapter 8.

Inflammatory Cells

Inflammatory lesions may result from trauma, infections, foreign bodies, neoplasia, immune-mediated disease (pemphigus, etc), uremia and the eosinophilic granuloma complex. Inflammation is characterized by the presence of inflammatory cells, *ie*, neutrophils, eosinophils, macrophages, lymphocytes and plasma cells. The proportion of the different types of inflammatory cells depends upon the etiology of the inflammatory condition. Chart 1 presents an algorithm to assist in interpretation of samples from the oropharynx.

Neutrophils are present in nearly all inflammatory responses and usually predominate. Occasionally, with mycoses, allergic inflammatory responses and the eosinophilic granuloma complex, other inflammatory cell types (macrophages and/or eosinophils) may predominate. The general interpretation suggested by finding the different inflammatory cell types is discussed below for each cell type.

Marked Predominance of Neutrophils

Inflammatory lesions caused by trauma, uremia or infection yield samples composed primarily of inflammatory cells, with an occasional squamous epithelial cell and fibrocyte/fibroblast. Usually, the inflammatory cell population is comprised of >90% neutrophils (many of which are degenerate if a Gram-negative bacterium is involved) and <10% of an admixture of macrophages, lymphocytes, eosinophils and/or plasma cells in variable proportions. Often, a homogeneous population of bacteria is seen if the inflammatory lesion is caused by a primary bacterial infection or with secondary bacterial infection. A heterogeneous population of bacteria suggests secondary bacterial overgrowth.

Macrophages

The population of inflammatory cells expected from lesions caused by mycotic infections and foreign body reactions is usually composed of >50% neutrophils, but on occasion may contain a predominance of macrophages. Occasionally, mycotic inflammatory lesions may also contain many eosinophils. Lymphocytes and plasma cells are present at variable levels, depending on the extent of cell-mediated response and/or chronicity of the inflammatory response. Samples from eosinophilic granuloma complex lesions may contain increased numbers of macrophages also.

Eosinophils

Allergic inflammatory lesions and the eosinophilic granuloma complex usually yield samples containing many eosinophils and variable numbers of other inflammatory cells. A few squamous epithelial cells and fibrocytes/fibroblasts may be present also. Eosinophils usually compose >20% of the inflammatory cell population, sometimes >80%. Rarely, an eosinophilic granuloma complex lesion may yield a cytologic preparation devoid of eosinophils. Histopathologic examination is needed to definitively diagnose these lesions. Samples from eosinophilic granuloma complex lesions may contain moderate numbers of fibroblasts that may have some atypical characteristics (Fig 7, Chapter 2). These fibroblasts may have large nuclei with multiple prominent nucleoli and an increased nucleus:cytoplasm ratio. Occasionally, the eosinophilic granuloma also contains moderate numbers of macrophages. On the other hand, allergic inflammatory responses usually contain only a few fibroblasts and/or macrophages. Seldom are reactive or atypical fibroblasts associated with allergic inflammatory responses. Both allergic inflammatory responses and the eosinophilic granuloma complex may contain a few mast cells and basophils, and variable numbers of lymphocytes and plasma cells. Mycotic infections and foreign body reactions occasionally contain numerous eosinophils. These 2 conditions usually contain numerous macrophages and sometimes also contain inflammatory giant cells.

Neoplasia

The oral cavity is the fourth most common site of neoplasia in dogs and cats.[1-3] Squamous-cell carcinoma, malignant melanoma and fibrosarcoma are the most common malignant tumors of the oral cavity in dogs.[1,4-6] Whether squamous-cell carcinoma or malignant melanoma is more common in dogs has not been well established.[7] However, squamous-cell carcinoma, which comprises 50% or more of the malignant tumors of the oropharynx in cats, is the most common malignant tumor of the feline oropharynx.[1,4,6,8,9] Benign epulides are the most common benign neoplasm of the canine oropharynx.[7] Studies comparing the frequency of benign and malignant neoplasms of the canine oropharynx indicate benign epulides are less common than malignant melanoma, but more common than squamous-cell carcinoma.[7] The common tumors of dogs and cats are listed in Table 1 according to the area of the oropharynx in which they tend to occur.

Definitive diagnosis of neoplasms of the oropharynx and tonsils can be made by cytologic examination for some tumors, such as lymphosarcoma. Other tumors, such as odontogenic tumors, require histopathologic evaluation for definitive diagnosis. Often, cytologic evaluation of oropharyngeal and tonsillar lesions indicates whether the lesion is inflammatory or neoplastic, is of epithelial or mesenchymal origin, and displays sufficient criteria of malignancy to be classified as malignant; sometimes, however, the specific cell of origin cannot be predicted. In these cases, histopathologic evaluation to determine the specific cell of origin may be important, since prognosis, treatment modalities and responsiveness to therapy may vary for different types of tumors. Lesions that cytologically appear to be neoplastic, but do not have cytologic criteria of malignancy, should not be classified as benign on the basis of cytologic findings alone. These lesions should be biopsied and submitted for histopathologic evaluation.

Table 1. Oropharyngeal tumors in dogs and cats listed by the location in which they tend to occur.

Location	Dogs	Cats
Lips and cheeks	Melanoma (usually malignant) Fibrosarcoma TVT	Tumors of the lips and cheeks are uncommon in cats
Gingivae	Epulis Melanoma (usually malignant) Squamous-cell carcinoma Fibrosarcoma TVT	Squamous-cell carcinoma Fibrosarcoma Adamantinoma (rare) Melanoma (rare, usually malignant) Adenocarcinoma (rare) Hemangiosarcoma (rare)
Palate	Melanoma (usually malignant) Fibrosarcoma Squamous-cell carcinoma Papilloma TVT	Fibrosarcoma Adenocarcinoma Melanoma (usually malignant)
Tongue	All except epulis	Squamous-cell carcinoma Fibrosarcoma
Tonsils	Squamous-cell carcinoma Lymphosarcoma	Squamous-cell carcinoma Lymphosarcoma

Squamous Epithelial Tumors: Invaginations of the squamous epithelium lining the buccal cavity give rise to the enamel caps of the teeth. Cytologically, neoplasms of enamel origin cannot be reliably differentiated from neoplasms arising from the squamous epithelium. Histopathologic examination is recommended when it is necessary to establish the specific cell of origin, *eg*, adamantinoma, etc.

Epulides: Epulides are the most common class of benign oral neoplasm. There are 3 general types of epulides: fibromatous, ossifying and acanthomatous.[7] Samples from fibromatous epulides usually are of low cellularity, consisting of spindle cells and a few squamous cells from the epithelium. Samples from ossifying epulides may contain pink-staining osteoid along with spindle cells. Acanthomatous epulides yield a predominance of squamous epithelial cells in various stages of maturation. Usually, criteria of malignancy are not prominent.

Squamous-Cell Carcinomas: Most carcinomas of the oral cavity are squamous-cell carcinomas. These neoplasms generally contain neoplastic squamous cells in all stages of development. Neoplastic squamous cells may be small to medium sized and round, and have very basophilic cytoplasm and round nuclei showing marked chromatin clumping and prominent nucleoli. Or they may be large, with a moderate to abundant amount of cytoplasm staining less intensely and may have a green tint. The nuclei of these cells tend to remain large instead of contracting and becoming pyknotic, as occurs with normal squamous-cell maturation. Squamous-cell carcinomas often show strong criteria of malignancy (Table 4, Chapter 1). Occasionally, squamous epithelial cells with clear rings around their nuclei and mildly to markedly basophilic cytoplasm are found. These cells are considered suggestive of squamous-cell carcinoma. If sufficient criteria of malignancy are not present to merit classification of the mass as a malignant tumor, histopathologic examination should be performed before the tumor is classified as benign. Because oral neoplasms often ulcerate, evaluation of oral neoplasms is often complicated by inflammation.

Glandular Tumors: Adenomas and adenocarcinomas of the oral cavity are rare. When they occur, they yield the cytologic characteristics described for adenomas and adenocarcinomas of salivary glands in Chapter 7.

Mesenchymal Tumors (Spindle-Cell Tumors): Fibrosarcomas and malignant melanomas (considered here under mesenchymal tumors because of their cytologic characteristics even though they arise from the neural crest) are by far the most common mesenchymal tumors of the oropharynx. Other mesenchymal tumors that have been identified in the oropharynx include fibromas, hemangiosarcomas and liposarcomas. These tumors are discussed in Chapter 2.

Fibrosarcomas: Fibrosarcomas usually yield a small to moderate number of cells by aspiration. Scrapings are much more productive. Fibrosarcoma cells may be fusiform to oval or round and may have 1-2 projections of cytoplasm streaming away from the nucleus (Plate 7). Depending on the differentiation of the tumor, sometimes only a few cells may be fusiform or spindle shaped. It is essential to evaluate all cells for tails of cytoplasm streaming away from the nucleus. The cytoplasm varies from mildly to markedly basophilic and sometimes contains small, clear or pink vacuoles. The cytoplasm boundaries may be indistinct.

Fibrosarcoma cell nuclei tend to be round to oval and centrally located, and contain single or multiple nucleoli. The nucleoli are often irregular in size and shape, and often very large. Fibrosarcoma cells occasionally are multinucleated. The chromatin of fibrosarcoma cells is usually much coarser than the chromatin of normal fibrocytes/fibroblasts.

Malignant Melanomas: In dogs and cats, most oropharyngeal melanomas are malignant. Melanoma cells (Plate 8) may be spindle or epithelioid in shape. Because some cells can usually be found with the characteristics of spindle cells and because melanoma cells tend to exfoliate as individual cells instead of in groups, clumps and sheets as epithelial cells do, they tend to have the appearance of spindle-cell tumors on cytologic preparations even though they arise from the neural crest (an ectodermal origin tissue). Melanocytes/melanoblasts are medium-sized cells with scanty to abundant cytoplasm, depending upon the level of cellular differentiation. Histopathologically, some melanomas are classified as amelanotic. However, cytologically, melanin granules can invariably be found. Because mast-cell tumors are also granulated, melanocytes/melanoblasts must be differentiated from mast-cell tumor cells (Plates 7 and 8). This differentiation is based upon the morphology of the cytoplasmic granules as well as on the morphology of the cells. Mast-cell granules are blue to red-purple, usually uniform in size, and round to oval. Melanin granules, however, are brown-black to green-black (this is their natural pigment color and does not depend on staining) and tend to be irregular in size and shape.

Melanomas classified histologically as amelanotic melanomas may yield a few cells devoid of granules, but many cells have a few fine granules. In general, since melanin production is an indication of differentiation, the less pigmented the cells, the more malignant the neoplasm. Preparations from melanomas usually contain both epithelioid-appearing cells and spindle cells, but mast cells are only round to oval. Malignant melanoma cells are often of bizarre shape, and multinucleated forms may occur. Generally, a few to many eosinophils are found in samples from mast-cell tumors, but not in samples from melanomas.

Melanocytes/melanoblasts must also be differentiated from macrophages containing melanin and from macrophages containing hemosiderin. Chronic irritation can result in increased dermal pigmentation and increased numbers of macrophages containing melanin, whereas local hemorrhage can result in numerous macrophages containing hemosiderin. Therefore, spindle-shaped melanocytes/melanoblasts should be identified to establish the diagnosis of melanoma. As with most, if not all, cytologic interpretations, if any question (that would affect management of the case) exists, the slides should be referred for interpretation, another cytologic preparation collected and perused, or other diagnostic procedures, such as radiography or histopathologic examination, should be implemented.

Discrete Round-Cell Tumors: The discrete round-cell tumors, lymphosarcoma (Plate 7), transmissible venereal tumor (Plate 7), histiocytoma (Fig 12, Chapter 2) and mast-cell tumor (Plate 7), all may develop in the mouth. Lymphosarcoma is by far the most common discrete round-cell tumor occurring in the mouth. In areas where transmissible venereal tumor (TVT) is enzootic, these tumors may occasionally be found in the oropharynx. Histopathologically, TVT may be misidentified as lymphoreticular tumors. Because of the difference in biologic behavior and therapy of lymphosarcoma and TVT, differentiating these tumors is important. Lymphosarcoma tends to occur in the tonsils, whereas TVT tends to occur on the buccal surface.

Cytologic preparations of lymphosarcoma yield a predominance of lymphoid cells, though in the oropharynx secondary inflammation is common and neutrophil numbers may be increased. With lymphosarcoma, usually >50% of the lymphoid cells are lymphoblasts and can be recognized by their size (larger than neutrophils). Also, they usually contain prominent multiple nucleoli and have a scant to moderate amount of light to moderately blue cytoplasm that is devoid of vacuoles. With lymphosarcoma, occasionally some lymphoblasts may be vacuolated. Generally, the nuclear chromatin of lymphoblasts has a smudged, stippled pattern. In contrast, though TVT cells are also larger than neutrophils, they have a moderate to abundant amount of cytoplasm that stains smoky gray to blue and contains numerous distinct vacuoles. The nuclei of TVT cells have a distinct ropy or cord-like chromatin pattern and contain 1-2 large, prominent nucleoli. Chapter 2 contains a further discussion of the differentiation of lymphosarcoma from TVT and descriptions of mast-cell tumors and histiocytomas.

Algorithmic Interpretation of Samples

Chart 1 presents a logical, methodical approach to evaluation of oropharyngeal and tonsillar cytologic samples. Certainly, there are other approaches and, hence, other algorithms can be designed for evaluation of oropharyngeal and tonsillar cytologic samples. Regardless of the approach used, a logical and methodical process allows efficient and thorough evaluation of the sample. Use of an algorithm reminds the evaluator of the changes in cell populations that should be studied, integrates the various changes in cellular characteristics in cell populations that can occur, and allows the evaluator to recognize when evaluation of the preparation is complete. If a logical and methodical approach is not taken, exorbitant amounts of time may be spent perusing the slide without any diagnostic reward because there is no diagnostic information present on the slide. This inefficiency in evaluation of cytologic preparations is very frustrating and has caused many people to stop or curtail their use of cytologic evaluation.

The Oropharynx and Tonsils

Chart 1. An algorithm for cytologic evaluation of oropharyngeal lesions.

Aspirate, imprint or scraping → Sufficient cells collected for evaluation
- No: See "A"
- Yes → Inflammatory cells are present
  - No → Some cells show criteria of malignancy
    - Yes → See "F" and the discussion of neoplasia of the oropharynx and tonsils
    - No: See "E"
  - Yes → ≤90% of the cells collected are inflammatory cells and the remaining cells are cells that normally occur in the area, and they do not show criteria of malignancy
    - No: See "D"
    - Yes — Fungi or yeast are found
      - Yes: See "B"
      - No → <85% of the cells are neutrophils
        - Yes—Bacteria are found
          - Yes: Homogeneous population
            - Yes → Bacterial infection most likely. Culture and treat. See "C"
            - No → Probably contaminated unless the sample was collected by deep aspiration. Culture and treat. See "C"
          - No: Infection, foreign body, neoplasia; see "G"
        - No — ≤15% macrophages
          - Yes → Culture for fungi, bacteria
            - Positive culture: treat and see "C"
            - Negative culture: see "A"
          - No — ≤10% eosinophils
            - Yes: Fungal culture
              - Negative culture → Adequate: Probably eosinophilic granuloma. Finish therapy.
              - Probably eosinophilic granuloma. Response to corticosteroid therapy
              - Inadequate: See "A"
              - Positive culture: Treat and see "C"
            - No → Culture for fungi, bacteria
              - Negative culture: See "A"

A. Repeat cytologic examination, radiograph the area, or biopsy the lesion and submit the biopsy for histopathologic evaluation.

B. Identify as:
   Blastomyces dermatitidis (Plate 4)
   Histoplasma capsulatum (Plate 4)
   Cryptococcus neoformans (Plate 4)
   Sporothrix schenckii (Plate 4)
   Coccidioides immitis (Plate 5)

Culture, or refer the slide if unsure of the organism or if specific identification of a hyphating fungus is needed.

C. If there is no response to therapy, the patient should be re-evaluated. Occasionally, tumors become infected and yield cytologic samples containing inflammatory cells and bacteria, but not cells from the tumor. In these cases, antibiotic therapy often eliminates the infection, and subsequent cytologic samples contain sufficient tumor cells to diagnose neoplasia.

D. When there is an admixture of inflammatory cells and noninflammatory cells, the lesion should be evaluated for causes of inflammation and for indications of neoplasia. The more the shift of the admixture is in one direction, the more likely that process is occurring, ie, if 85% of the cells are inflammatory cells, then inflammation is very likely and neoplasia is less likely. On the other hand, if 15% of the cells are inflammatory and 85% are noninflammatory cells, neoplasia with secondary inflammation is more likely.

Also, the greater the proportion of inflammatory cells, the stronger the criteria of malignancy must be in cells suspected to be neoplastic for neoplasia to be diagnosed.

Re-evaluation by cytologic, radiographic and/or histopathologic examination after treatment of the inflammatory condition may be necessary.

E. If no inflammatory cells are present and no cells show criteria of malignancy, the lesion is probably due to hyperplasia, benign neoplasia, cyst formation (such as salivary cysts) or collection from normal tissue surrounding the lesion, but malignant neoplasia cannot be ruled out. Re-evaluation by cytologic, radiographic and/or histopathologic examination may be necessary.

F. If no inflammatory cells are present and some of the cells show criteria of malignancy, neoplasia is likely. The morphology of the cells collected should be evaluated to determine, if possible, the tumor cell type and the level of criteria of malignancy. Depending on the tumor cell type and level of criteria of malignancy present, a prediction of the malignant potential of the tumor may be possible. However, histopathologic examination may be necessary for definitive diagnosis.

G. Infection (mycotic or bacterial), neoplasia or foreign body are all possible. At this time, the cytologic preparation may be referred for interpretation, another sample may be collected, the lesion may be cultured and treated accordingly, or radiographic examination or biopsy with histopathologic examination may be performed. If the patient is treated, a cytologic sample collected 1-2 weeks after therapy is begun may reveal the true nature of the lesion.

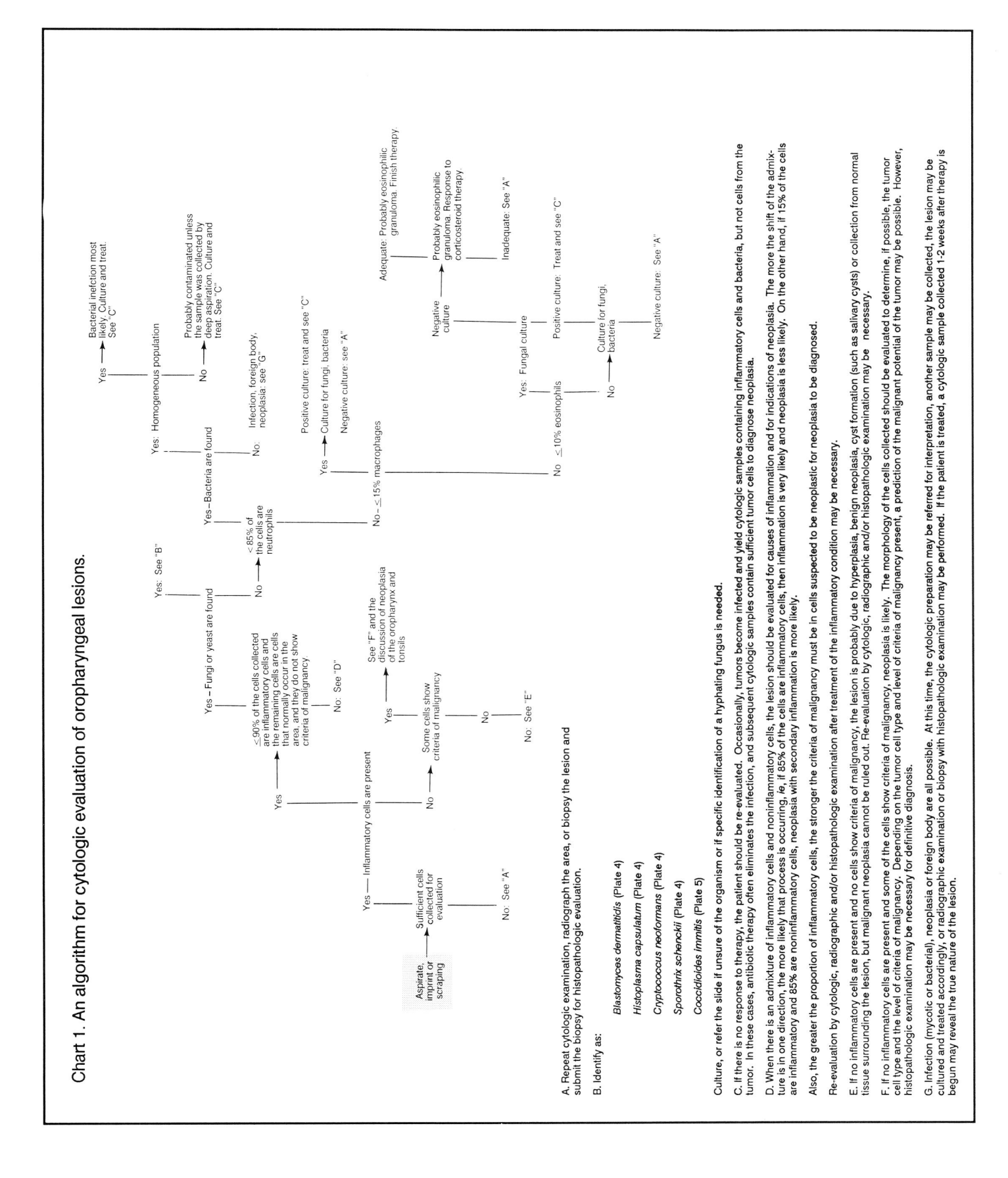

References

1. Theilen and Madewell: *Veterinary Cancer Medicine*. 2nd ed. Lea & Febiger, Philadelphia, 1987. pp 499-534.

2. Dorn *et al*: Survey of animal neoplasms in Alameda and Contra Costa counties, California. I. Methodology and description of cases. *J Natl Cancer Inst* 40:295-305, 1968.

3. Dorn *et al*: Survey of animal neoplasms in Alameda and Contra Costa counties, California. II. Cancer morbidity in dogs and cats from Alameda County. *J Natl Cancer Inst* 40:307-318, 1968.

4. Moulton: *Tumors in Domestic Animals*. 2nd ed. Univ California Press, Berkeley, 1978. pp 240-272.

5. Todoroff and Brodey: Oral and pharyngeal neoplasia in the dog: a retrospective survey of 361 cases. *JAVMA* 175:567-571, 1979.

6. Dubielzig: Proliferative dental and gingival diseases of dogs and cats. *JAAHA* 18:577-584, 1982.

7. Richardson *et al*: Oral neoplasms in the dog: A diagnostic and therapeutic dilemma. *Comp Cont Ed Pract Vet* 5:441-446, 1983.

8. Brodey: Alimentary tract neoplasms in the cat: A clinicopathologic survey of 46 cases. *Am J Vet Res* 27:74-80, 1966.

9. Cotter: Oral pharyngeal neoplasms in the cat. *JAAHA* 17:917-920, 1981.

10. Patnaik and Mooney: Feline melanomas: A comparative study of ocular, oral, and dermal neoplasms. *Vet Pathol* 25:105-112, 1988.

5

The Eyes and Associated Structures

K.W. Prasse and S.M. Winston

Cytologic examination of the eye and adnexa in dogs and cats is an important diagnostic adjunct for the general practitioner, as well as the specialist in ophthalmology. In this chapter, cytologic findings are reviewed by anatomic location. Where appropriate, closely related techniques that require the same or similar types of samples are mentioned, such as fluorescent antibody staining of conjunctival scrapings. Special considerations for sample collection from the various ocular structures are included. Chapter 1 contains a general discussion of fine-needle aspiration technique and slide preparation. Certain lesions, particularly of the eyelids and orbit, are common to other body systems, and illustrations may appear elsewhere in the text.

The Eyelids

The eyelid is comprised of layers of skin and mucous membrane (palpebral conjunctiva) separated by muscle and specialized glands, particularly of the sebaceous type. Lesions of the eyelids for which cytologic evaluation is useful include ulcerative and exudative lesions of the epidermal surface (blepharitis) and discrete masses on either the epidermal or conjunctival surface. (Conjunctivitis and conjunctival cytology are described later.)

Fine-needle aspiration usually provides diagnostic specimens on ulcerated lesions and discrete masses. Scraping may be a reasonable means of sample collection for diffuse exudative epidermal lesions of the eyelid, such as parasitic blepharitis. Touch impressions are not recommended for exudative skin lesions because these samples contain surface debris and may not reflect the true extent of the lesion.

Blepharitis

Blepharitis may be focal or diffuse and acute or chronic. Causes may be bacterial, mycotic, parasitic, allergic or autoimmune (pemphigus). The objectives in cytologic examination of blepharitis are to characterize the type of exudate (neutrophilic, lymphocytic-plasmacytic, eosinophilic or granulomatous) and look for the causative agent. *Demodex folliculorum* causes minimal exudation. Bacterial blepharitis, particularly staphylococcal, has a neutrophilic exudate. Certain fungi, such as *Blastomyces dermatitidis*, cause a primarily neutrophilic exudate, whereas others cause a granulomatous exudate (macrophages, epithelioid cells and giant cells).

Allergic and autoimmune causes of blepharitis are less well defined, and the type of exudate may vary with the cause and/or stage of the disease. The presence of either bacteria or a primarily neutrophilic exudate may not exclude allergic and autoimmune causes, especially if the lesion is ulcerated. The eosinophilic granuloma complex may be manifested as periocular blepharitis in cats.[1] A fine-needle aspirate reveals primarily eosinophils, some mast cells and a mixture of other WBC types.

Chapter 5

Figure 1. Sebaceous-gland epithelial cells from a well-differentiated sebaceous-gland tumor on a canine eyelid.

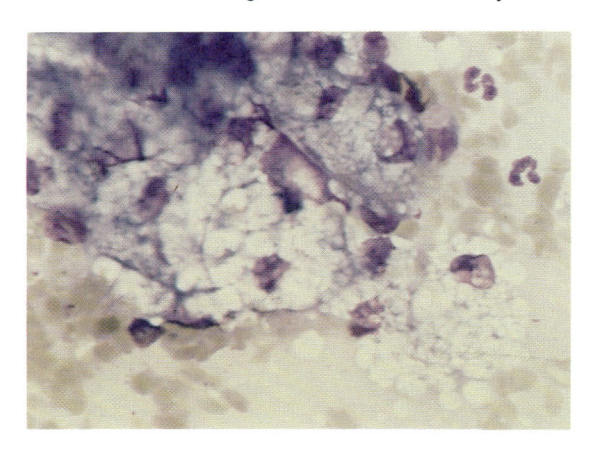

Discrete Masses

Discrete masses on the eyelids may be nonneoplastic or neoplastic (benign or malignant). Among neoplasms, benign sebaceous-gland tumors (sebaceous adenoma, sebaceous epithelioma) are the most common type on canine eyelids.[2] The glands of Zeis and Moll at the eyelid margin and the Meibomian glands, which lie beneath the palpebral conjunctiva and open at the lid margin, are all of the sebaceous type; tumors arising from them are similar to all cutaneous sebaceous-gland tumors. The cells are readily recognized by their voluminous vacuolated cytoplasm that nearly obscures small rounded nuclei (Fig 1).

Figure 2. Giant cell, macrophages, lymphocytes and a sebaceous-gland epithelial cell (lower left) from a chalazion on a canine eyelid.

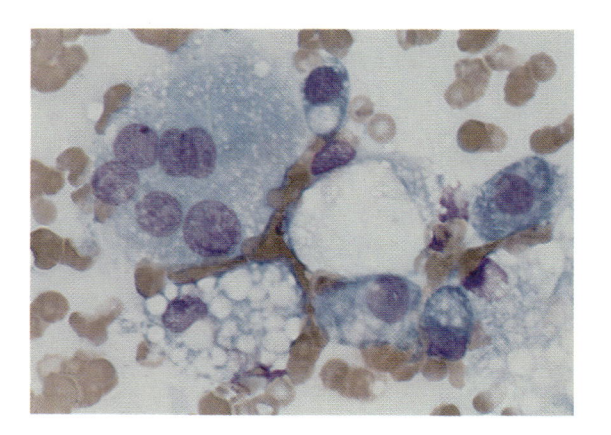

The malignant counterpart of these tumors is rare on the eyelids.

Other tumors commonly encountered on the eyelids and readily diagnosed by cytologic examination include melanomas (benign and malignant) (Plate 8), histiocytomas, mast-cell tumors (benign and malignant) (Plate 7), papillomas, squamous-cell carcinomas (Plate 6), and infrequently spindle-cell types of connective tissue tumors (Plate 7).[2,3] These are further discussed in Chapter 2.

Nonneoplastic discrete masses unique to the eyelid include the hordeolum, a localized purulent lesion of sebaceous glands at the lid margin, and the chalazion, a similar lesion that involves the Meibomian gland. Fine-needle aspiration of these lesions yields nu-

Figure 3. Canine conjunctival scraping contains palpebral columnar ciliated cells and goblet cells (upper right).

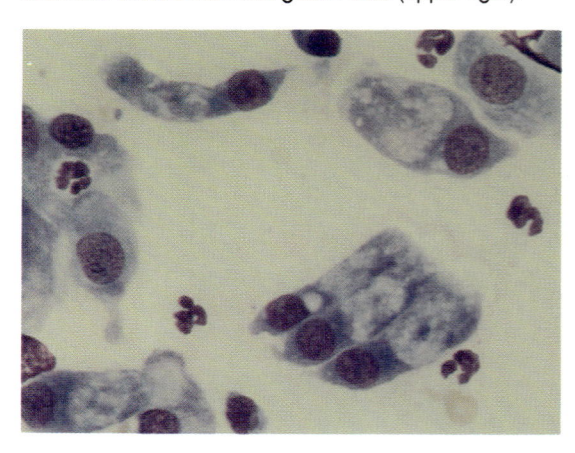

merous foamy macrophages and a few giant cells and lymphocytes. The macrophages are apparently phagocytosing glandular secretory product; cytophagia is not prominent. Variable numbers of sebaceous-gland epithelial cells also are found (Fig 2).

Differentiating a hordeolum or chalazion from a sebeceous-gland adenoma by cytologic examination may be difficult if the latter has internally ruptured and caused secondary inflammation. Hordeolum or chalazion may contain inspissated secretory product or mineralized debris that appears as amorphous granular material on cytologic preparations.

The Conjunctiva

The primary indications for conjunctival cytologic evaluation are to characterize an exudate and to attempt to identify the cause of conjunctivitis. Certain anatomic structures affect the types of cells found on all preparations from normal and diseased eyes. The conjunctiva is composed of 2 continuous layers of epithelium that lie in apposition. The inner epithelial layer of the eyelid, called the palpebral conjunctiva, is composed of pseudostratified columnar epithelium and interspersed goblet cells (Fig 3). Cilia may be found on the columnar cells. At the fornix deep within the conjunctival sac, the epithelium reflects back over the globe. This bulbar conjunctiva is composed of stratified squamous epithelium (Fig 4). Bulbar conjunctiva is continuous with the corneal epithelium at the limbus. The squamous cells are noncornified and often contain melanin granules (Fig 5).

Figure 4. Basal, intermediate and mature noncornified squamous cells typical of bulbar conjunctival epithelium, from a canine conjunctival scraping.

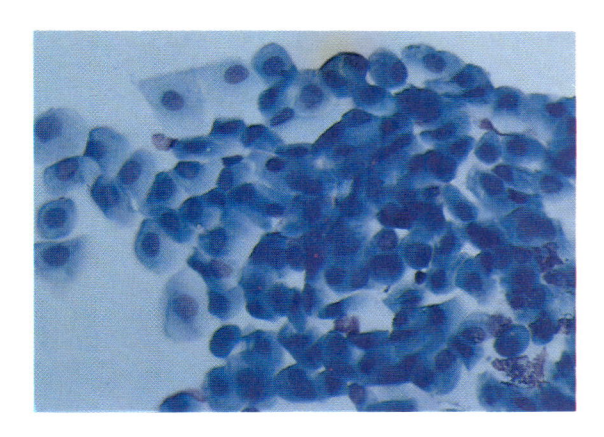

In most conjunctival scrapings, squamous cells are more numerous than columnar cells. In animals that have been treated with ophthalmic ointments (particularly neomycin), epithelial cells may contain dense basophilic cytoplasmic inclusions (Fig 6).[4] Such inclusions must be differentiated from infectious agents. At the fornix, conjunctival lamina propria contains lymphoid tissue; various types of lymphoid cells may be found in any conjunctival scraping (Fig 5). Without clinical signs of conjunctivitis, little emphasis should be placed on the observation of lymphocytes or plasma cells among epithelial cells.

Cytologic preparations from the conjunctiva should include freshly derived cells. External debris within the conjunctival sac should be removed before scraping. The con-

Figure 5. Conjunctival scraping from a dog with chronic conjunctivitis shows a melanin-laden squamous cell, plasma cells, neutrophils (lysed), RBC and a lymphocyte.

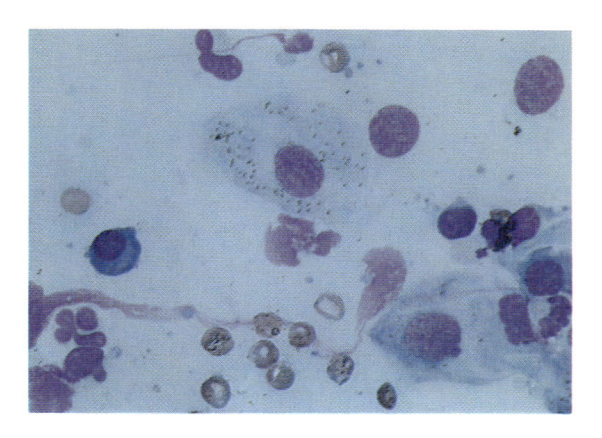

junctival scraping is made with a flat, round-tipped spatula 5-7 mm wide. A topical anesthetic is applied, and the spatula is extended into the conjunctival sac and scraped 2-3 times in one direction, thereby harvesting material from both bulbar and palpebral surfaces. Several smears should be made. Examine all prepared slides because findings may vary dramatically from slide to slide on the same eye.

Neutrophilic Conjunctivitis

Exudate in which neutrophils predominate is very common in canine and feline conjunctivitis. This type of exudate occurs regardless of cause: bacterial, viral, allergic or other.

Figure 6. A canine conjunctival scraping contains squamous cells with dense, homogeneous, blue cytoplasmic bodies (center), believed to be a consequence of treatment with ophthalmic ointments.

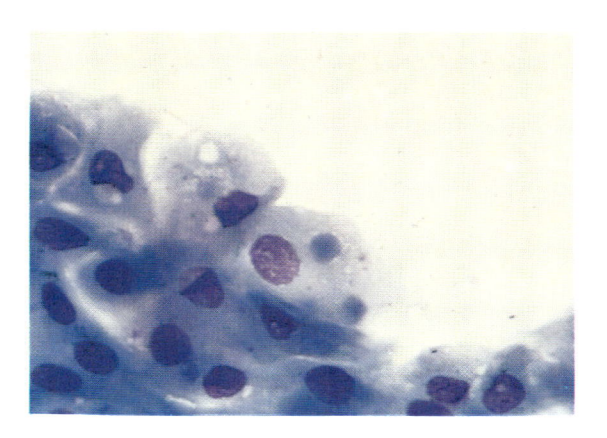

Figure 7. Nondegenerate neutrophils, squamous cells, 2 plasma cells (top left center) and a lymphocyte (lower right) from a cat with neutrophilic conjunctivitis. Other smears were fluorescent antibody-positive for *Herpes felis*.

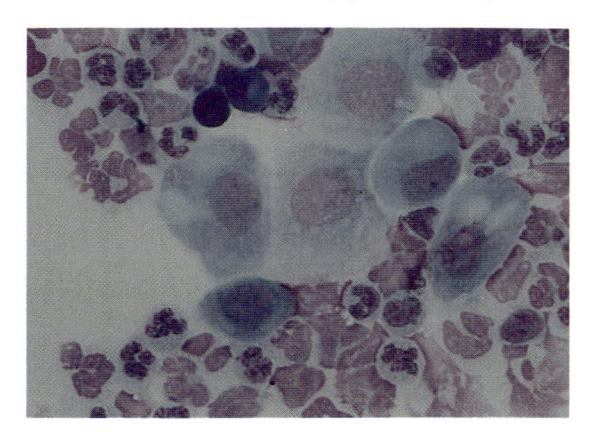

Figure 8. Conjunctival smear from a dog with neutrophilic conjunctivitis shows autophagy of neutrophils by a squamous cell (center), numerous neutrophils and lymphocytes, and a goblet epithelial cell (lower left center).

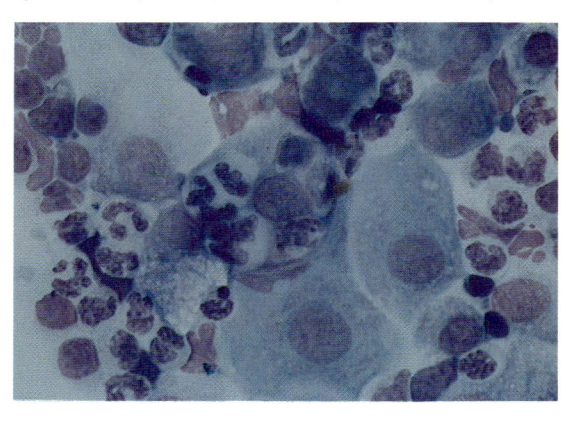

Figure 9. Initial body of *Chlamydia psittaci* in the cytoplasm of a squamous cell in a conjunctival scraping from a cat.

Figure 10. Initial body of *Chlamydia psittaci* in the cytoplasm of a squamous cell (lower center), with neutrophils, in a conjunctival scraping from a cat with chlamydial conjunctivitis.

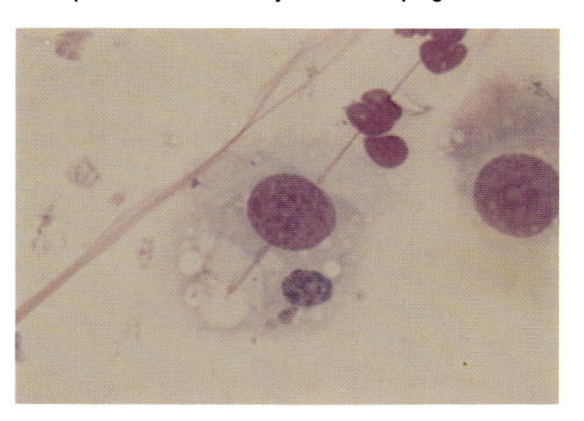

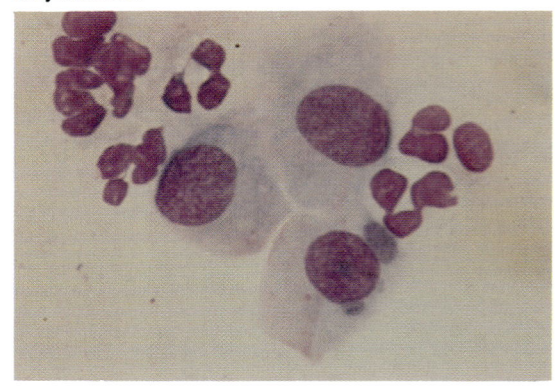

Neutrophilic exudate may have nondegenerate or karyolytic neutrophils (Fig 7). In cats, the latter are rarely encountered. In both species autophagy of neutrophils by squamous cells is common, though no causal relationship has been established (Fig 8). Mucus is a common component of neutrophilic exudates and may cause cells to appear in rows on the smear. Establishing the cause of neutrophilic conjunctivitis may be difficult, and the factors to consider are different between dogs and cats.

The exudate of canine neutrophilic conjunctivitis almost always contains bacteria, regardless of primary cause. The bacteria are often large and/or small cocci and less frequently rods (Plate 3). The dilemma is whether the bacteria are of primary importance or merely opportunistic. Normal bacterial flora of the canine conjunctival sac has been described.[5] Keratoconjunctivitis sicca is a common canine disorder causing neutrophilic exudate in which bacteria are commonly encountered. The disease is diagnosed readily by the Schirmer tear test.

Distemper is the most important viral cause of canine neutrophilic conjunctivitis. Canine distemper is diagnosed by its classic clinical signs and fluorescent antibody staining of conjunctival smears. Searching for canine distemper inclusion bodies on conjunctival scrapings by routine or special stains has very limited diagnostic value.

In contrast to that of dogs, the exudate of feline neutrophilic conjunctivitis only rarely contains bacteria. When observed, bacteria should always be considered clinically significant in feline conjunctivitis.

A common cause of feline neutrophilic conjunctivitis is herpesvirus infection (Fig 7). Diagnosis is confirmed by positive results on fluorescent antibody staining of conjunctival smears; a negative result, however, does not exclude feline herpesvirus. Inclusion bodies are not seen in conjunctival smears in feline herpesvirus infection.[6]

Neutrophils predominate also in the conjunctival exudate of feline chlamydial infection. In experimental *Chlamydia psittaci* infections, organisms were found by postinoculation day 6, on which clinical signs first appeared.[7] Solitary, large (3-5µ), basophilic particulate forms initially are found in the cytoplasm of squamous cells (Figs 9-11). The particulate nature of the initial body is an important observation to distinguish *Chlamydia*

Figure 11. Conjunctival scraping from a cat with chlamydial conjunctivitis shows initial bodies of *Chlamydia psittaci* in 2 squamous cells (center and right center), and neutrophils.

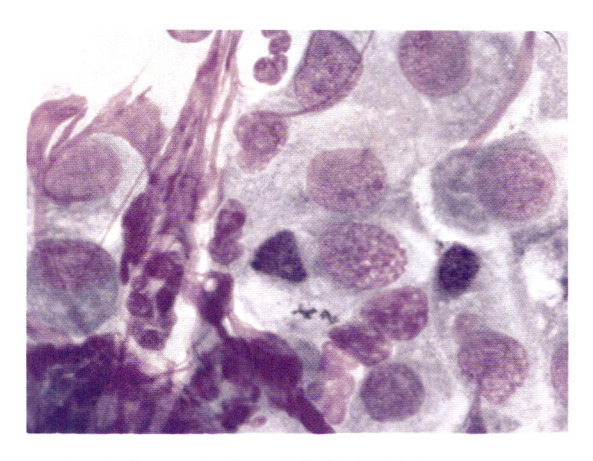

Figure 12. Elementary bodies of *Chlamydia psittaci* adjacent to the nucleus in cytoplasm of a squamous cell in a conjunctival scraping from a cat with chlamydial conjunctivitis.

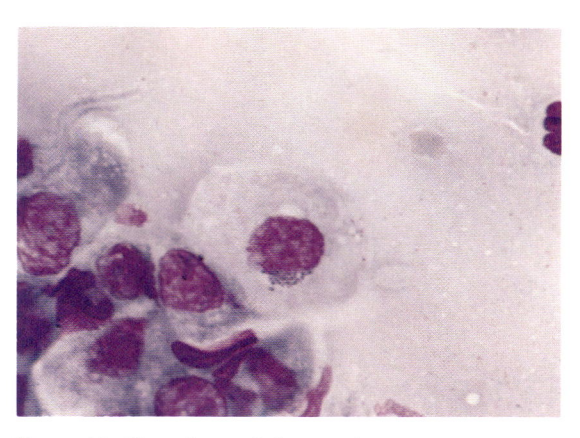

Figure 13. *Mycoplasma felis* organisms adherent to the surface of a squamous cell (center), a melanin-laden squamous cell (left center), and numerous nondegenerative neutrophils in a conjunctival scraping from a cat with mycoplasmal conjunctivitis.

psittaci from incidental foci of homogeneous cytoplasmic basophilia found in squamous epithelial cells (Fig 6).[4] Organisms also may appear as aggregates of coccoid basophilic bodies (elementary bodies), 0.5-1µ in diameter (Fig 12). By the 14th postinoculation day of experimental infections, organisms were rarely found.[7] The infection is often well established, and the organisms are no longer present when an affected cat is first examined by a veterinarian. Consequently, identification of the organisms is rarely used for definitive diagnosis in feline chlamydial infection.

Feline mycoplasmosis, another cause of neutrophilic conjunctivitis, may be diagnosed by finding the organisms on routinely stained smears. In one study, mycoplasmosis was diagnosed in 9 naturally infected cats by isolation and identification of *Mycoplasma* spp. Of

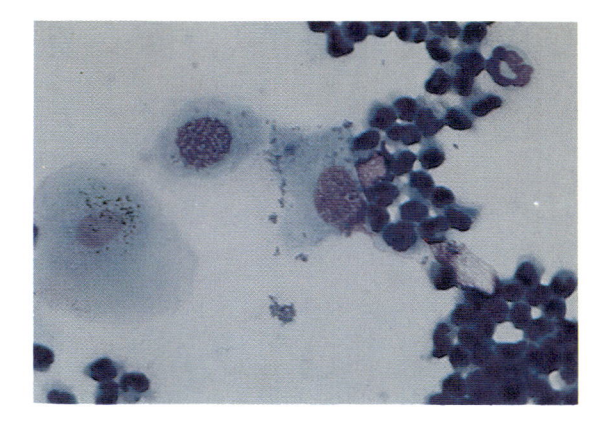

Figure 14. *Mycoplasma felis* organisms in a squamous cell (right center), neutrophils and RBC in a conjunctival scraping from a cat with mycoplasmal conjunctivitis.

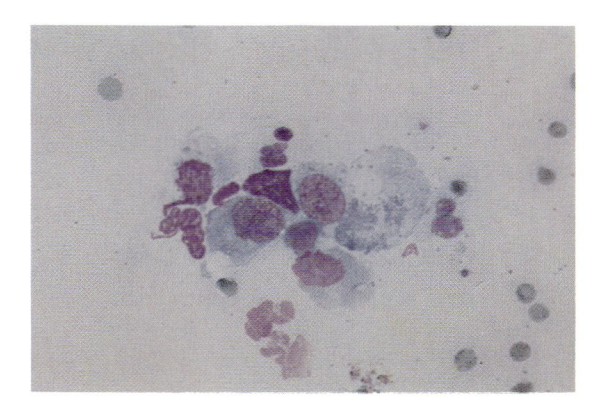

Figure 15. Numerous lymphocytes, a plasma cell (top left center) and squamous cells in a conjunctival scraping from a dog with lymphocytic-plasmacytic conjunctivitis.

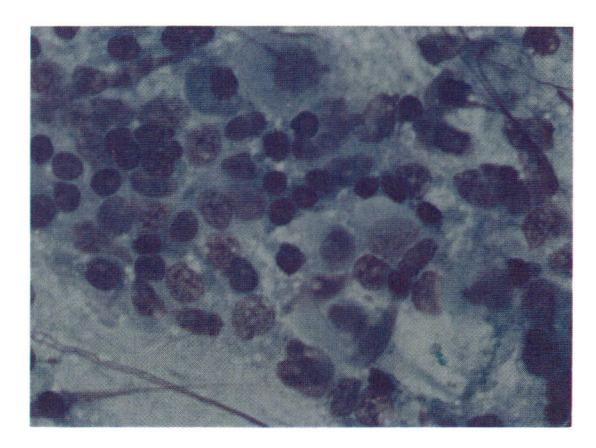

samples from 16 eyes, the organisms were found on Romanowsky-stained smears from 15 eyes. This suggests a high degree of diagnostic sensitivity for routine cytologic evaluation in *Mycoplasma* infection.[8] The basophilic organisms, 0.2-0.8 μ long, may be found in clusters adherent to the outer limits of the plasma membrane or over the flattened surface of squamous epithelial cells (Figs 13,14). They also may be seen in clusters between cells. Though the organisms are relatively easily found on conjunctival scrapings, we rarely encounter this disease.

Lymphocytic-Plasmacytic Conjunctivitis

Conjunctivitis in which lymphoid cells predominate is less common than purulent conjunctivitis. As noted previously, lymphocytes and a few plasma cells may be found among epithelial cells from normal eyes. Discussions on infectious conjunctivitis in cats and dogs state that lymphocytes and perhaps monocytes predominate in the early stages of viral infection.[5,6,9] We encounter lymphocytic-plasmacytic conjunctivitis infrequently in our practice (Fig 15). In the diseases described above that cause primarily neutrophilic conjunctivitis, the exudate may have a few lymphocytes, plasma cells and monocytes or macrophages. Follicular conjunctivitis yields cells typical of lymphoid hyperplasia.

Eosinophilic and Mast-Cell Conjunctivitis

Eosinophilic conjunctivitis is encountered primarily in cats (Fig 16). It has been observed in cats concomitant with eosinophilic keratitis, as a component of eosinophilic granuloma complex, and as a disease unto itself.[1] In conjunctival smears from both dogs and cats, mast cells may be the predominant inflammatory cell. Whereas the pathogenesis is presumably allergic, the cause of these conditions remains obscure.

Noninflammatory Lesions of Conjunctiva

Neoplasms that may involve conjunctiva include papillomas, squamous-cell carcinomas, melanomas, lipomas and others. A unique form of mast-cell neoplasia may involve the canine conjunctiva. It is manifested as severe diffuse swelling of the conjunctiva. Cytologic examination of mast-cell tumors is further discussed in Chapter 2.

Cyst-like swellings of the conjunctiva are uncommon. One example is the zygomatic mucocele, which may occur in various locations, from the top of the head, ventral to the eye, to the roof of the mouth.[10] The cytologic findings with these lesions are identical to those of other salivary cysts described in Chapter 7.

The Nictitating Membrane

The nictitating membrane, or third eyelid, is composed of a T-shaped cartilage covered by conjunctiva that is continuous with the bulbar and palpebral conjunctiva on its inner and outer surfaces. The gland of the third eyelid, a seromucous gland, envelops the base of the cartilage. Lymphoid tissue is located on the bulbar surface superior to the gland. Consequently, cells found on nictitans scrapings are determined by which surface is sampled.

Figure 16. Mast cell (top right), eosinophils, free eosinophilic granules, neutrophils, a squamous cell and columnar epithelial cells (lower left) in a cat with eosinophilic conjunctivitis.

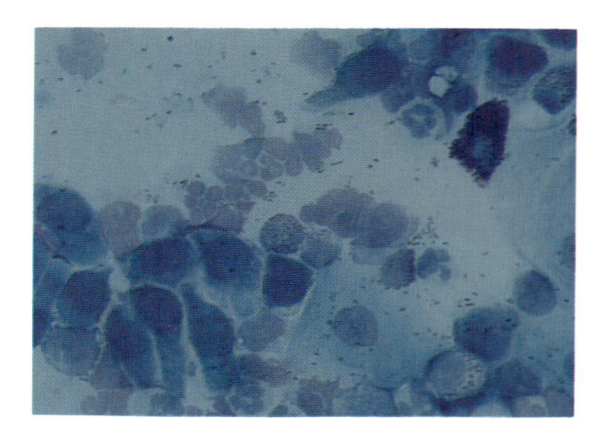

Scrapings of the bulbar surface of the membrane in normal or diseased eyes may resemble cytologic preparations from lymph nodes, with all expected types of lymphoid cells.

As a conjunctival surface, the nictitating membrane may be affected by most of the diseases of the conjunctiva described in the previous section. Only a few specific lesions of the membrane require cytologic evaluation for differential diagnosis. Feline follicular conjunctivitis frequently involves the bulbar surface of the membrane, and cytologic examination reveals lymphoid hyperplasia (Fig 17). A specific lesion in German Shepherds is called plasma-cell infiltration or plasmoma, in which scrapings of the third eyelid reveal plasma cells and other WBC.[11] Hyperplasia of the gland of the third eyelid, called cherry eye, should not be a diagnostic problem that requires cytologic examination. The nictitating membrane may be the site of primary or metastatic tumors, such as squamous-cell carcinoma (Plate 6), or other tumors common to conjunctiva; cytologic examination is helpful to distinguish these lesions.

The Nasolacrimal Apparatus

Dacryocystitis

Dacryocystitis is inflammation of the lacrimal sac. Inflammatory exudates composed primarily of neutrophils and macrophages and usually accompanied by bacteria may obstruct the puncta, canaliculi or nasolacrimal sac. Exudates may be retrieved by flushing the upper or lower punctum with saline through a blunt 22- to 23-ga needle. Either the initial plug of material or particularly flocculent material should be examined.

Figure 17. Numerous small lymphocytes, a lymphoblast (top left), a macrophage (center) and a neutrophil (lower right) in a scraping from the inner surface of the third eyelid of a cat with follicular hyperplasia.

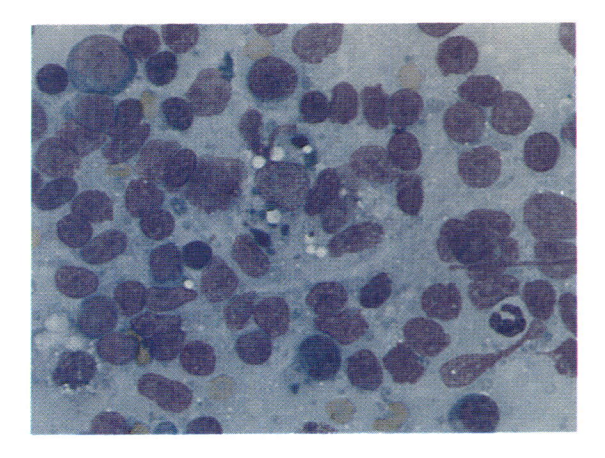

Figure 18. A large globule of mucus (top center), macrophages and RBC arranged in rows (caused by mucus content) in an aspirate of a lacrimal duct cyst in a young Basset Hound.

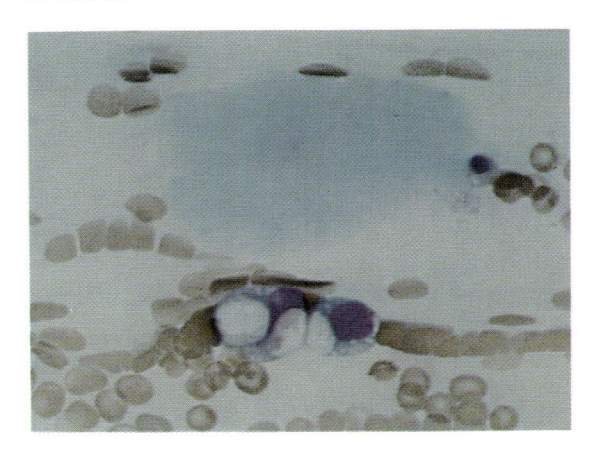

Lacrimal Duct Cyst

A lacrimal duct cyst (dacryops) causes swelling of the medial canthus. The serosanguineous cyst fluid has low cellularity.[10] On smears, RBC and small numbers of neutrophils, monocytes and other WBC without bacteria are found. Mucus is usually present and may cause the cells to appear in rows (Fig 18). There may be a breed predisposition in young Basset Hounds.

Parotid Transposition Cysts

A unique noninflammatory cystic lesion may occur in the lateral canthus as a complication of parotid duct transposition. The cyst may occur if the orifice of the transplanted duct becomes occluded. Cyst contents are similar to those of a naturally occurring salivary mucocele and include large foamy macrophages and exfoliated salivary epithelial cells (Fig 19). Variable numbers of neutrophils also may be found; bacteria are absent.

The Sclera and Episclera

The sclera is the noncorneal fibrous tunic of the eye. The scleral stroma is continuous with the corneal stroma. The fibrovascular episclera overlies the scleral stroma. It is located between the limbus and insertions of the extraocular muscles, and is covered in part by bulbar conjunctiva. These tissues are rich in collagen and nearly free of cells. Fibrocytes

Figure 19. Foamy exfoliated salivary epithelial cells, a single melanophage (top left), neutrophils and hematoidin crystals superimposed on some cells in a smear of an aspirate from a parotid duct cyst that occluded the opening into the conjunctival sac of a dog.

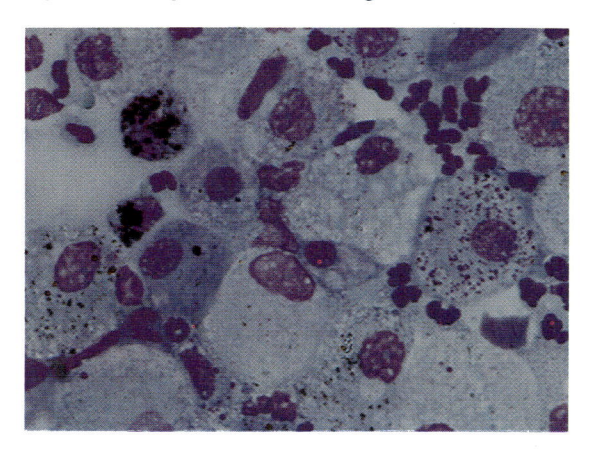

and melanocytes increase in number in the inner scleral layers, which merge with the choroid.

A nodular or dome-shaped chronic inflammatory lesion affects the episclera and sclera of dogs.[12] It has been called nodular fasciitis, nodular episcleritis, fibrous histiocytoma and proliferative keratoconjunctivitis, among other terms. It primarily involves the episclera and sclera, most often near the limbus deep to the bulbar conjunctiva. Fine-needle aspiration yields lymphocytes, plasma cells, macrophages and a few neutrophils. These findings serve to differentiate the lesion from neoplasms, such as lymphosarcoma (Plate 7), mast-cell tumor (Plate 7) and melanoma (Plate 8), that also may involve the sclera.

The Cornea

The cornea is composed of a thick collagenous stroma covered by noncornified stratified squamous epithelium on the outer surface and a thick basal lamina (Descemet's membrane) deep to a single layer of flattened epithelial cells (endothelium) on the inner surface. The cornea is subject to a wide variety of lesions, including congenital malformation, opacifications, proliferative changes, ulcerations, and exudative keratitis.[13] Many corneal

Figure 21. Squamous cells, mast cells and free eosinophilic granules in a corneal scraping from a cat with eosinophilic keratitis.

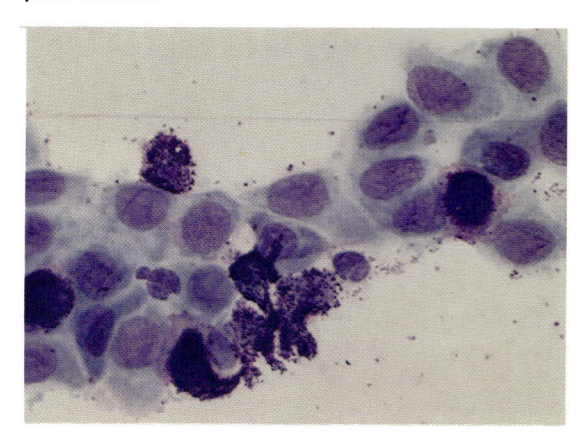

lesions have a classic appearance, and diagnosis is made from the history and by gross examination.

Cytologic examination is most useful to characterize exudative lesions and may aid in differentiation of certain proliferative lesions. After applying a topical anesthetic, samples are most often acquired by scraping or may be obtained with a hypodermic needle if the lesion is very small or focal. Several diseases may concurrently affect the cornea and conjunctiva; these were described in the previous section on the conjunctiva.

Corneal Ulcers

Ulcerative corneal lesions with exudation should be cytologically examined for organisms. Any exudate is usually purulent. Certain Gram-negative rods, such as *Pseudomonas* spp, produce collagenase, which causes

Figure 20. A giant cell containing a chain of spherules of *Cladosporium* sp (a pigmented fungus) in a corneal scraping from a cat with mycotic keratitis.

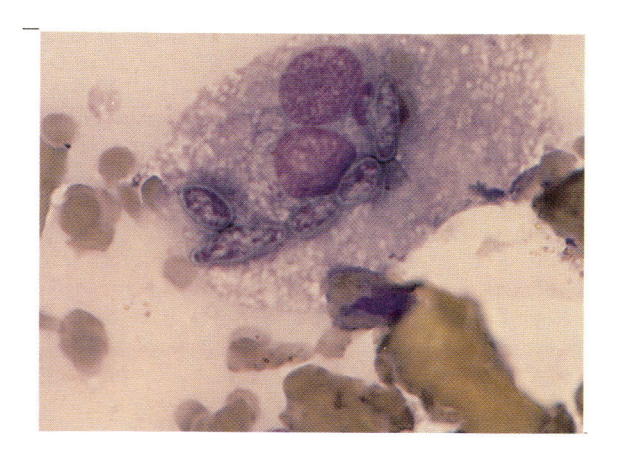

a rapidly progressing, so-called "melting" ulcer.

Exudates in keratomycosis may vary in character from nearly devoid of WBC to a neutrophilic or granulomatous composition. Scrapings may reveal such organisms as *Aspergillus* or *Candida*, which are the most common species involved in keratomycosis (Plate 5). Pigmented fungi are rare (Fig 20). In corneal scrapings with few WBC, large clumps of corneal epithelium should be closely studied because hyphae may be embedded in the epithelium. Special stains for fungi (periodic acid-Schiff and Gomori's methenamine silver) may be useful.

Eosinophilic Keratitis

Eosinophilic keratitis is a corneal disease of cats, and cytologic examination is usually diagnostic.[14] The raised granular vascular lesion is usually not ulcerated and has small foci of gray-white deposits on the surface. Scrapings reveal an impressive number of mast cells among corneal epithelial cells, and variable numbers of eosinophils or free eosinophilic granules may be seen (Fig 21). When the gray-white surface deposits are lifted off with a hypodermic needle and smeared, cell debris composed primarily of nucleic acid streams and numerous free eosinophilic granules are found. In scrapings from ulcerated lesions or more deeply scraped nonulcerated lesions, eosinophils predominate, and lymphocytes and plasma cells also may be numerous (Fig 22).

Figure 22. Eosinophils, neutrophils, lymphocytes and squamous cells in a corneal scraping from a cat with eosinophilic keratitis.

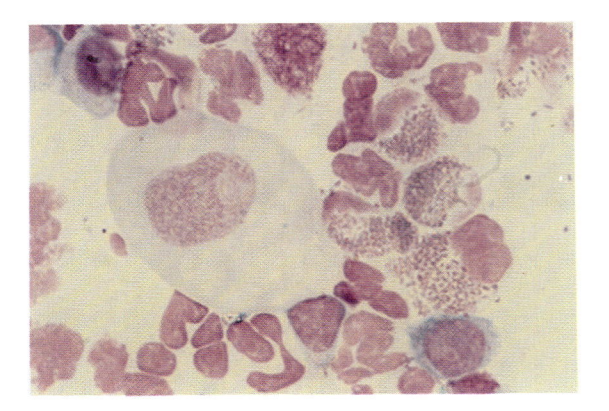

Figure 23. Amorphous nonstaining crystalline material and cell debris in a corneal scraping from a dog with mineralizing corneal degeneration.

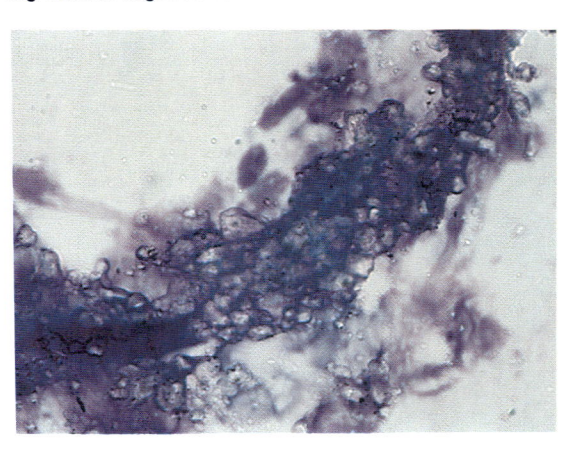

Chronic Superficial Keratitis

Chronic superficial keratitis, or pannus, is a common proliferative canine corneal lesion seen predominantly in German Shepherds. Scrapings, though not necessary for diagnosis, reveal a mixture of WBC types, including lymphocytes, plasma cells, macrophages and neutrophils. Lipid corneal degeneration and mineralizing corneal degeneration are 2 common opacifying corneal lesions of dogs. Each lesion may cause plaque-like or granular thickening of the cornea. Scraping of lipid corneal degeneration is nondiagnostic because the lipid does not readily exfoliate. Scraping of mineralizing corneal degeneration may reveal crystalline unstained granules (Fig 23). The granules show a positive reaction with von Kossa stain, a method of demonstrating calcium.

Corneal Tumors

Tumors of the cornea are rare in dogs and cats. Fine-needle aspiration, rather than scraping, is recommended. Melanomas (Plate 8), papillomas, squamous-cell carcinomas (Plate 6), and various sarcomas have been described.[13] The cytologic characteristics of these tumors are further described in Chapter 2.

Epithelial Inclusion Cyst

A raised solitary stromal epithelial inclusion cyst occurs in the canine cornea.[15] The cyst is thought to be secondary to trauma. A clear acellular fluid may be aspirated from such cysts.

Aqueous Humor

Aspiration of aqueous humor for cytodiagnostic purposes may be indicated when the fluid is cloudy or opaque. Though the technique is relatively simple, we rarely perform aqueous centesis because it is usually not helpful in diagnosis. Hyphema, hypopyon, flare, and the presence of lipid are determined by clinical examination, and cytologic examination is noncontributory. For example, in feline anterior uveitis, there are no distinguishing cytologic features among the various causes. Most intraocular tumors, either primary or secondary, do not exfoliate into aqueous humor; lymphosarcoma is a rare exception (see the following section on the iris and ciliary body). In most cases of infectious endophthalmitis, recovery of organisms from vitreous body aspirates is more productive (described later in this chapter).

Under general anesthesia, aspiration of aqueous humor is done with a 25-ga hypodermic needle attached to a 3-ml syringe. The cornea is penetrated near the limbus, and the needle tip is placed over the pupil.[16] With the exception of hyphema, the protein content of aqueous humor is very low; consequently, *in vitro* disintegration of cells may be rapid. Sediment smears should be made soon after aspiration. Whereas total cell counts and protein concentration may be determined, we have not practiced these techniques.[16]

Neutrophilic infiltration of aqueous humor is characteristic of most causes of anterior uveitis, including lens-induced uveitis and viral infections. A few lymphocytes and monocytes may be found. In cases of hypopyon, bacteria may or may not be found among the neutrophils. *Blastomyces dermatitidis* (Plate 4), *Prototheca* spp (Plate 5), and *Leishmania donovani* (Plate 5) may be found in aqueous humor in certain cases.[17] Phagocytosis of melanin by neutrophils is an infrequent finding of unknown significance (Fig 24). Hyphema is characterized either by cells typical of fresh blood or, in protracted cases, blood with a few erythrophages and hemosiderophages. Tumors metastatic to the anterior uvea include carcinomas (Plate 6), sarcomas (Plate 7), lymphosarcomas (Plate 7), canine transmissible venereal tumors (Plate 7), and feline myeloproliferative tumors.[18] Cytologic examination of aqueous humor may on rare occasions distinguish these disorders.

The Iris and Ciliary Body

Space-occupying masses on the anterior uvea may be an indication for cytologic examination of fine-needle aspirates. Aspiration is accomplished under general anesthesia as described above for aqueous humor.

Melanoma

Melanoma is the most common primary intraocular tumor in this location (Plate 8). The preparation should contain melanocytes that exhibit cytomorphologic features of malignancy to be diagnostic, since free melanin and some melanocytes are a component of all uveal aspirates.

Lymphosarcoma

Lymphosarcoma (Plate 7) also occurs here. Whereas lymphoblasts, mitotic cells and lymphoid cells with broad pseudopodia are present, normal small lymphocytes and plasma cells also may be seen (see Chapter 8 for further discussion and additional photographs of lymphosarcoma). Ocular lymphosarcoma is rarely primary. When it is suspected, the animal should be thoroughly examined for systemic lesions that may be more easily sampled for diagnostic purposes.

Metastatic Carcinomas

The anterior uvea also is a site for metastasis of systemic carcinomas.[17] Adenomas and adenocarcinomas may originate from ciliary body epithelium. Among primary intra-

Figure 24. Free melanin granules and phagocytized melanin granules in neutrophils in a sediment smear of aqueous fluid from a dog.

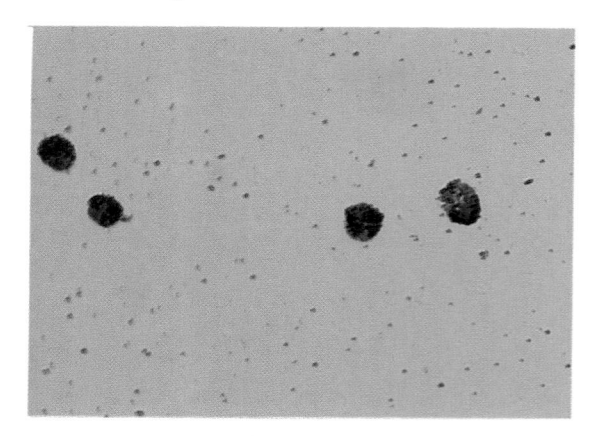

Figure 25. Lens fibers in the sediment of a vitreous body aspirate from a dog. Several RBC provide a size reference.

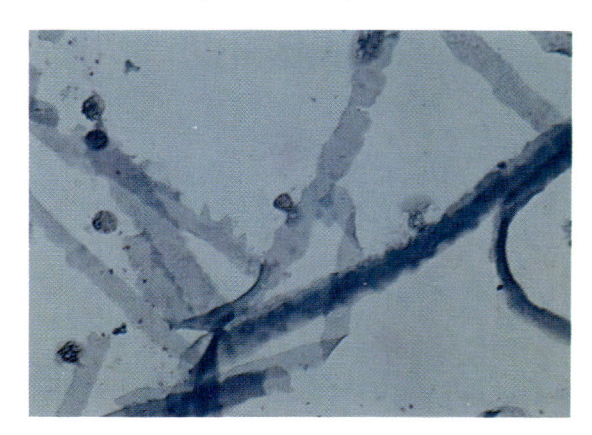

ocular tumors, these are second to melanomas in frequency.[19] Cytologic features of benign and malignant epithelial tumors are further described in Chapter 1.

The Vitreous Body

Opacity in the vitreous body is an indication for centesis and cytologic examination. The diagnostic yield is quite good in our experience. Aspiration of the vitreous body is not an innocuous procedure. It is normally only done on an irrevocably blind eye. If a potentially visual eye is aspirated, extreme care must be taken not to cause hemorrhage or other sequelae that could jeopardize vision. Aspiration is done under general anesthesia. A 25-ga needle is used to penetrate the eye 6-8 mm caudal to the limbus, directing the needle toward the retina. The lens must be avoided to prevent disruption of the lens capsule and induction of lens-induced uveitis.

Aspirate 0.5-1.0 ml of fluid. Sediment smears should be made immediately after aspiration and centrifugation. After air drying and before staining, heat the underside of the glass slide by passing it through the tip of a small flame 2 or 3 times. Heat fixation helps prevent vitreous body material from washing off the slide, a common problem with unfixed smears.

Vitreous body material is normally acellular, though most samples contain a few RBC and scattered melanin granules which, in this location in dogs, are oblong with pointed ends. Lens fibers may be found in sediment smears in cases of lens-induced endophthalmitis or inadvertent damage of the lens during sample aspiration (Fig 25). Microfilariae may be found in samples that contain blood from microfilaremic dogs but they are not associated with ocular disease. Melanin-laden cells may be found in samples from normal or diseased eyes.

Endophthalmitis

Bacterial endophthalmitis is purulent, and organisms are usually demonstrable in the exudate on vitreous smears. Neutrophilic exudate without organisms can be seen in lens-induced endophthalmitis and trauma. Mycotic endophthalmitis with opacification of the vitreous body is relatively common in dogs. Ocular lesions were found in 41% of canine blastomycosis cases.[20] Affected dogs had a neutrophilic exudate and *Blastomyces dermatitidis* yeasts (Plate 4) in vitreous body smears. Empty capsules of dead yeast organisms may be the only indication of the infection in some animals. Other fungi that may be found in the vitreous body include *Cryptococcus neoformans* (Plate 4) and *Histoplasma capsulatum* (Plate 4).[21]

Prototheosis may also affect the vitreous body.[22] The organisms are usually systemic, though ocular manifestations due to chorioretinitis may be the initial clinical problem. A neutrophilic exudate and *Prototheca* organisms (Plate 5) may be found on vitreous smears.

Figure 26. Macrophages, erythrophages and RBC in a vitreous body aspirate from a dog with intraocular hemorrhage.

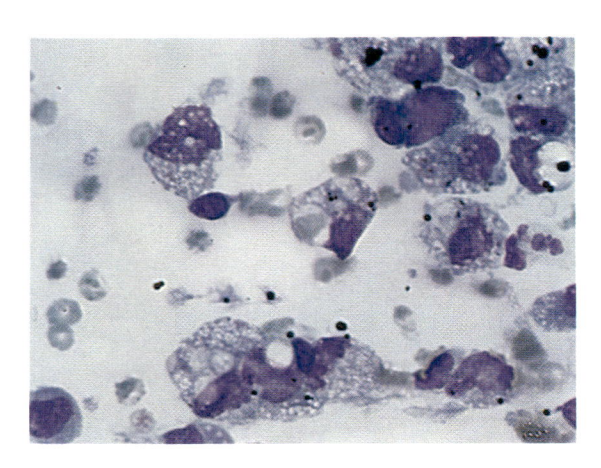

Figure 27. Angular cells exhibiting anisocytosis, anisokaryosis and binucleation, indicating neoplasia of connective tissue type, in a retrobulbar aspirate from a dog. Chondrosarcoma was confirmed by histopathologic examination.

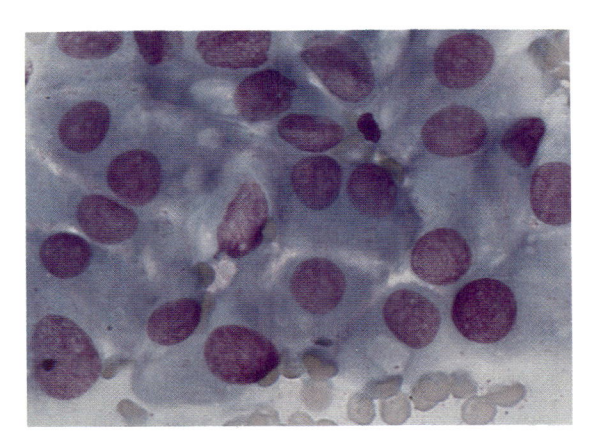

Hemorrhage

With hemorrhage, cytologic findings in vitreous smears are similar to those in hematomas or other sites of hemorrhage. In addition to RBC, monocytes and macrophages exhibiting erythrophagia and hemosiderin predominate (Fig 26). Causes of hemorrhage can be systemic or local ocular diseases, such as bleeding disorders, retinal detachment, intraocular tumor, hypertension, hyperthyroidism or rickettsial disease.

Intraocular Tumors

Posterior-segment intraocular tumors can be diagnosed on cytologic examination of

Figure 28. Variably sized noncornified squamous cells, RBC and cellular debris aspirated from a dog with a postenucleation orbital cyst.

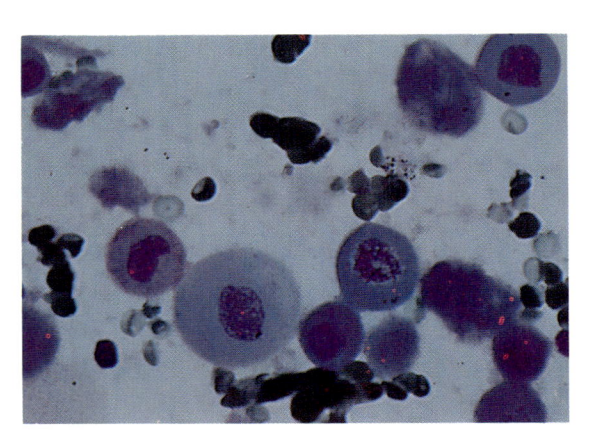

vitreous smears. Absence of neoplastic cells does not exclude intraocular tumor from consideration.

The Orbit

Exophthalmos

Exophthalmos often results from a space-occupying lesion in the orbit. Retrobulbar fine-needle aspiration and cytologic examination are indicated. These techniques may be the only way to acquire diagnostic specimens from lesions in the orbit and caudal to the eye. Traumatic proptosis is not an indication for retrobulbar aspiration.

The aspiration needle is placed in the opposite direction to which the globe is displaced and extended toward the orbital bone. Aspiration also can be done through the mouth, plac-

Figure 29. Degenerating squamous cells and a large foamy macrophage aspirated from a dog with a postenucleation orbital cyst.

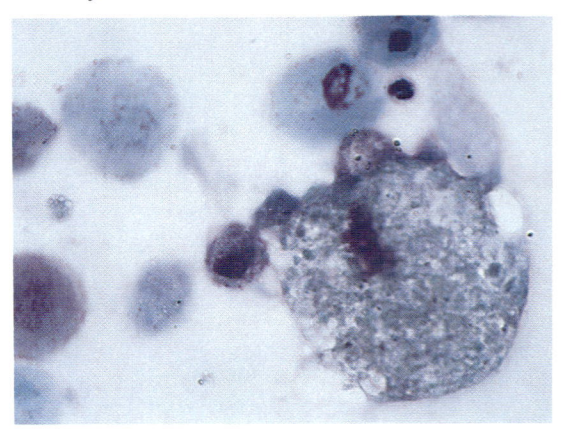

ing the needle caudal to the last molar. The critical structures to avoid are the optic nerve and the globe itself. Inflammatory lesions of infectious or foreign body causes, hematomas, and benign or malignant neoplasms are all possible in this location. The various principles of diagnostic cytology described throughout the text and in detail in Chapter 1 are applicable in their differentiation.

Orbital Tumors

Whereas aspiration of retrobulbar abscesses and hematomas yields much material, the yield from retrobulbar tumors is usually sparse. Orbital neoplasms we have encountered include lymphosarcomas, plasmacytomas, carcinomas of unknown types, squamous-cell carcinomas, salivary-gland carcinomas, sarcomas of unknown type, fibrosarcomas and chondrosarcomas (Fig 27).

Postenucleation Orbital Cyst

Orbital cysts are an infrequent complication of enucleation.[23] A possible mechanism of cyst formation is implantation or incarceration of conjunctival epithelium or glandular tissue at the time of enucleation. Cytologic examination reveals basal, intermediate and mature noncornified squamous cells, large foamy macrophages, and abundant mucus (Figs 28, 29).

References

1. Latimer and Dumstan: Eosinophilic plaque involving eyelids of the cat. *JAAHA* 23:649-652, 1986.

2. Krehbiel and Langham: Eyelid neoplasms of dogs. *Am J Vet Res* 36:115-119, 1975.

3. Carlton, in Peiffer: *Comparative Ophthalmic Pathology*. Charles C Thomas, Springfield, IL, 1983. pp 64-86.

4. Streeten and Streeten: "Blue body" epithelial cell inclusions in conjunctivitis. *Ophthalmol* 92:575-579, 1985.

5. Gelatt, in Gelatt: *Textbook of Veterinary Ophthalmology*. Lea & Febiger, Philadelphia, 1981. pp 206-261.

6. Peiffer, in Gelatt: *Textbook of Veterinary Ophthalmology*. Lea & Febiger, Philadelphia, 1981. pp 699-723.

7. Hoover et al: Experimentally induced feline chlamydial infection (Feline pneumonitis). *Am J Vet Res* 39:541-547, 1978.

8. Campbell et al: *Mycoplasma felis* associated conjunctivitis in cats. *JAVMA* 163:991-995, 1973.

9. Lavach et al: Cytology of normal and inflamed conjunctivas in dogs and cats. *JAVMA* 170:722-727, 1977.

10. Martin et al: Cystic lesions of the periorbital region. *Comp Cont Ed Pract Vet* 9:1022-1029, 1987.

11. Helper, in Gelatt: *Textbook of Veterinary Ophthalmology*. Lea & Febiger, Philadelphia, 1981. pp 330-342.

12. Fischer, in Peiffer: *Comparative Ophthalmic Pathology*. Charles C Thomas, Springfield, IL, 1983. pp 272-288.

13. Dice, in Gelatt: *Textbook of Veterinary Ophthalmology*. Lea & Febiger, Philadelphia, 1981. pp 343-374.

14. Paulsen et al: Feline eosinophilic keratitis: A review of 15 cases. *JAAHA* 23:63-69, 1986.

15. Schmidt and Prasse: Corneal epithelial inclusion cyst in a dog. *JAVMA* 168:144, 1976.

16. Hazel et al: Laboratory evaluation of aqueous humor in the healthy dog, cat, horse, and cow. *Am J Vet Res* 46:657-659, 1985.

17. Keller, in Gelatt: *Textbook of Veterinary Ophthalmology*. Lea & Febiger, Philadelphia, 1981. pp 375-389.

18. Carlton, in Peiffer: *Comparative Ophthalmic Pathology*. Charles C Thomas, Springfield, IL, 1983. pp 289-298.

19. Peiffer, in Peiffer: *Comparative Ophthalmic Pathology*. Charles C Thomas, Springfield, IL, 1983. pp 183-212.

20. Legendre et al: Canine blastomycosis: A review of 47 clinical cases. *JAVMA* 178:1163-1168, 1981.

21. Carlton, in Peiffer: *Comparative Ophthalmic Pathology*. Charles C Thomas, Springfield, IL, 1983. pp 299-317.

22. Buyukimihci et al: Protothecosis with ocular involvement in a dog. *JAVMA* 167:158-161, 1975.

23. Hanig and Hornblass: Treatment of postenucleation orbital cysts. *Ann Ophthalmol* 18:191-193, 1986.

The External Ear Canal

R.L. Cowell, R.D. Tyler and C.J. Baldwin

Causes of Otitis

Otitis externa is commonly encountered in veterinary practice. It may be unilateral, bilateral, acute or chronic.[1] While dogs and cats of all ages and breeds can be affected, otitis externa most frequently affects middle-aged dogs and young cats. Otitis externa in some form is reported to affect 5-20% of the canine and 2-6.6% of the feline population at any one time.[2-4] These animals generally show one or more of the following signs: head shaking, pain, pruritus, otic discharge, malodor, alopecia, excoriation and pyotraumatic dermatitis.[1-5] Conformation, habits, skin diseases, organisms, tumors and trauma are some of the factors thought to initiate, predispose or perpetuate otitis externa. Each is briefly addressed below.[1-4,6]

Conformation

A long, relatively narrow ear canal tends to trap moisture, foreign debris and glandular secretions. Excessive hair in the external ear canal tends to inhibit ventilation and increase retention of cerumen. Also, dogs with pendulous ears have decreased ventilation, which increases humidity within the ear canal. Such a moist environment can destroy the protective barrier of the epidermis and allow infection.

Habits

Dogs housed outside and hunting dogs are more likely to have foreign bodies lodge in the ear canal, such as grass awns, dirt or twigs. Dogs that swim or are frequently bathed may develop otitis externa due to stimulation of ceruminous gland activity resulting in overproduction of secretions. Moisture trapped in the ear canal may also affect the protective function of the epidermis.

Skin Diseases

Generalized skin disease may affect the ear canal epithelium (eg, immune-mediated, contact allergy) or cause overproduction of cerumen (eg, seborrhea complex, endocrinopathies, allergy). Remember that the ears are one of the "pruritic zones" with allergic diseases.

Organisms

Bacteria, yeasts and parasites may cause otic disorders. Small numbers of bacteria and yeast organisms are present in the ear canals of many clinically normal dogs and cats. These organisms can quickly overgrow and infect the ear canal when conditions permit. Ear mites are one of the major causes of otitis externa in cats, and also in dogs in certain regions of the country. Larval and nymph stages of the spinous ear tick, *Otobius megnini*, can cause acute otitis externa.

Tumors

Any cutaneous neoplasm can occur in the ear canal. Ear tumors are more common in dogs than cats.

Trauma

Traumatic use of cotton-tipped swabs or irritating solutions can damage the epithelial lining and allow organisms to colonize and infect the ear canal.

Diagnosis

Most cases of acute otitis externa can be readily managed using the information gained by a thorough history, physical examination, otoscopic examination and cytologic evaluation of ear canal secretions.[1,3,7] Careful evaluation of the patient's skin is also important because ear disease is often associated with generalized skin disease.[6] Foreign bodies, tissue masses, abnormal ear canal conformation, mites, ticks and other abnormalities can be detected during otoscopic examination, and any infectious agents present can be identified cytologically.[1,3] The algorithm in Chart 1 can be used to aid in evaluation of ear canal secretions. Additional diagnostic tests, such as culture, thyroid evaluation, intradermal skin testing and biopsy are generally needed to determine the underlying cause of chronic or recurrent otitis externa.[1,3,7]

Collection of Samples

Smears of ear canal secretions for cytologic evaluation are best collected with cotton-tipped swabs. Samples may be collected by passing a cotton-tipped swab through the cone of an otoscope (Fig 1). This works well in larger dogs, in which a large cone can be used. Another method is to carefully pass a swab into the ear canal without the aid of an otoscope after performing otoscopic examination to be sure the tympanic membrane is intact, because the swab may compress debris in the horizontal canal and obscure the tympanum. Passing a cotton-tipped swab through the cone

Figure 1. Smears of horizontal ear canal secretions may be collected by passing a cotton-tipped swab through the cone of an otoscope after otoscopic examination.

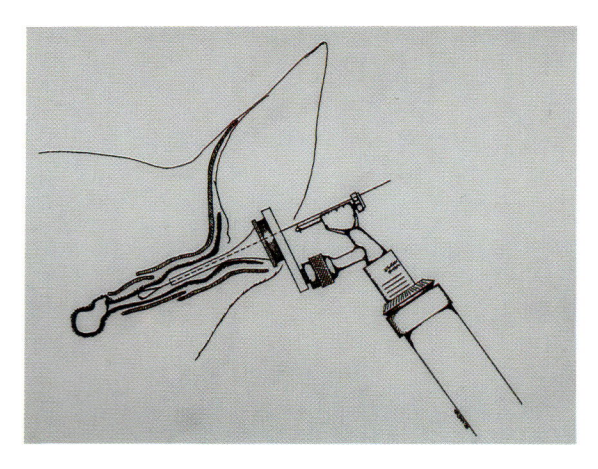

Figure 2. Ear swab from a normal dog shows some staining and nonstaining epithelial cells and debris. Note the absence of inflammatory cells and bacteria. (Wright's stain, original magnification 25X)

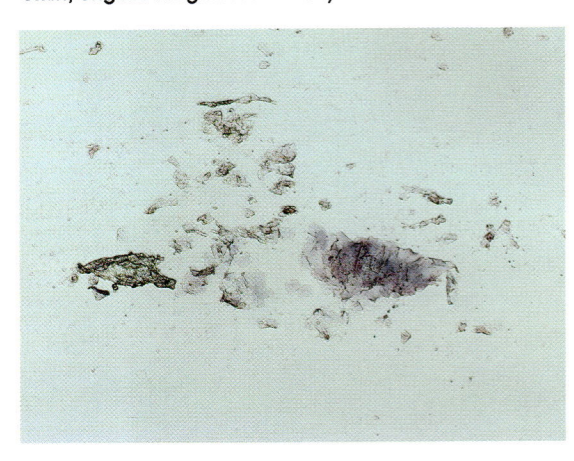

of an otoscope allows the operator to visualize the horizontal ear canal and be sure the specimen is collected from that area. Collecting ear swabs from the horizontal ear canal is desirable since most bacterial ear infections begin in this area.[8]

After ear canal secretions have been collected on a cotton-tipped swab, the swab is rolled on a clean, dry glass slide. Freshly made slides can be examined microscopically for ear mites before the material has dried. With experience, yeast (*Pityrosporum* spp) organisms can also be easily identified on unstained smears. After the material on the slide is allowed to air dry, it is stained with any of the usual hematologic stains. Some slides should always be stained and examined microscopically for organisms and WBC.

Cytologic Examination

Smears of external ear canal secretions should be evaluated for the different types and relative numbers of bacteria (rods, cocci), yeasts (*Pityrosporum* spp), fungal hyphae (*eg, Candida*), mites, neutrophils, cerumen and neoplastic cells.

Bacteria

The ear canals of clinically normal dogs often contain small numbers of bacteria.[8] The bacterial concentration typically is low enough that one sees only occasional or no bacteria on cytologic preparations (Fig 2). Many of these bacteria are potentially pathogenic and can colonize the ear canal when normal conditions are altered.[1-3,7] With bacterial infections, cytologic evaluation of ear canal secretions generally reveals large numbers of bacteria free in the smear, and often phagocytized bacteria in neutrophils. Otitis externa may be associated with large numbers of bacterial cocci (Plate 3), usually *Staphylococcus* or *Streptococcus* spp, which tend to induce a creamy, dark-yellow or light-brown otic discharge. Large numbers of bacterial rods (Plate 3), usually *Pseudomonas aeruginosa* or *Proteus mirabilis*, tend to elicit a thick, sweet-smelling, pale-yellow exudate. A combination of rods and cocci may also be found.[1,3,7] When routine therapy is ineffective, culture and sensitivity tests are indicated because of the high incidence of antimicrobial resistance associated with otitis externa.[9]

Fungi

Pityrosporum pachydermatis (Malassezia canis) is by far the most common cause of mycotic otitis externa in dogs and cats.[3,5] *Pityrosporum* (Fig 3) is a broad-based, budding, Gram-positive, nonmycelioid yeast that is frequently a normal inhabitant of the canine and feline external ear canal.[2,5,7,10] *Pityrosporum* organisms have been found cytologically in ear swabs of up to 49% of normal dogs and 23% of normal cats evaluated.[11]

Finding >10 *Pityrosporum* organisms per high power field (40X objective) suggests a yeast overgrowth. In this situation, *Pityrosporum* should be considered as contributing to the otitis externa.[10] Pure *Pityrosporum* infections tend to develop copious, dark-brown exudate with a sweet odor.[1-3,7] However, bacterial infections, especially those caused by Gram-positive cocci, concurrent with *Pityro-*

Figure 3. *Pityrosporum* infections are characterized by large numbers of broad-based, budding yeast organisms. (Wright's stain, original magnification 50X (insert, original magnification 250X))

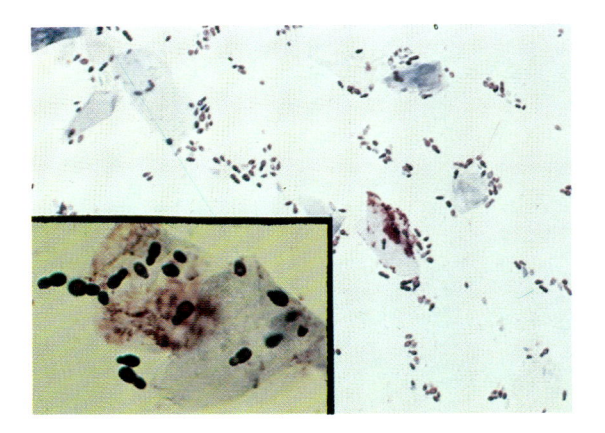

Figure 4. Mixed infection characterized by large numbers of bacterial rods and cocci. Some *Pityrosporum* organisms are also present. (Wright's stain, original magnification 250X)

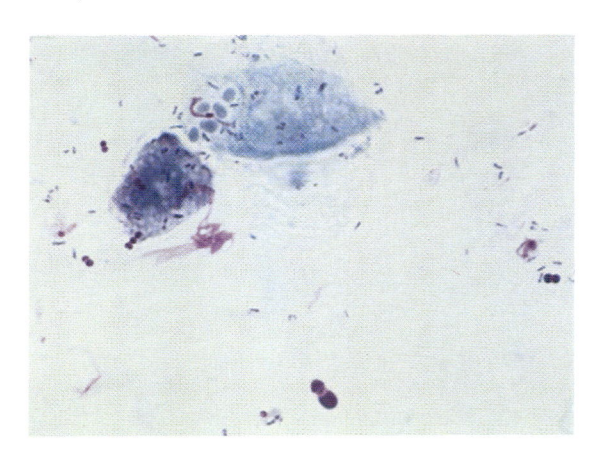

sporum infections (Fig 4) are reportedly common.[7] *Pityrosporum* organisms can be readily identified as dark-staining, budding yeasts. With practice, *Pityrosporum* organisms are readily identified on unstained smears.

Other fungi, such as *Candida* spp, *Aspergillus* spp and *Microsporum* spp, only rarely cause otitis externa. When unidentified yeasts or hyphae (Plate 5) are observed cytologically, culture is indicated for identification.

Mites

Otitis externa secondary to ear mites (Fig 5) is a common problem in dogs and cats. In animals hypersensitized to mite antigens, clinical signs of otitis externa may develop with as few as 2-3 mites in the ear canal.[2,3] *Otodectes cynotis* reportedly accounts for 50% of feline and 5-10% of canine cases of otitis externa.[3] Typically, a dry reddish-brown or black, granular discharge is seen. The discharge consists of cerumen, epidermal cells and inflammatory cells.[1-4,6,7] Secondary bacterial and/or yeast infections often coexist. This can cause the discharge to become moist.[6]

Because small numbers of mites may not be visualized on otoscopic examination, careful cytologic evaluation of unstained exudate for eggs, larvae or adult mites should be undertaken. Both unstained and stained slides of ear canal secretions should be evaluated. Mites readily wash off slides during the staining process; therefore, they are seldom seen on stained slides. Hence, unstained slides are best for finding mites, while stained slides are best for recognizing increased numbers of bacteria and/or yeast.

Figure 5. Ear mite (*Otodectes cynotis*) on an unstained smear of ear canal secretions. (Original magnification 25X).

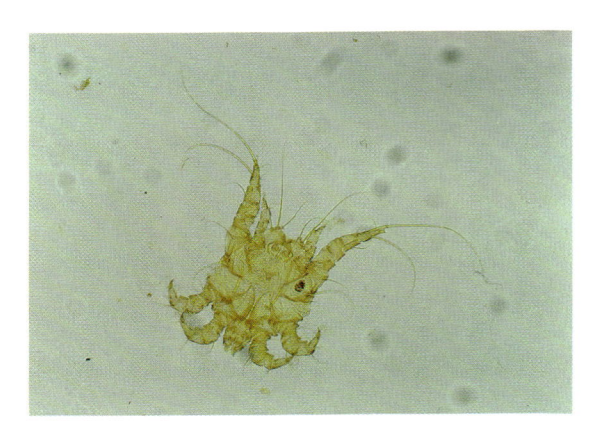

Demodex canis infection of the external ear canal is a rare cause of otitis externa.[2,6] Demodectic otoacariasis usually is not associated with lesions on other areas of skin.[2,7] Large numbers of adult demodectic mites are typically seen in cerumen smears.[2,7]

Neoplasia

The ear canal can potentially develop any of the tumors that occur on skin, as well as ceruminous-gland tumors. However, neoplastic cells are only rarely seen on cytologic evaluation of external ear canal secretions. Many tumors are covered by normal epithelium and their neoplastic cells are not available for collection by an ear swab. These tumors may alter the ear canal condition and allow secondary in-

Chart 1. Flow chart for evaluation of smears of ear canal secretions.

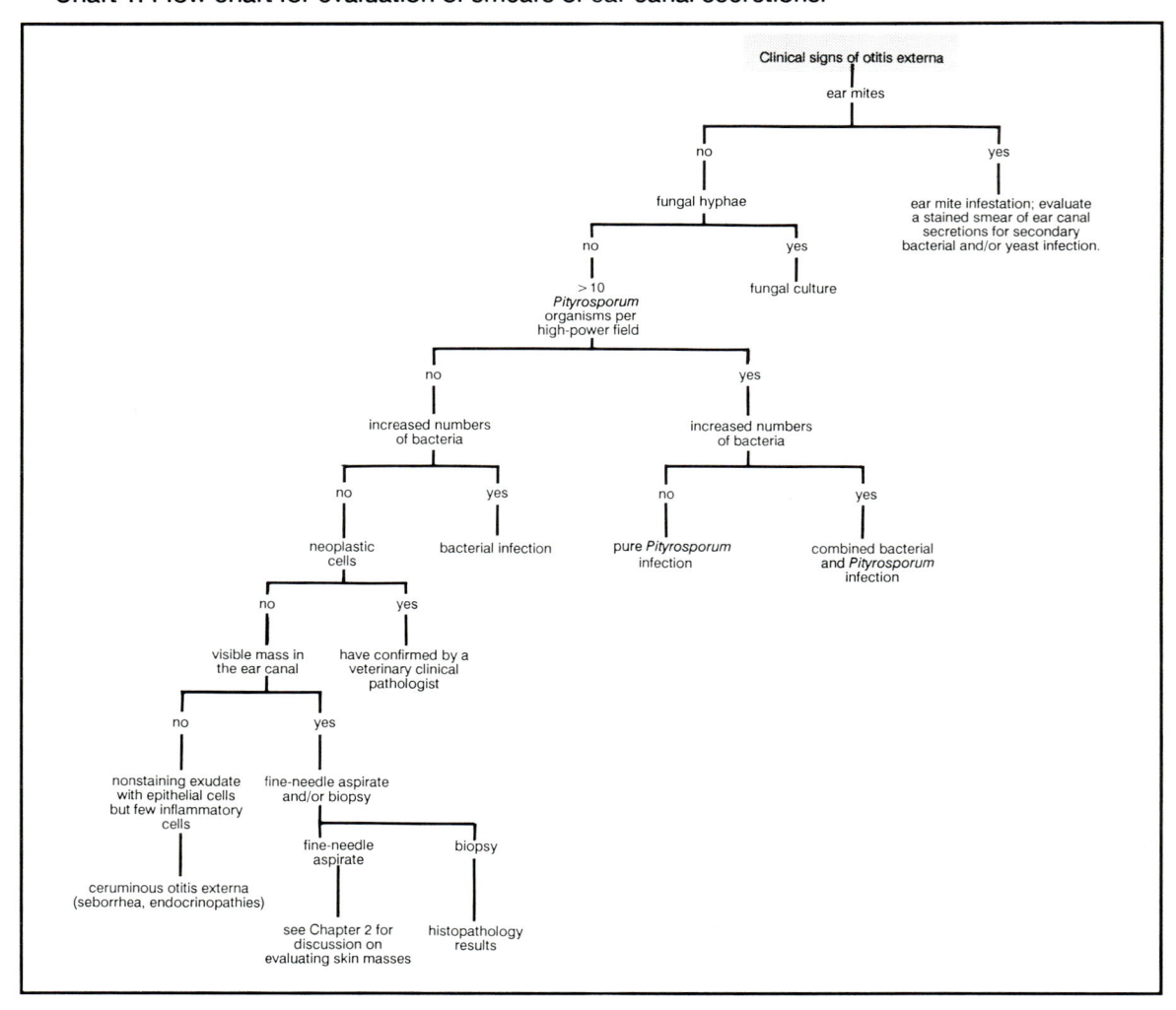

fection to develop. Cytologically, inflammation may be all that is observed. If a mass is observed on otoscopic examination of the ear canal and cytologic examination of ear swabs does not establish the cause of the mass, fine-needle aspiration or biopsy should be performed to help identify the mass. See Chapter 2 for a discussion on evaluation of cutaneous and subcutaneous masses.

Miscellaneous

Ceruminous otitis externa is associated with some seborrheic diseases. The characteristic oily, yellow discharge may grossly resemble purulent exudate.[2,6] However, because these secretions contain very few inflammatory cells and cerumen fails to take stain, very little material is visible on microscopic examination of the discharge.[2]

References

1. August: Otitis externa in the dog and cat. *Proc 53rd Ann Mtg AAHA*, 1986. pp 201-204.

2. August: *The Complete Manual of Ear Care*. Veterinary Learning Systems, 1986. pp 37-51.

3. Griffin: Otitis externa. *Comp Cont Ed Pract Vet* 3:741-749, 1981.

4. Grono, in Kirk: *Current Veterinary Therapy VII*. Saunders, Philadelphia, 1980. pp 461-466.

5. Gedek *et al*: The role of *Pityrosporum pachydermatis* in otitis externa of dogs: evaluation of a treatment with miconazole. *Vet Record* 104:138-140, 1979.

6. Harvey: Ear canal disease in the dog: medical and surgical management. *JAVMA* 177:136-139, 1980.

7. August: *The Complete Manual of Ear Care*. Veterinary Learning Systems, 1986. pp 53-60.

8. Dickson and Love: Bacteriology of the horizontal ear canal of dogs. *J Small Anim Pract* 24:413-421, 1983.

9. Blue and Wooley: Antibacterial sensitivity patterns of bacteria isolated from dogs with otitis externa. *JAVMA* 171:362-363, 1977.

10. Rausch and Skinner: Incidence and treatment of budding yeasts in canine otitis externa. *MVP* 53:914-915, 1978.

11. Baxter: The association of *Pityrosporum pachydermatis* with the normal external ear canal of dogs and cats. *J Small Anim Pract* 17:231-234, 1976.

7

Subcutaneous Glandular Tissue:
Mammary, Salivary, Thyroid and Parathyroid

J.M. Maddux and R.M. Shull

The mammary, salivary, thyroid and parathyroid glands are located in the subcutaneous fat layer. Knowledge of normal microanatomy of these glands and of other structures in close proximity is important for accurate cytologic interpretation. Except for the thyroid and parathyroid glands, regional locations of these glands differ considerably. Cytologically, normal exocrine glands (mammary and salivary) may appear similar, and differ from normal endocrine glands (thyroid and parathyroid). Lymphoid and adipose tissues may be found near any of these glands. Thymic tissue may be near the thyroid and parathyroid, especially in young animals or when any of these tissues exist in ectopic locations.

Cytologic evaluation of subcutaneous glandular tissue is a valuable extension of clinical examination. Collection of samples by fine-needle aspiration biopsy is simple and rapid, and avoids the trauma and anesthetic risk of surgical biopsy. Most lesions are readily palpable and therefore easily aspirated. Though aspiration is the usual means of obtaining specimens, cytologic evaluation may also be performed on imprints of excised tissue, scrapings of ulcerated surface lesions, and mammary secretions. Many publications on cytologic examination of subcutaneous glandular tissue exist in the human medical literature, but information dealing with its application in veterinary medicine is sparse.[1-6]

The primary goal of aspiration cytology is to distinguish inflammatory from neoplastic lesions and to differentiate, when possible, benign neoplasms from malignant neoplasms. Diagnostic accuracy for cytologic differentiation of benign from malignant mammary neoplasms in dogs varies from 33% to 79%.[7,8] However, differentiation of inflammation from neoplasia is more reliable. A high rate of false negatives in cases of malignancies may result from several factors. Sampling errors occur if the needle is not directed into a representative area of the tumor. This problem is proportional to tumor size, and sampling of multiple sites in large tumors may increase the likelihood of aspirating neoplastic cells. Multiple mammary tumors in an animal may be of different types, thus requiring examination of all lesions. A grading system for differentiation of benign from malignant mammary tumors in dogs based on 10 important criteria of malignancy has been proposed.[7] Some criteria of malignancy were best appreciated in smears prepared with wet fixation and Papanicolaou type stains, which are less frequently used in general veterinary practice. Accuracy of evaluation may also depend on the experience of the cytologist. Samples yielding equivocal results, such as cyst fluid, nonseptic inflammatory changes or those cytologically positive for neoplasia but without sufficient criteria to establish malignancy, should be evaluated histologically. Samples yielding definitive nonneoplastic diagnoses and samples yielding definitive diagnoses of malignant neoplasia may not need to be evaluated histologically.

Figure 1. Neutrophils and foamy macrophages in secretions from an inflamed mammary gland. (Wright's stain, 1000X)

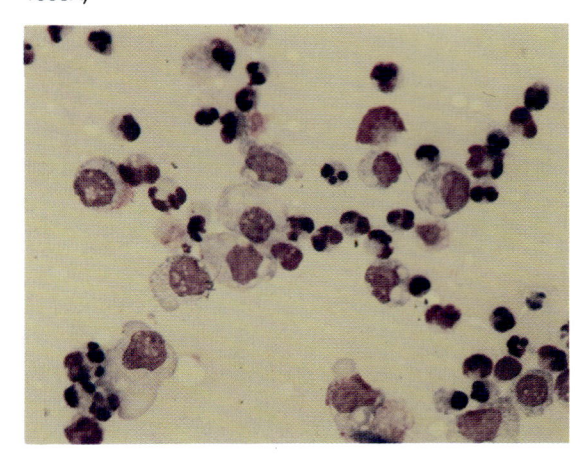

Chart 1 presents an algorithm for cytologic evaluation of mammary, salivary, thyroid and parathyroid tissue.

The Mammary Glands

Normal Cytologic Appearance

Mammary tissue of dogs and cats consists of 5 pairs of modified sweat glands that extend along the ventral body wall from the cranial thorax to the inguinal region. Glands consist of secretory acini and a series of excretory ducts. Myoepithelial cells lie between glandular epithelial cells and the basement membrane. During lactation the glands undergo marked hypertrophy to produce colostrum and then milk. Normal mammary secretions contain large amounts of protein and lipid droplets, and are of low cellularity. The predominant cell type in milk is the "foam cell," a large, vacuolated epithelial cell that resembles an active macrophage. These cells usually occur singly. Small numbers of lymphocytes and neutrophils may also be present.

Aspirates of normal mammary tissue are frequently acellular or contain only blood. When mammary tissue is present, secretory cells are arranged in an acinar pattern. Individual cells have moderate amounts of basophilic cytoplasm and round, dark nuclei of uniform size. Duct epithelial cells have basal, ovoid nuclei and scanty cytoplasm, and are arranged in small sheets or fragments of ductules.[9] Myoepithelial cells appear as dark-staining, naked, oval nuclei or as spindle-shaped cells. Adipocytes and lipid droplets may be present.

Benign Lesions

Mastitis: Mastitis, or inflammation of the mammary glands, may occur either as a diffuse form involving 1 or more mammae or as a focal lesion. Mastitis is usually associated with postpartum lactation or pseudopregnancy and may result from ascending or hematogenous infections.

Mammary secretions are usually adequate for diagnosis in cases of diffuse inflammation, while aspirates may be required for diagnosis of focal lesions. Smears are very cellular and contain large amounts of debris. Inflammatory cells may include neutrophils, lymphocytes, macrophages and foam cells in variable numbers, depending on the causative agent (Fig 1). Bacteria may be seen within phagocytes (Plate 3). Offending agents are usually coliforms, streptococci and staphylococci, though other bacteria and fungi may occasionally be isolated. Focal, nonseptic "inflammatory nodules" may occur secondary to lobular hyperplasia.[10] These are characterized cytologically by epithelial-cell metaplasia, pigment-laden macrophages, nondegenerate neutrophils, lymphocytes and plasma cells.

Cysts: Mammary cysts result from a dysplastic process in which dilated ducts expand to form large cavitations.[10] Cyst linings may consist of single layers of flattened epithelium or may have papillary overgrowth. Cysts may be present as single nodules or multinodular masses that grow slowly and have a bluish surface. Cysts are common in middle-aged and older bitches, but may occasionally appear in

Figure 2. Sheet of glandular cells exhibiting little nuclear or cytoplasmic pleomorphism and a fine granular chromatin pattern characteristic of a mammary adenoma. A large, pigment-laden macrophage is present. (Wright's stain, 1250X)

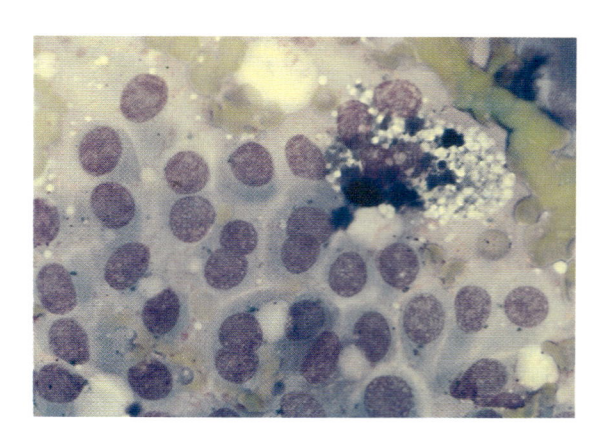

Subcutaneous Glandular Tissue

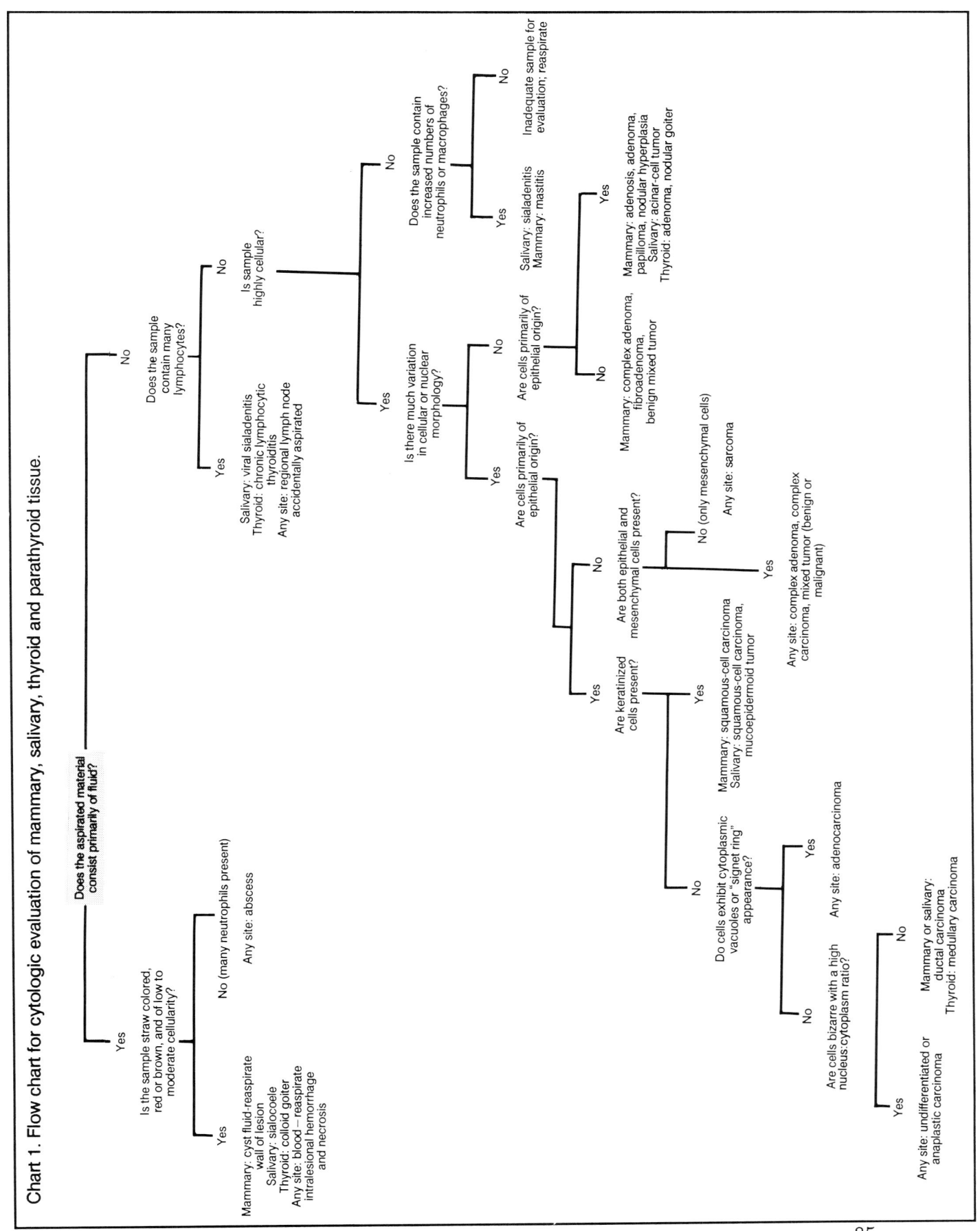

Chart 1. Flow chart for cytologic evaluation of mammary, salivary, thyroid and parathyroid tissue.

Does the aspirated material consist primarily of fluid?

- **Yes** → Is the sample straw colored, red or brown, and of low to moderate cellularity?
  - **Yes** → Mammary: cyst fluid-reaspirate wall of lesion; Salivary: sialocoele; Thyroid: colloid goiter; Any site: blood – reaspirate intralesional hemorrhage and necrosis
  - **No** (many neutrophils present) → Any site: abscess

- **No** → Does the sample contain many lymphocytes?
  - **Yes** → Salivary: viral sialadenitis; Thyroid: chronic lymphocytic thyroiditis; Any site: regional lymph node accidentally aspirated
  - **No** → Is sample highly cellular?
    - **No** → Does the sample contain increased numbers of neutrophils or macrophages?
      - **Yes** → Salivary: sialadenitis; Mammary: mastitis
      - **No** → Inadequate sample for evaluation; reaspirate
    - **Yes** → Is there much variation in cellular or nuclear morphology?
      - **No** → Are cells primarily of epithelial origin?
        - **Yes** → Mammary: adenosis, adenoma, papilloma, nodular hyperplasia; Salivary: acinar-cell tumor; Thyroid: adenoma, nodular goiter
        - **No** → Mammary: complex adenoma, fibroadenoma, benign mixed tumor
      - **Yes** → Are cells primarily of epithelial origin?
        - **No** → Are both epithelial and mesenchymal cells present?
          - **Yes** → Any site: complex adenoma, complex carcinoma, mixed tumor (benign or malignant)
          - **No** (only mesenchymal cells) → Any site: sarcoma
        - **Yes** → Are keratinized cells present?
          - **Yes** → Mammary: squamous-cell carcinoma; Salivary: squamous-cell carcinoma, mucoepidermoid tumor
          - **No** → Do cells exhibit cytoplasmic vacuoles or "signet ring" appearance?
            - **Yes** → Any site: adenocarcinoma
            - **No** → Are cells bizarre with a high nucleus:cytoplasm ratio?
              - **Yes** → Any site: undifferentiated or anaplastic carcinoma
              - **No** → Mammary or salivary: ductal carcinoma; Thyroid: medullary carcinoma

85

young dogs. Though considered benign, mammary cysts may be precancerous. Fluid aspirated is usually yellow, brown, green or blood-tinged, and of low cellularity unless there is concurrent inflammation. Cells are primarily "foam cells" and pigment-laden macrophages. Epithelial cells aspirated from cysts lined by papillary projections may occur in dense clusters and exhibit a minor degree of nuclear pleomorphism.

Solid Masses: Dysplastic lesions and benign neoplasms of mammary tissue include lobular hyperplasia, adenosis, adenomas and papillomas, all of which may appear similar cytologically.[10] Smears made from aspirates contain many epithelial cells occurring singly or arranged in sheets and clusters. These cells exhibit little or no pleomorphism. Chromatin is evenly dispersed, and single, small, round nucleoli may be visible. Pigment-laden macrophages may be present (Fig 2).

Benign tumors involving stromal and epithelial elements, such as complex adenomas, fibroadenomas and benign mixed tumors, are common in dogs.[10] Smears of aspirates from these lesions contain spindle-shaped cells of connective tissue origin in addition to clusters of epithelial cells similar to those described above (Fig 3). Spindle-shaped cells, however, are not a definitive cytologic characteristic of complex or mixed tumors, as they may also be found in some simple tumors.[7]

Malignant Neoplasms

Mammary-gland tumors are common in both dogs and cats; however, the biologic behavior of the tumors varies greatly between these species. Mammary tumors comprise up to 50% of neoplasms in the bitch.[11,12] About 50% of mammary tumors are classified histologically as "mixed" and 40% are adenocarcinomas. Adenocarcinomas are considered malignant, and about 10-20% of other mammary tumor types are malignant. Mammary tumors are the third most common neoplasm in cats and account for about 17% of all neoplasms in queens.[13] Most feline mammary tumors are adenocarcinomas and the overall malignancy rate is above 80%. Mammary tumors are rare in males of both species.

Various carcinomas are recognized histologically and often have similar cytologic characteristics. Most of these tumors arise from glandular epithelium and thus are adenocarcinomas. Ductal carcinomas, anaplastic carcinomas and squamous-cell carcinomas are less common. Adenocarcinomas are usually discrete masses that do not adhere to the overlying skin. Smears of aspirates from adenocarcinomas generally contain epithelial cells occurring singly and in clusters of variable size. Cellular pleomorphism and mitotic activity are variable and related to the tumor's degree of malignancy.

Adenocarcinoma cells are usually round, with round to oval, eccentrically placed nuclei and variable quantities of basophilic cytoplasm that occasionally contains vacuoles filled with secretory product (Fig 4). Cell borders are usually distinct. Other cytologic criteria that best correlate with malignancy include variable nuclear size, nuclear giant

Figure 3. Mixture of epithelial and mesenchymal cells from a benign mixed mammary tumor. (Wright's stain, 1000X)

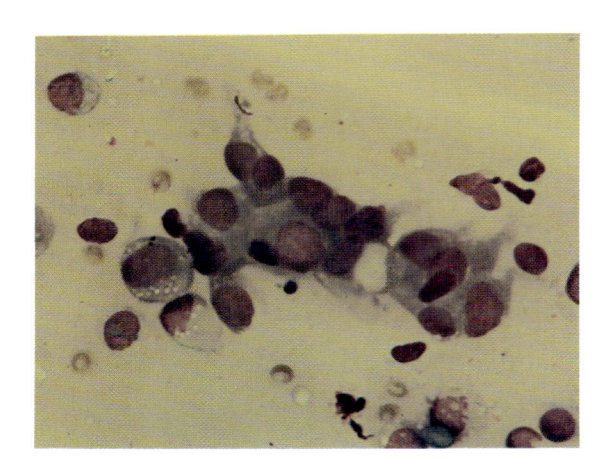

Figure 4. Cluster of epithelial cells from a mammary carcinoma. Marked variation in cell and nuclear morphology, basophilic cytoplasm with secretory product in vacuoles, and macronucleoli characterize this tumor. (Wright's stain, 1250X)

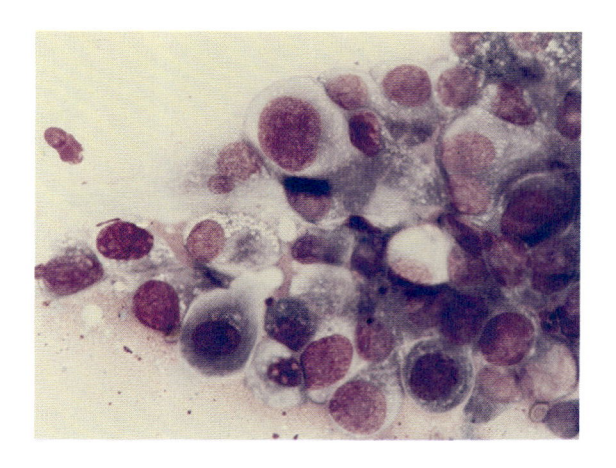

Figure 5. Cluster of foamy secretory cells from a normal salivary gland. Erythrocytes assume a linear pattern due to the mucin content of the sample. (Wright's stain, 800X)

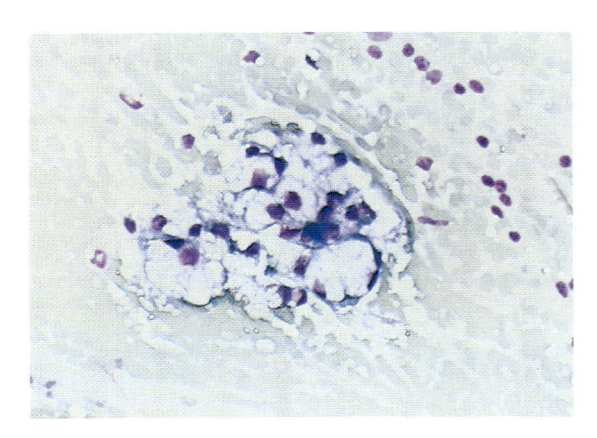

forms, high nucleus:cytoplasm ratio, variable nucleolar number, abnormal nucleolar shape and the presence of macronucleoli.

Anaplastic carcinomas are diffuse, red, swollen lesions that must be differentiated from mastitis.[10] Cytologically, they exhibit an array of very large, very pleomorphic epithelial cells. These cells occur singly and in small clusters, and have a high nucleus:cytoplasm ratio, and bizarre nuclear and nucleolar forms. Multinucleate forms and mitotic figures are common.

Nonglandular carcinomas may be simple, with only epithelial proliferation, or complex, with cells of epithelial and myoepithelial origin. Malignant epithelial cells are highly pleomorphic, with a high nucleus:cytoplasm ratio. They usually do not contain intracytoplasmic vacuoles, as do adenocarcinomas.

Squamous-cell carcinomas in mammary glands appear cytologically similar to those in other body regions (Plate 6). Tumor cells occur singly or in small sheets, and may be keratinized or nonkeratinized. Large keratinized epithelial cells have pyknotic or inapparent nuclei, a low nucleus:cytoplasm ratio, and abundant, pale-staining cytoplasm. Nonkeratinized cells have large, vesicular nuclei, a high nucleus:cytoplasm ratio, and deeply basophilic cytoplasm (see Chapter 2 for further discussion). These tumors frequently adhere to the overlying dermis and may be ulcerated, leading to the presence of many inflammatory cells and bacteria in samples taken from ulcerated areas.

Mammary sarcomas are less common than carcinomas. Histologically recognized mesenchymal tumors include osteosarcoma, fibrosarcoma, liposarcoma, combined (osteo-fibrolipo-) sarcoma, reticulum-cell sarcoma and mast-cell tumors.[12] Cells of sarcomas are often irregular or spindle shaped, occur singly or in small sheets, and have indistinct cell borders. Degree of pleomorphism and mitotic activity is variable and indicative of tumor malignancy. In general, cytologic criteria of malignancy described for carcinomas apply to sarcomas. Mast-cell tumors in mammary tissue are clinically and cytologically similar to those in other body regions (Plate 7, see Chapter 2 for further discussion).

Carcinosarcomas are relatively uncommon tumors of mixed origin. Cytologically they may contain both epithelial and mesenchymal populations. The presence of both cell types and predominance of 1 type over the other depend on the area of the tumor aspirated. The cytologic criteria of malignancy described above apply to these tumors.

The Salivary Glands

Normal Cytologic Appearance

Major salivary glands in dogs and cats are the parotid, mandibular, sublingual and zygomatic glands. Minor, or buccal, salivary glands are spread over the oral mucosa. Salivary glands are comprised of secretory cells arranged in acini and an extensive ductular network. A layer of myoepithelial cells lies between the glandular cells and basement membrane. Aspirated samples from normal salivary glands reveal secretory epithelial cells with small, round nuclei and abundant cytoplasm distended with clear vacuoles.[9] Acinar cells usually occur in clusters (Fig 5). Ductal epithelial cells are small cells arranged in sheets, with uniform round nuclei and scanty cytoplasm. Single cells of acinic or ductal origin are rare. Samples may also include occasional spindle-shaped myoepithelial cells, adipocytes, and lipid droplets. Hemorrhage is frequent upon aspiration of salivary glands. RBC in smears assume a characteristic linear pattern due to the mucin content of the sample.

Nonneoplastic Lesions

Sialoceles: The most common salivary gland disorder in dogs is the sialocele.[14] These are nonepithelial-lined cavities filled with salivary secretions. Leakage of salivary secretions into fascial tissues usually follows blunt trauma but may occasionally be secondary to calculi or duct obstruction by bite wounds, abscesses and ear canal surgery. Swellings occur most commonly on the floor of the mouth (ranulae) or the cranial cervical area, and less frequently in pharyngeal or retrobulbar areas. Aspirated fluid is viscous, clear or blood tinged, and contains small to moderate numbers of nucleated cells.

Cytologic evaluation of sialocele aspirates usually reveals diffuse or irregular clumps of homogeneous pink- to violet-staining mucin. Large phagocytic cells with small round nuclei and abundant foamy cytoplasm may be found individually or in small clusters (Fig 6). Salivary-gland epithelial cells may be intermixed but are not easily distinguished cytologically from macrophages.[15] Nondegenerate neutrophils are often present in small numbers but may be present in large numbers due to tissue inflammation without infection. Lobulation of neutrophil nuclei may not be distinct, since the cells often do not spread out well in the viscous fluid. RBC often occur in linear patterns due to the mucin content. Neutrophils may increase in numbers as the duration of the lesion progresses. Macrophages with phagocytosed debris or exhibiting erythrophagocytosis may also be present. Golden, rhomboidal hematoidin crystals within macrophage cytoplasm result from RBC degradation and suggest chronicity (Plate 2).

Sialadenitis: Sialadenitis, inflammation of salivary glands, is uncommon but may be associated with trauma, infarction, canine distemper virus, rabies virus, paramyxovirus or bacteria, or secondary to sialoceles.[14,16] Cytologic evaluation of inflamed salivary glands reveals populations of cells similar to these in inflammatory lesions in other locations. Some variation in inflammatory cell population may occur with different causative agents. Nonseptic lesions contain many nondegenerate neutrophils, moderate to many active macrophages, and variable amounts of hemorrhage, necrotic cells and debris. Viral lesions, such as those resulting from canine distemper virus infections, may have significant numbers of lymphoid cells. Lesions caused by bacterial infections contain numerous degenerate neutrophils and variable numbers of active macrophages and bacteria (Plates 1-3).

Neoplasia: Salivary-gland neoplasia is uncommon in dogs and cats.[14,17] It occurs most frequently in aged animals without breed or sex predilection, and often involves the parotid gland. Carcinomas and adenocarcinomas occur more often than mixed tumors or sarcomas. A variety of carcinomas may be recognized histologically, including acinar-cell tumors, adenocarcinomas, squamous-cell carcinomas, mucoepidermoid tumors and undifferentiated carcinomas; however, cytologic distinction of type may not be possible, especially with poorly differentiated tumors.

Acinar-cell carcinomas are the most common salivary gland neoplasm in dogs. These tumors are of low-grade malignancy. Needle aspirates reveal cells with round nuclei of uniform size. Cells exhibit minimal pleomorphism. Distinction of acinar-cell tumors from nonneoplastic swelling may be difficult, and is based on such characteristics as lack of well-defined acinar structures, absence of ductal epithelium and increased cellularity in aspirates of neoplasms. Cystic lesions require aspiration of the wall of the structure for cytologic diagnosis.

Salivary-gland adenocarcinomas consist of cells with abundant basophilic cytoplasm, often distended with secretory product, giving cells a "signet-ring" appearance due to peripheral nuclear displacement. Nuclei are round, with mild pleomorphism. Squamous-cell carcinomas of salivary glands appear cytologically similar to squamous-cell carcinomas in other body regions (Plate 6; see Chapter 2 for further discussion). Tumor cells may occur in rafts or clusters and vary from large keratinized epithelial cells with pyknotic nuclei, a low nucleus:cytoplasm ratio and abundant pale-staining cytoplasm, to small, nonkeratinized cells with large vesicular nuclei, a high nucleus:cytoplasm ratio and deeply basophilic

Figure 6. Cluster of foamy macrophages, few nondegenerate neutrophils, and erythrocytes from a sialocele. (Wright's stain, 1250X)

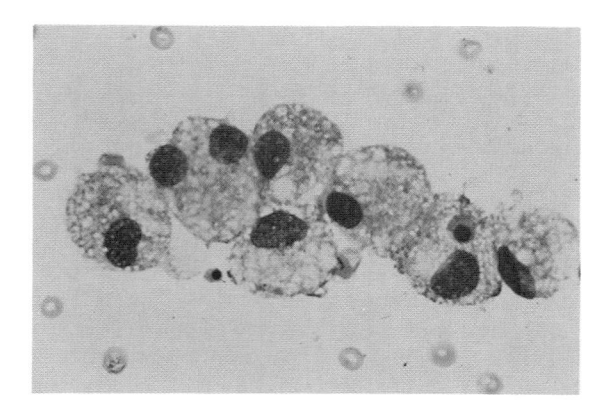

cytoplasm. Mucoepidermoid tumors have cell populations representing both mucus-secreting adenocarcinomas and squamous-cell carcinomas.

Undifferentiated carcinomas consist of epithelial cells with round nuclei, a high nucleus: cytoplasm ratio and well-defined cell borders. These tumors may not be distinguishable cytologically from histiocytic lymphomas and other metastatic tumors.[17]

Mixed tumors of salivary glands are rare. Cytologically they have characteristics of both mesenchymal and epithelial neoplasms. Epithelial populations have characteristics similar to those of previously described carcinomas. Mesenchymal populations are pleomorphic, with irregular or spindle-shaped cells and indistinct borders. These cells usually occur individually but may be found in sheets. Sarcomas are also rare and have cells with characteristics of a mesenchymal cell population.

The Thyroid Glands

Normal Cytologic Appearance

The thyroid glands of dogs and cats are paired endocrine glands in the ventral cervical region. Their exact location may vary from the laryngeal region to the thoracic inlet. Ectopic thyroid tissue may also occur in the cranial mediastinum near the heart base. The normal thyroid gland is not readily palpated and is, therefore, not usually aspirated for cytologic examination. Palpable abnormalities may occur unilaterally or bilaterally as diffuse swelling, multinodular swelling or solitary nodular masses. Aspiration cytology may help differentiate benign from malignant lesions and help rule out other causes of cervical masses, including abscesses, lymphadenopathy, sialoceles and nonthyroid neoplasms.

Thyroid tissue consists of numerous follicles lined by cuboidal to polygonal epithelial cells and filled with colloid. Each gland is enclosed in a connective tissue capsule and has a rich vascular supply. Fine-needle aspirates of normal thyroid tissue contain large quantities of colloid that appears as grayish-purple amorphous background material. Numerous blood cells are often present as a result of hemorrhage during aspiration. Thyroid epithelial cells are generally scarce and occur in small sheets with a monolayer appearance (Fig 7). Nuclei are of uniform size, with hyperchromatic, clumped chromatin, and are located centrally in a moderate amount of basophilic cytoplasm.[9] Identification of these cells as thyroid epithelium is aided by the presence of intracytoplasmic perinuclear blue-black granules representing tyrosine accumulation.[15] Many naked nuclei from these cells may be scattered through the specimen. Large macrophages containing variable amounts of pigment believed to be digested colloid are occasionally seen.

Benign Lesions

Inflammation: Chronic lymphocytic thyroiditis is an immune-mediated lesion that rarely causes enlargement of the thyroid gland in dogs.[18,19] Dogs with this syndrome usually have no signs of disease in early stages when the thyroid gland is most likely to be enlarged. When clinical signs of hypothyroidism appear, the thyroid gland has usually atrophied, is not palpable, and is therefore difficult to aspirate. Cytologically, affected thyroid glands contain numerous lymphocytes, plasma cells and macrophages in addition to normal and degenerating follicular cells.

Hyperplasia: Hyperplastic enlargement of the thyroid can occur secondary to iodine deficiency, iodine excess or inability to synthesize either thyroglobulin or thyroxine.[20] Clinically affected animals may be young or adults and appear hypothyroid or euthyroid. Early follicles contain hyperplastic cells with little or no colloid, while later follicles become involuted and are filled with colloid. Enlargement is generalized. Cytologic patterns may depend on the duration of the lesion.

Figure 7. Sheet of normal thyroid-gland epithelial cells. Cells have centrally located nuclei, with clumped chromatin and a small rim of basophilic cytoplasm. (Wright's stain, 1250X)

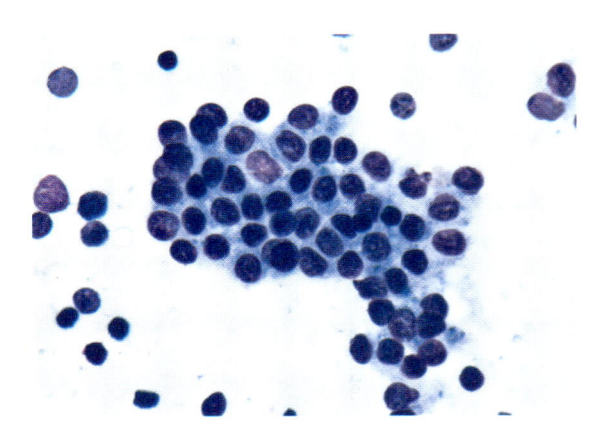

with clusters of follicular cells and scattered naked nuclei as the predominant finding. Follicular cells are uniform in appearance, with small round nuclei placed centrally in a moderate amount of basophilic cytoplasm. Aspirates are often bloody due to extensive vascularity. Cystic lesions, clinically termed "colloid goiter," are more common. Aspirated fluid may appear serous but is more commonly brown and turbid due to previous hemorrhage and necrosis. Cytologic examination reveals individual cells or small clusters of follicular cells on a dense colloid background. Foamy, pigment-laden macrophages, lymphocytes and RBC are also present.

Adenoma: Adenomas of the thyroid gland are benign tumors. Clinically detectable adenomas are uncommon in dogs and generally occur as single, focal nodules. Functional thyroid adenomas in cats with clinical hyperthyroidism have been recognized frequently since the syndrome was first reported in 1978.[21] Adenomatous hyperplasia and focal adenomas may be solid cellular masses or may develop a central cavity filled with colloid, blood and cholesterol crystals. In smears of aspirates, follicular cells occur in small clusters and are monomorphic, resembling normal follicular cells (Fig 8). The presence of blue-black intracytoplasmic tyrosine granules is variable. Aspirates of cystic adenomas contain pigment-laden macrophages, lymphocytes and RBC, with stained colloid in the background. Cholesterol crystals may be seen (Fig 15, Chapter 2).[29] Adenomas may be difficult to distinguish from well-differentiated carcinomas.

Figure 8. Cluster of cells from a thyroid adenoma. Cells have monomorphic nuclei, with fine granular chromatin and abundant basophilic cytoplasm containing small vacuoles and numerous blue-black granules. (Wright's stain, 1000X)

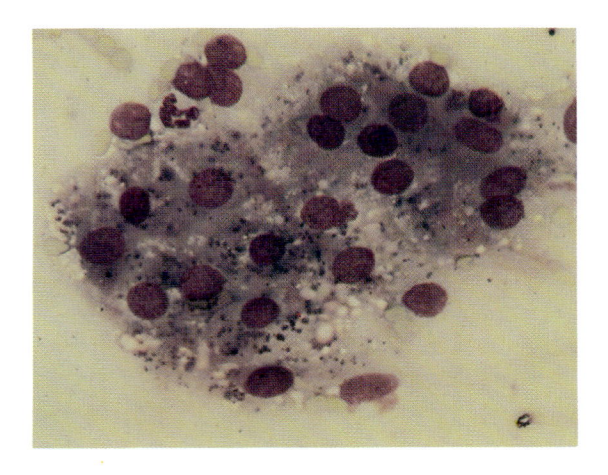

Figure 9. Cluster of cells from a follicular-compact thyroid carcinoma. Cells exhibit characteristics of malignancy, including extreme cytoplasmic basophilia and variation in cell size, nuclear size and nucleus:cytoplasm ratio. Several cells have abundant secretory material that displaces nuclei peripherally. (Wright's stain, 800X)

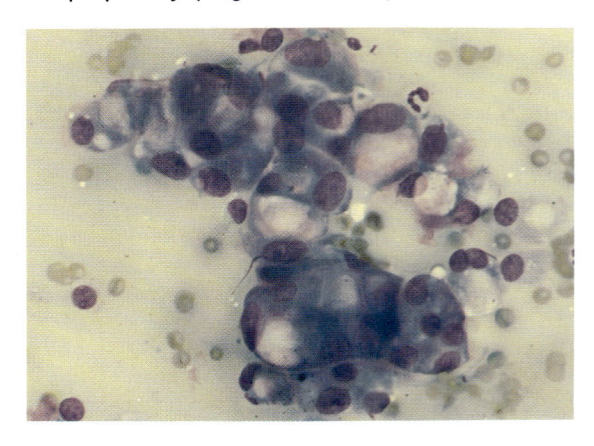

Malignant Neoplasms

Thyroid carcinomas are not common in dogs, but they account for about two-thirds of clinically detectable thyroid enlargements.[20,22] Tumors usually occur in older dogs, with no sex predilection. A breed predisposition has been shown for Boxers, Beagles and Golden Retrievers.[20] Thyroid carcinomas are rare in cats. Most affected cats are euthyroid. Tumors are usually tightly adherent to underlying tissues due to extensive local invasion. Metastasis correlates with increased tumor size.

A good correlation between results of aspiration cytology and histopathologic examination has been found with thyroid carcinomas.[23] The problem of excessive blood contamination in many specimens may require repeated aspirations. In the absence of excessive blood contamination, smears tend to be highly cellular and may or may not contain colloid. Follicular and papillary carcinomas yield cells that occur both singly and in dense clusters (Fig 9). Nuclear and cell pleomorphism is variable. Nuclei are mildly enlarged and have a fine granular chromatin clumping and prominent nucleoli; mitotic figures are not frequent. Well-differentiated tumors may be difficult to distinguish from adenomas. Cystic areas secondary to tumor necrosis and hemorrhage may contain RBC, neutrophils, foam cells, degenerating tumor cells and cholesterol crystals.

Medullary carcinomas are tumors of parafollicular C cells. These tumors are much less common than follicular or papillary carcinomas. Aspirates are very cellular, with cells occurring singly or in clusters, but follicular or papillary patterns are not present. Cells are relatively uniform in size and shape. Nuclei have a coarse, granular chromatin pattern and are placed eccentrically within the cell. Fine eosinophilic granules may be present within the cytoplasm.[24]

Undifferentiated carcinomas of the thyroid are rare in dogs and cats.[25] Cells are oval to spindle shaped, with bizarre, pleomorphic nuclei. Cells may occur either as multinucleated giant cells or as small cells with a high nucleus:cytoplasm ratio. Malignant mixed thyroid tumors are also rare, being composed of epithelial and mesenchymal elements (Fig 10).

Figure 10. Cells of epithelial and mesenchymal origin from a mixed thyroid tumor exhibit characteristics of malignancy. Many erythrocytes, nondegenerate neutrophils and active macrophages are present, suggesting hemorrhage and necrosis within the tumor. (Wright's stain, 800X)

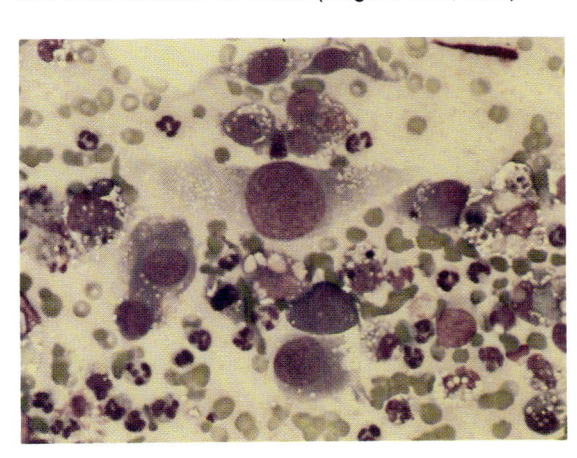

The Parathyroid Glands

The parathyroid glands are located adjacent to the thyroid glands. Tumors of the parathyroid glands are rare in animals.[26] Affected animals show clinical signs of primary hyperparathyroidism. Adenoma of the chief cells occurs as a single nodule that is freely movable under the skin. Carcinomas are usually larger than adenomas and are fixed to underlying tissues due to local infiltration. Adenomas consist of a monomorphic population of cuboidal or polyhedral cells, with pale-staining cytoplasm. Carcinomas show more pleomorphism within the cell population.

References

1. Soderstrom, in Linsk and Franzen: *Clinical Aspiration Cytology.* Lippincott, Philadelphia, 1983. pp 9-24.

2. Koss: *Diagnostic Cytology and Its Histopathologic Basis.* 3rd ed. Lippincott, Philadelphia, 1979. pp 989-1000.

3. Linsk and Franzen: *Clinical Aspiration Cytology.* Lippincott, Philadelphia, 1983. pp 105-137.

4. Linsk et al, in Linsk and Franzen: *Clinical Aspiration Cytology.* Lippincott, Philadelphia, 1983. pp 85-104.

5. Lowhagen and Linsk, in Linsk and Franzen: *Clinical Aspiration Cytology.* Lippincott, Philadelphia, 1983. pp 61-83.

6. Zajicek, in Koss: *Diagnostic Cytology and Its Histopathologic Basis.* 3rd ed. Lippincott, Philadelphia, 1979. pp 1001-1104.

7. Allen et al: *Vet Pathol* 23:649-655, 1986.

8. Griffiths et al: Fine needle aspiration cytology and histologic correlation in canine tumors. *Vet Clin Pathol* 13:13-17, 1984.

9. Rebar: *Handbook of Veterinary Cytology.* Ralston Purina, St. Louis, 1980. p 17.

10. Brodey et al: Canine mammary gland neoplasms. *JAAHA* 19:61-90, 1983.

11. Ferguson: Canine mammary gland tumors. *Vet Clin No Am* 15:501-511, 1985.

12. Madewell and Theilen: *Veterinary Cancer Medicine.* 2nd ed. Lea & Febiger, Philadelphia, 1987. pp 327-344.

13. Hayes and Mooney: Feline mammary tumors. *Vet Clin No Am* 15:512-520, 1985.

14. Harvey et al, in Ettinger: *Textbook of Veterinary Internal Medicine.* 2nd ed. Saunders, Philadelphia, 1983. pp 1126-1191.

15. Perman et al: *Cytology of the Dog and Cat.* American Animal Hospital Association, Denver, CO, 1979.

16. Kelly et al: *Vet Record* 104:268, 1979.

17. Moulton: *Tumors in Domestic Animals.* 2nd ed. Univ California Press, Berkeley, 1978. pp 249-252.

18. Belshaw, in Ettinger: *Textbook of Veterinary Internal Medicine.* 2nd ed. Saunders, Philadelphia, 1983. pp 1592-1614.

19. Gosselin et al: Autoimmune lymphocytic thyroiditis in dogs. *Vet Immunol Immunopathol* 3:185-201, 1982.

20. Capen, in Moulton: *Tumors in Domestic Animals.* 2nd ed. Univ California Press, Berkeley, 1978. pp 392-399.

21. Holzworth et al: Hyperthyroidism in the cat: Ten cases. *JAVMA* 176:345-353, 1980.

22. Sullivan et al: Thyroid tumors in the dog. *J Small Anim Pract* 28:505-512, 1987.

23. Thompson et al: Fine needle aspiration cytology in the diagnosis of canine thyroid carcinoma. *Can Vet J* 21:186-188, 1980.

24. Kini *et al*: Cytopathologic features of medullary carcinoma of the thyroid. *Arch Pathol Lab Med* 108:156-159, 1984.

25. Anderson and Capen: Undifferentiated spindle cell carcinoma of the thyroid in a dog. *Vet Pathol* 23:203-204, 1986.

26. Capen and Martin, in Ettinger: *Textbook of Veterinary Internal Medicine*. 2nd ed. Saunders, Philadelphia, 1983. pp 1550-1592.

8

The Lymph Nodes

J.R. Duncan

Lymph nodes, because of their function in lymphatic drainage, antigen processing and cellular and humoral immunity, are involved in a variety of local and systemic disease processes. The superficial, subcutaneous location of some lymph nodes (mandibular, superficial cervical, inguinal, popliteal) allows easy detection of enlargement visually or by palpation. These lymph nodes can be readily positioned for fine-needle aspiration (see Chapter 1). Any enlargement of a lymph node is justification for aspiration biopsy and cytologic examination.[1] Lymph nodes draining areas affected by neoplasia may also be aspirated to detect metastasis even when they are not enlarged.

Figure 1. Aspirate from a hyperplastic lymph node. Small lymphocytes (arrows) and plasma cells characterize the reaction. Note that small lymphocytes are smaller than neutrophils and their nuclei are about the size of an RBC. Many free nuclei, identified by pink, homogeneous chromatin and absence of cytoplasm, are evident.

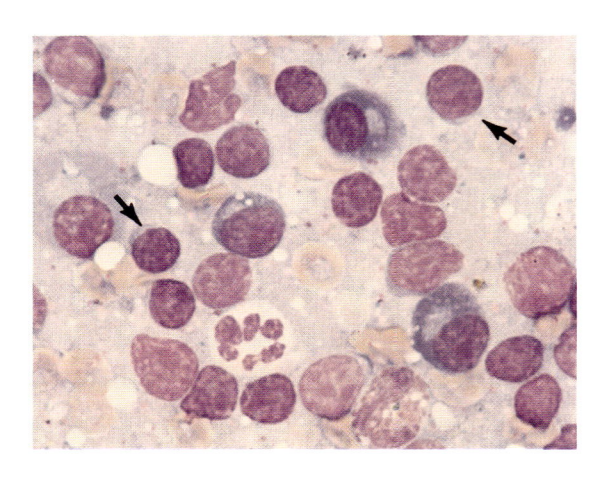

Three general processes cause lymph node enlargement: hyperplasia, inflammation and neoplasia. Cytologic examination of fine-needle aspirates of enlarged nodes usually allows differentiation of these processes. Because of its great convenience, lymph node aspiration biopsy has become a popular procedure in human medicine in recent years.[2] Similarly, this high-yield diagnostic technique is frequently used in veterinary medicine.[3-5]

Fine-needle aspirates of *in-situ* lymph nodes or touch imprints of excised nodes are the usual means of obtaining cells for examination (see Chapter 1). Lymphocytes are very fragile; therefore, care must be taken to prevent excessive lysis of cells. Smears can be made in traditional blood smear fashion, but excessive pressure must not be applied when making the smear. Drawing the aspirate across the slide with a needle, needle holder or other blunt object is an alternative method.

Cytologic Findings

Normal Lymph Nodes

Small lymphocytes comprise 75-95% of the total cell population (Figs 1-5).[3] They have round nuclei, about the size of a canine RBC, with densely aggregated chromatin forming large chromocenters. The cell has scant, pale-blue cytoplasm and is smaller than a neutrophil.

Medium and large lymphocytes (often called lymphoblasts) are the size of a neutrophil or larger and up to 4 times the size of an RBC (Figs 3,5). Their chromatin is less aggregated, and nucleoli may be visible. The

Figure 2. Small lymphocytes, plasma cells and a large transformed lymphocyte (arrow) characterize this aspirate from a hyperplastic lymph node. Irregular, pink nuclei from lysed cells are seen.

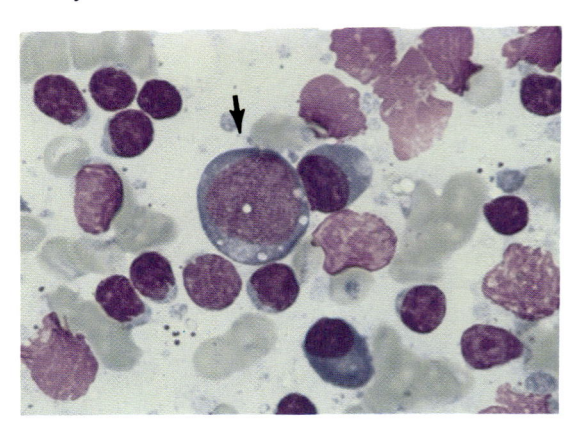

cytoplasm is pale blue and more abundant than in small lymphocytes. These larger lymphocytes comprise only a small percentage of the population of a normal lymph node.

Plasma cells have small, round, eccentric nuclei with condensed chromatin (Figs 1-4). Their abundant cytoplasm is deep blue and has a prominent clear Golgi zone. Immature plasma cells (transformed B-lymphocytes) are larger and have less aggregated chromatin and a higher nucleus:cytoplasm ratio (Fig 2). Their very blue cytoplasm often contains vacuoles. Plasma cells in various stages of development are seen in small numbers in normal lymph nodes.

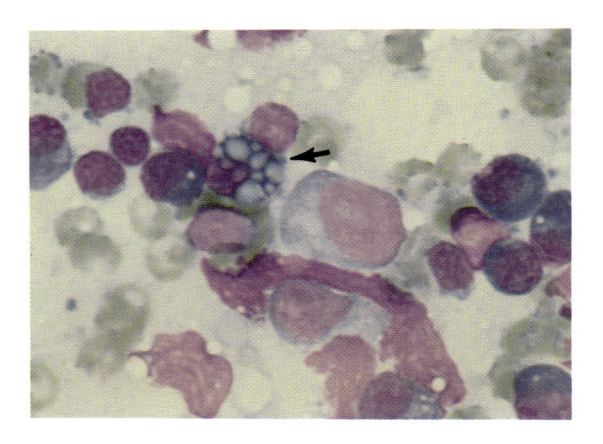

Macrophages, characterized by abundant cytoplasm often containing vacuoles and granular debris, also are found in small numbers (Fig 5). Macrophages from areas of intense lymphopoiesis and cellular turnover may contain prominent basophilic nuclear debris (tingible bodies) (Fig 6).

Reticular cells and endothelial cells are common in lymph nodes, but these tissue-bound cells are rarely aspirated intact. They usually appear as large swollen nuclei, often devoid of cytoplasm.

Figure 4. Small lymphocytes, plasma cells, neutrophils and a single mast cell are present in this aspirate from a hyperplastic lymph node.

Figure 3. Plasma cells, small lymphocytes and 2 large lymphocytes (lymphoblasts) characterize this aspirate from a hyperplastic lymph node. The plasma cell with the vacuolated cytoplasm is a Russell cell (arrow). The pink, amorphous structures are free nuclear material.

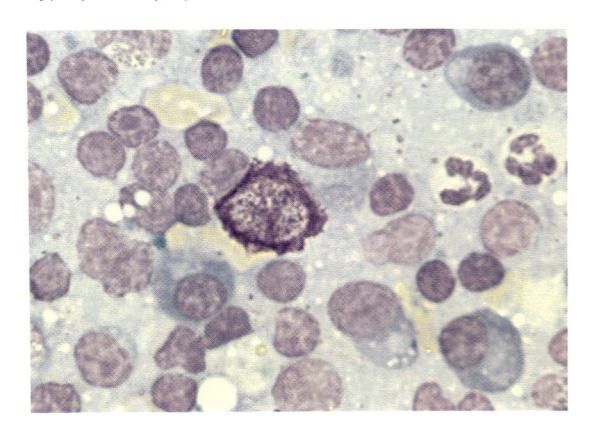

Occasionally, small numbers of neutrophils, eosinophils and mast cells are observed in a normal node (Fig 4).

Lymphoglandular bodies are cytoplasmic fragments and are highly characteristic of lymphoid tissue (Figs 6,7). They are round, homogeneous, basophilic structures similar in size to platelets.

Because of the pressures of the aspiration technique, lymphocytes, which are very fragile, may rupture and release their nuclei.

Free nuclei are swollen and uniformly pink in contrast to the blue blocky or granular pattern of intact lymphocyte nuclei (Figs 1-3). Blue nucleoli are often exposed in the nuclear chromatin of ruptured cells. These free nuclei carry no diagnostic significance and should not be confused with large immature lymphocytes.

Reactive Hyperplasia

Cytologically, no clear line of separation exists between a normal lymph node and a hyperplastic one (Figs 1-4). Differentiation, however, is probably a moot point, since most lymph nodes are reactive to some degree. A heterogeneous cell population is usually obtained as the needle is directed through follicular centers, paracortical area, medullary cords and medullary sinuses. The small lymphocyte is the predominant cell type in both normal and hyperplastic lymph nodes. Plasma cell numbers vary from none to >5-10% of the population in some areas of the smear. They occasionally are filled with vacuoles (Russell's bodies) (Fig 3). Numbers of medium and large lymphocytes may be increased; they may constitute up to 15% of the total cell population in hyperplasia.[5] Immature plasma cells or transformed lymphocytes, which are medium to large in size, also may be observed. Macrophages may on occasion represent >2% of the population, particularly with hyperplasia of sinus macrophages. Any enlarged lymph node with the above cytologic findings should be considered hyperplastic, since a normal node should not be enlarged.

Hyperplasia occurs when antigens in high concentration reach the draining lymph node and stimulate the immune system. In some instances, these antigens also cause inflammation and attract inflammatory cells to the node (lymphadenitis). In many cases, reactions causing hyperplasia are localized, but they may be systemic and affect all nodes. Generalized lymphadenopathy with a hyperplastic cytologic picture may occur in feline leukemia virus infection, Rocky Mountain spotted fever and ehrlichiosis.

Lymphadenitis

Inflammation is characterized cytologically by accumulation of inflammatory cells. Neutrophils (Plate 3), eosinophils and macrophages occur singly or in combination. Inflammation is probably present when the population is >5% neutrophils or >3% eosinophils. Macrophage numbers can increase in inflammation but also in hyperplasia

Figure 5. Seen among small and medium-sized lymphocytes is a large macrophage containing phagocytized debris.

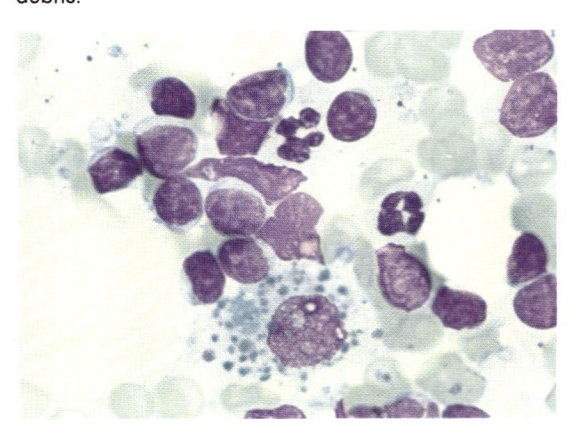

Figure 6. In this aspirate from a lymphomatous lymph node are large immature lymphocytes with prominent nucleoli, dispersed chromatin and abundant blue cytoplasm. The large cell in the center with bluish cytoplasmic globules is a tingible-body macrophage. The small blue structures (arrow) are lymphoglandular bodies.

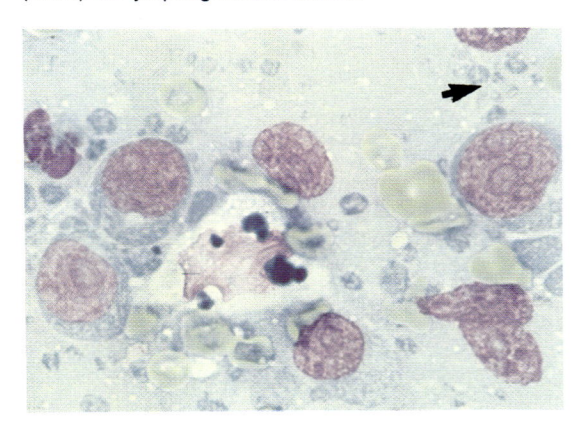

Figure 7. Immature, neoplastic lymphocytes characterize this smear from a dog with lymphosarcoma. Note that the cells are much larger than RBCs. The pink structures lacking cytoplasm and containing prominent nucleoli are nuclei from lysed cells. Small blue lymphoglandular bodies are numerous.

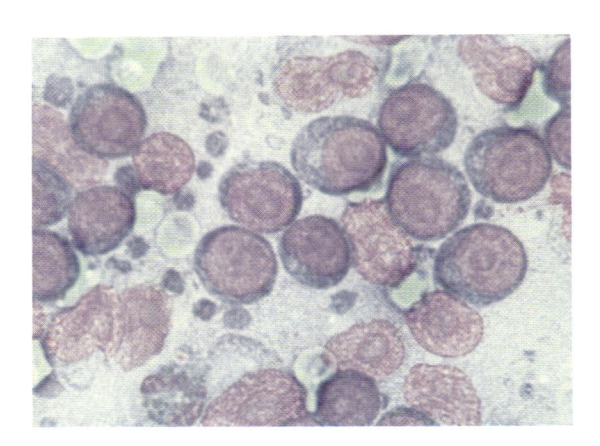

Figure 8. This aspirate from an animal with blastomycosis is characterized by pyogranulomatous inflammation. Neutrophils, epithelioid macrophages and a single multinucleated giant cell are present.

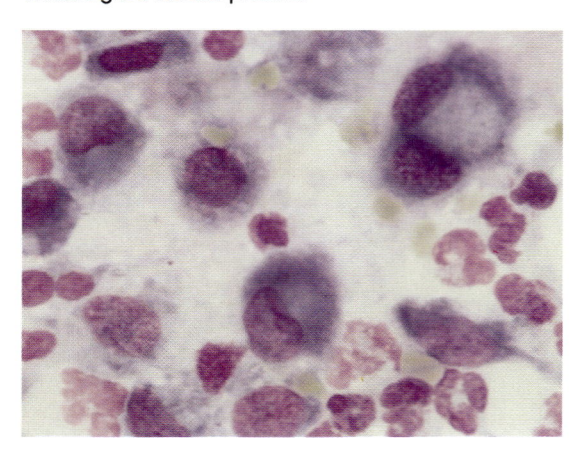

and sometimes in neoplasia. Macrophages also may appear as epithelioid cells and multinucleated giant cells in granulomatous inflammation.

Epithelioid cells are characterized by blue cytoplasm with minimal vacuolation, and contain very little phagocytic debris (Fig 8). Organisms may, however, be present within the cytoplasm. These cells may occur in aggregates. Inflammatory cells may represent only a small portion of the total cell population that otherwise suggests lymphoid hyperplasia, or they may completely replace the normal cell population.

Most bacterial infections (Plate 3) elicit a neutrophilic or purulent response (Plate 3), but *Mycobacterium* spp (Plate 4) can cause a granulomatous response. An eosinophilic exudate of varying degree is common in lymph nodes draining allergic inflammations of the skin, respiratory tract and digestive tract. Such systemic fungal infections as histoplasmosis (Plate 4), blastomycosis (Plate 4), coccidioidomycosis (Plate 5) and cryptococcosis (Plate 4), protozoal infections as cytauxzoonosis (Plate 5), toxoplasmosis (Plate 5) and leishmaniasis (Plate 5), and algal infections as prototheocosis (Plate 5) characteristically evoke a granulomatous or pyogranulomatous response (Plate 3) in lymph nodes. In salmon disease, there is lymphoid depletion and sinus macrophage hyperplasia (Fig 9).

Lymphosarcoma

Lymphosarcoma is characterized by immature lymphocytes that eventually replace the entire normal cell population (Figs 6,7). When immature cells comprise >50% of the cell population, a diagnosis of lymphosarcoma can be reliably made, but smaller numbers may be present in early stages, which makes diagnosis by cytologic examination alone more difficult. Usually these neoplastic lymphocytes are larger than neutrophils and have granular dispersed chromatin, nucleoli, a lower nucleus:cytoplasm ratio, and basophilic cytoplasm. Mitoses may be more numerous than in hyperplasia and "tingible-body" macrophages may indicate intense lymphopoiesis and cell turnover; but neither alone is a reliable indicator of neoplasia. Lymphoglandular bodies are more numerous than in hyperplasia.

Occasionally, lymphosarcoma is manifested as the small, well-differentiated lymphocyte type. This form is very difficult to distinguish from hyperplasia because small lymphocytes predominate in each.

If a diagnosis is equivocal, the entire lymph node should be removed with the capsule intact and fixed in 10% buffered formalin. A complete cross section should then be examined histologically for architectural obliteration by a homogeneous population of neoplastic cells.

Figure 9. Aspirate of a lymph node from a dog with salmon disease. Large macrophages contain the causative agent, *Neorickettsia helminthoeca*.

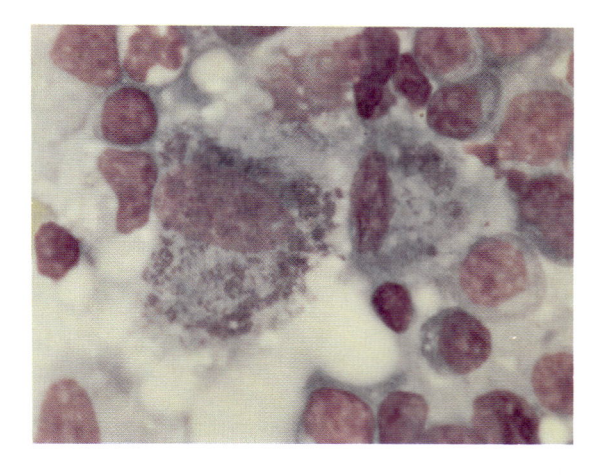

Metastatic Neoplasia

The presence of cells not normally found in lymph nodes or an increase in numbers of certain cell types normally present (*ie*, mast cells) may suggest metastatic neoplasia (Figs 10-12 and Plates 6 and 7). Carcinomas frequently metastasize to lymph nodes. Metastatic epithelial cells (Fig 10 and Plate 6) can occur singly or in groups. They are very large and bear no resemblance to cellular constituents of normal or hyperplastic nodes.

Epithelial cells of any type in a lymph node aspirate indicate neoplasia, but these cells must be differentiated from epithelioid cells of granulomatous inflammation, described previously. Salivary epithelial cells (Chapter 7, Fig 5) from the submandibular salivary gland may be accidentally aspirated. These cells are uniform in size and have round to oval nuclei and abundant blue foamy cytoplasm, and should not be confused with carcinoma cells.

Malignant melanomas metastasize to lymph nodes. The melanocyte usually can be identified by its granular brown-black cytoplasmic pigment (Fig 11). Do not confuse pigment in melanocytes with that in melanophages that have phagocytized melanin originating from pigmented structures or lesions in the area drained by the node. Melanophages also phagocytize pigment released by melanocytes. Differentiation may be difficult, but melanocytes usually have more attenuated and less vacuolated cytoplasm. Hemosiderin, carbon, bile and other pigments in macrophages must not be confused with melanin.

Figure 10. An epithelial cell cluster from a transitional-cell carcinoma that metastasized to a lymph node.

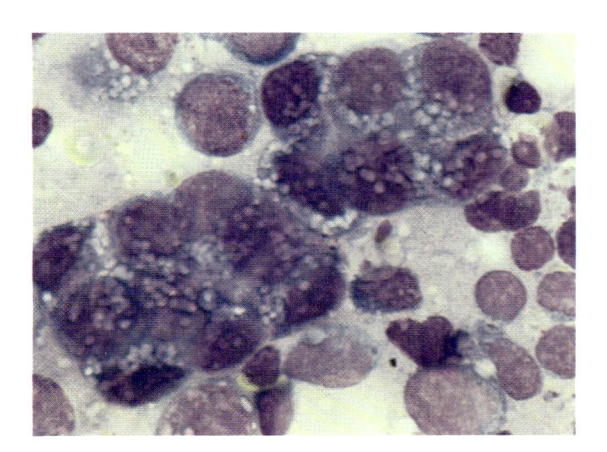

Figure 11. An aspirate containing malignant melanocytes that have metastasized to the lymph node. Greenish-black cytoplasmic granules characterize these cells.

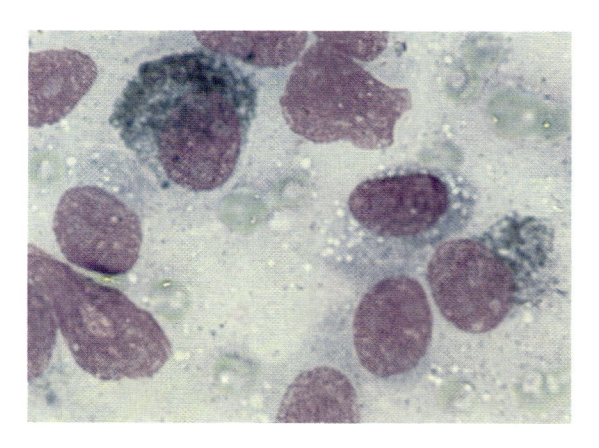

Though sarcomas do not metastasize to lymph nodes as frequently as carcinomas, spindle cells in significant numbers should suggest a sarcoma of some type. Malignant mast-cell tumors can metastasize to lymph nodes. The tumor cells may be well differentiated and distinguished from normal mast cells only by the large number of cells present (Plate 7). Greater than 3% mast cells suggests neoplasia. Undifferentiated tumors have larger cells with fewer, less prominent granules (Plate 7). Transmissible venereal tumors (Plate 7) may metastasize to lymph nodes.

In cases of neoplasia, one is usually specifically looking for metastatic neoplastic cells because the justification for lymph node aspiration was a malignant tumor identified in the area drained by the particular node. Tumor cells are usually obtained if metastasis has progressed to cause clinically evident enlarged nodes; however, small foci in normal-sized nodes may be missed on aspiration. Negative findings in palpably enlarged nodes should always be subordinate to clinical findings.[6]

Various myeloproliferative disorders may result in a leukemic hemogram and neoplastic cells in the sinuses of lymph nodes. Cytologic examination of a fine-needle aspirate of a lymph node reveals the cell population of a normal or hyperplastic node and a population of leukemic cells (Fig 12). In acute leukemias, blast cells comprise the neoplastic cell population and may be difficult to differentiate from lymphoblasts of lymphosarcoma. In chronic leukemias, various maturation stages are present. Extramedullary hematopoiesis can occur in lymph nodes and contribute to cytologic findings of various stages of erythroid and myeloid cells and megakaryocytes. It is a rare occurrence in chronic anemias.

Lymph node aspiration is a valuable diagnostic aid. With some experience, one can usually determine the type of disease present and may even make a disease or etiologic diagnosis.

Chart 1 presents an algorithm for evaluation of lymph node aspirates or impression smears.

Figure 12. Among small lymphocytes and a plasma cell are very immature neutrophils. This lymph node aspirate is from an animal with granulocytic leukemia.

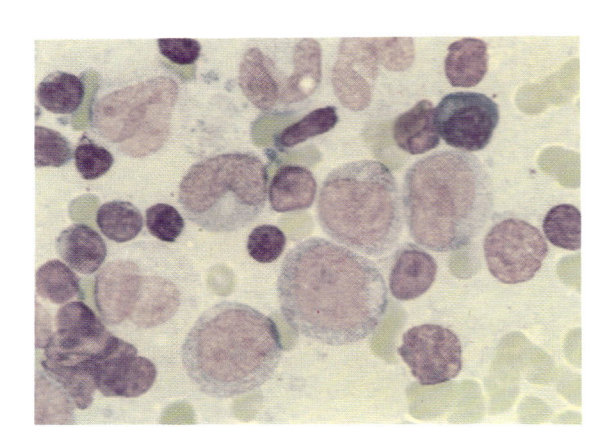

References

1. Soderstrom: *Fine-Needle Aspiration Biopsy*. Grune & Stratton, New York, 1966. pp 62-82.

2. Frable: Fine-needle aspiration biopsy: A review. *Human Pathol* 14:9-28, 1983.

3. Perman *et al*: *Cytology of the Dog and Cat*. American Animal Hospital Association, Denver, 1979. pp 11-13.

4. Rebar: *Handbook of Veterinary Cytology*. Ralston Purina, St. Louis, 1980. pp 37-39.

5. Thrall: Cytology of lymphoid tissue. *Comp Cont Ed Pract Vet* 9:104-111, 1987.

6. Lee *et al*: Lymph node examination by fine-needle aspiration in patients with known or suspected malignancy. *Acta Cytol* 31:563-572, 1987.

Chart 1. An algorithm for evaluation of lymph node aspirates or impression smears.

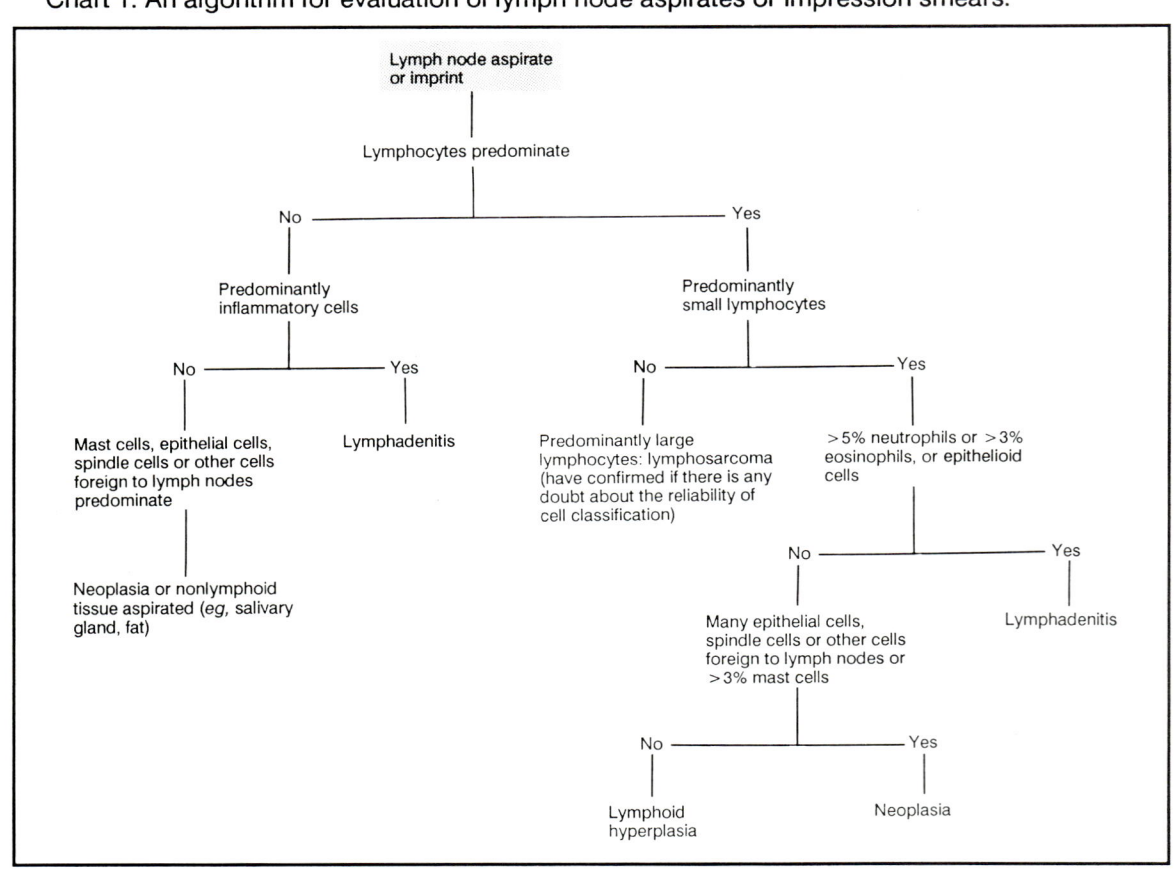

9

Bone Marrow

R.D. Tyler and R.L. Cowell

Bone marrow is the major hematopoietic organ of the body. In young animals, active hematopoietic tissue is found throughout both flat and long bones. As growth ceases, hematopoietic activity in the central areas of long bones regresses. In adults, most active hematopoiesis occurs in the flat bones and the extremities of long bones. The central area of long bones contains mostly fat, with very little active hematopoietic tissue.

Active hematopoietic tissue is very vascular. It consists of islands of hematopoietic tissue surrounded by vascular sinuses. The islands of hematopoietic tissue are composed of: erythroid, granulocytic, monocytic and thrombocytic series cells; marrow structural cells (adventitial cells); fat cells; and a few macrophages, lymphocytes, plasma cells and mast cells. The hematopoietic tissue islands are bounded by the endothelium lining the vascular sinuses.

Indications

The most common indication for bone marrow cytologic examination is recognition of hematologic abnormalities not readily explained by a good history, physical examination, chemistry profile and/or other clinical procedures. Bone marrow examination is often rewarding in evaluating animals with nonregenerative anemia, persistent neutropenia or persistent thrombocytopenia.

Also, bone marrow cytologic evaluation can be used to: assess the marrow's involvement in some neoplastic conditions, such as lymphoid neoplasia and mast-cell neoplasia; to identify suspected infectious agents, such as *Histoplasma capsulatum*, *Leishmania donovani* and *Toxoplasma gondii*; and for evaluation of patients with evidence of hyperproteinemic conditions, such as multiple myeloma, lymphoma, ehrlichiosis, leishmaniasis and disseminated histoplasmosis.

Contraindications

There are few significant contraindications for bone marrow biopsy. Restraint, sedation and anesthesia usually pose a greater risk to the patient than the biopsy procedure. However, bone aspiration biopsies can often be collected without sedation; general anesthesia is seldom necessary. Hemorrhage is a theoretical concern in thrombocytopenic animals, but significant bleeding rarely occurs, even in severely thrombocytopenic animals.[1-3] Iatrogenic marrow infection is possible, but the risk is miniscule, especially if the area of skin through which the aspirate is collected has been properly prepared.

Sample Collection and Preparation

Proper collection and preparation of marrow is necessary for maximum diagnostic usefulness. Bone marrow degenerates rapidly after collection or the animal's death. Therefore, bone marrow samples from dead animals should be collected immediately (within 30 minutes) after the animal's death. Regardless of whether the animal is alive or dead, bone marrow cytologic preparations should be prepared immediately after collection. Interestingly, granulocytes appear to be the first cells to undergo significant morphologic distortion after marrow sample collection or the animal's death. The granulocyte nucleus swells and, losing its contorted lobulated pattern, becomes large and round to ovoid. The nuclear chromatin pattern loses its dense clumped areas and stains less intensely and more uniformly. As a result, neutrophils that have undergone this alteration may be mistaken for blast cells. This error can lead to misdiagnosis of neoplasia. Extreme caution must be used when examining samples from animals dead for 30 minutes or more before slide preparation. These samples can be examined for cellularity, organisms, mast-cell infiltration, erythrophagocytosis, plasmacytosis and accumulation of iron-containing pigments, but examination for evidence of neoplasia can result in misdiagnosis. The same requirements and limitations apply for bone marrow samples submitted for histopathologic examination.

After bone marrow preparations are air dried, they should be stained as soon as possible. When submitting bone marrow cytologic preparations for consultation, several air-dried unfixed preparations, air-dried fixed preparations, and air-dried stained preparations should be submitted when possible.

Some techniques for collecting, preparing and staining bone marrow cytologic preparations are discussed below.

Instruments and Supplies

A 16- to 18-ga, 1- to 1 3/4-inch bone marrow aspiration biopsy needle, clear Petri dish or watch glass, 10- to 20-ml syringe, several clean microscope slides, several clean microscope slide coverslips, the supplies for a surgical prep and, optionally, EDTA/isotonic fluid solution are required for collecting and preparing bone marrow aspirate biopsies. These instruments and supplies should be located on a clean work counter in close proximity to the work area where the sample is to be collected. If anticoagulant is not used, smears must be prepared from the aspirate immediately (within 30 seconds of collection). Some acceptable bone marrow biopsy needles are the Rosenthal (Becton Dickinson, Rutherford, NJ), Illinois sternal (V. Mueller, Chicago) and Jamshidi (Kormed, Minneapolis) needles.

A sterile 2-3% EDTA/isotonic saline solution can be prepared using commercially available EDTA blood collection tubes. These tubes contain about 1.5 mg of EDTA (as a freeze-dried powder or liquid solution) per milliliter of blood to be added. Injecting 0.35 ml of sterile isotonic saline into a 7-ml EDTA tube produces about 0.35 ml of 3% EDTA or 0.42 ml of 2.5% EDTA, depending on whether the tube originally contained powdered or liquid EDTA.

Aspiration Biopsy

Site: Bone marrow aspiration biopsies may be collected from the iliac crest, trochanteric fossa of the femur, proximal humerus and sternebrae of dogs and cats (Fig 1). The iliac crest in large dogs and trochanteric fossa in small dogs and cats are the most accessible and require the least chemical restraint. As a result, they are the most commonly used sites. Because of the danger of penetration of the thoracic cavity, the sternebrae should be avoided in cats and small dogs. For the same reason, the ribs should be used only when incisional biopsies are performed. The trochanteric fossa may not be approachable in large, well-muscled or very obese patients. Also, in older dogs the cortical bone of the trochanteric fossa may be so dense that it prevents easy penetration of the marrow cavity. Due to the small diameter of the bones of cats and small dogs, the trochanteric fossa often supersedes the iliac crest as a site for bone marrow aspiration in these animals.

Collection: To aspirate bone marrow via the trochanteric fossa, the animal is placed in lateral recumbency. If the iliac crest is used, the animal can be standing, sitting or in sternal recumbency. Regardless of the site used, the hair is clipped from the skin several inches around the area where needle puncture is anticipated. The skin is then prepared as for surgery and 1.5-3 ml of a local anesthetic is injected into the skin and under the periosteum at the site of anticipated puncture.

A small stab incision is made at the biopsy site with a sterile scalpel blade. The greater trochanter is located by palpation and the biopsy needle is passed medial to the trochanter, with its long axis parallel to the long axis of the

Figure 1. Schematic of a dog skeleton showing sites for bone marrow collection. The trochanteric fossa and iliac crest are used most often (inset).

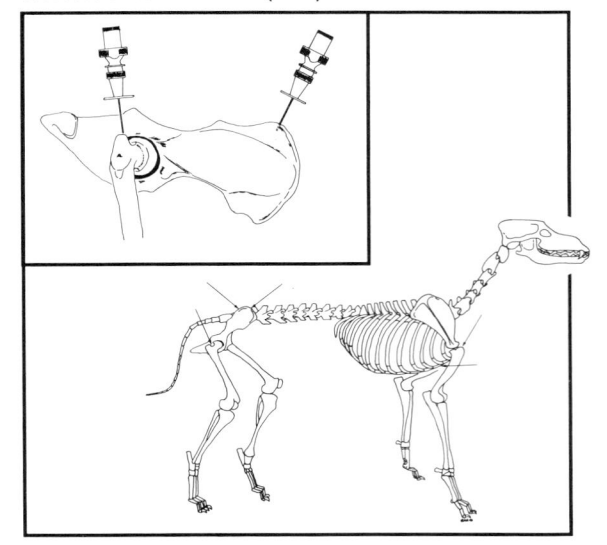

Figure 2. Smear preparation for bone marrow aspirates not collected in EDTA/isotonic saline solution. A. Some of the aspirate is expelled onto a tilted glass microscope slide. The slide can be propped up with another glass slide braced against the side of a Petri dish. Marrow flecks tend to adhere to the slide as the marrow runs down it. B. Another glass slide is placed over the slide containing the aspirate. This spreads the aspirate. C. The 2 slides are slid apart. D. This produces 2 preparations.

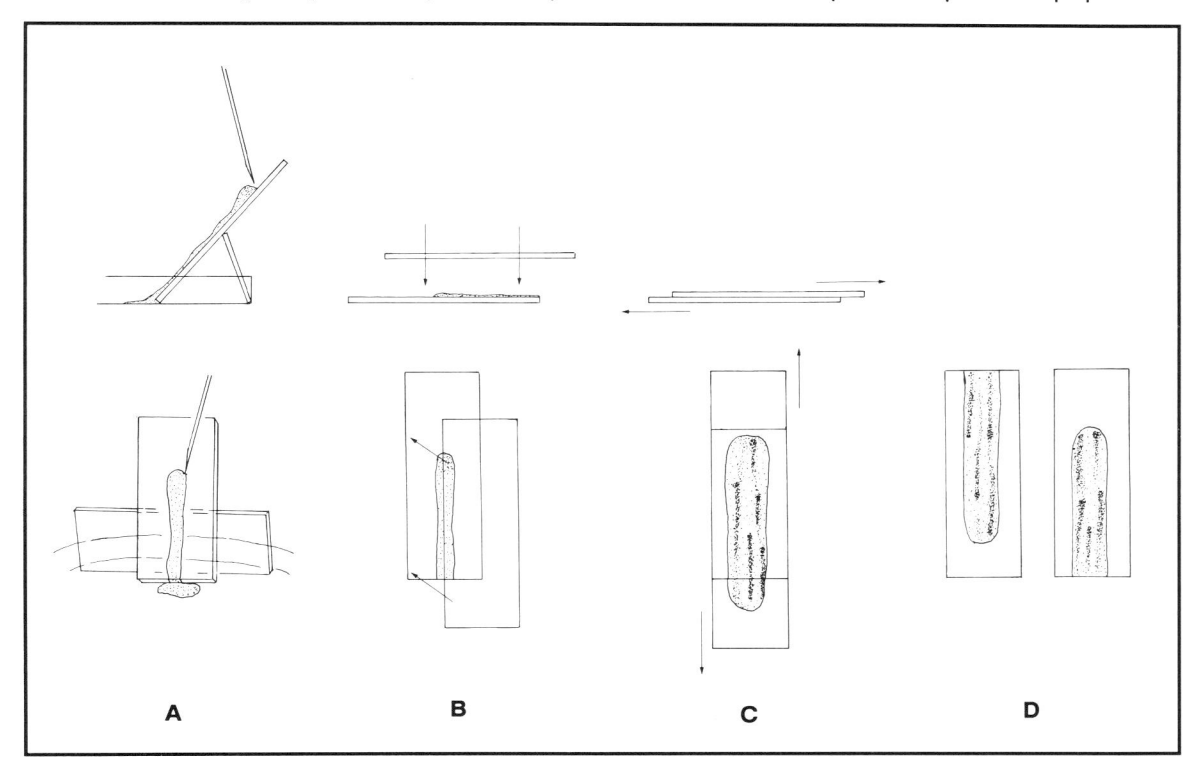

femur, until the needle reaches the trochanteric fossa. When bone is contacted, moderate pressure is applied and the needle is rotated in an alternating clockwise-counterclockwise motion. The operator usually feels the resistance decrease when the needle enters the bone marrow in the trochanteric fossa, but this sensation may not be as obvious for the iliac crest. In the iliac crest, once the needle is firmly in bone, it is probably in the marrow cavity.

When the marrow cavity has been entered, the stylet is removed and a 10- to 20-ml syringe containing 0.5-1 ml of sterile 2-3% EDTA/isotonic saline solution is attached to the needle. Strong negative pressure is applied by rapidly pulling the plunger back as far as possible (usually two-thirds to three-fourths the volume of the syringe). Most animals show evidence of pain when bone marrow aspiration begins. This is good evidence that the needle is in the marrow cavity. After a few drops of marrow are collected, the negative pressure is released. If EDTA is used, the volume of marrow collected should not exceed the volume of EDTA/isotonic saline solution in the syringe.

Continued negative pressure contaminates the marrow sample with blood. Whether marrow sample appears in the syringe or not, negative pressure should not be applied to the syringe twice in the same area. This causes aspiration of excessive amounts of blood.

If marrow is not collected at the first site, the syringe is removed, the stylet is replaced in the biopsy needle, the needle is repositioned by slight advancement and rotation, and negative pressure is reapplied. If marrow is still not collected, the negative pressure is maintained and the needle is slowly withdrawn until marrow is obtained or the needle exits the bone. If this fails to collect an adequate sample, aspiration can be attempted from another site in the same bone or from another bone. If a sample cannot be collected by aspiration, a core biopsy or incisional biopsy is necessary.

Smear Preparation without EDTA: If EDTA/isotonic saline is not used, as soon as a few drops of marrow sample appear in the syringe, the plunger is released, the syringe is detached from the needle, and the stylet is replaced in the needle. The needle remains embedded in the bone.

The sample is then immediately expelled directly onto a glass microscope slide that is tilted 45-70°, allowing the sample to drain from the slide into a watch glass or Petri dish (Fig 2). Marrow flecks tend to adhere to the glass microscope slide. A second glass microscope slide is placed perpendicularly across the marrow flecks adhered to the first slide. This causes the marrow flecks to spread. Then, the 2 slides are smoothly pulled apart in a horizontal plane, dispersing the flecks.

In Romanowsky-stained smears, the marrow flecks appear as blue-purple streaks. If the sample does not contain marrow flecks, the needle can be repositioned by slight advancement and rotation. The stylet is removed, another syringe is attached, and the aspiration procedure is repeated. After 2 aspiration attempts or when marrow flecks are recovered, the needle is removed.

Smear Preparation with EDTA: If EDTA/isotonic saline is used, once the marrow sample is collected, the plunger is released to relieve the negative pressure, and the needle is detached from the syringe. The stylet is replaced in the needle and the needle remains embedded in the bone. The contents of the syringe are thoroughly mixed and the anticoagulated marrow sample is expelled into a watch glass or clear Petri dish. If the sample does not contain marrow flecks, the needle can be repositioned by slight advancement and rotation. The stylet is removed, another syringe containing EDTA/saline solution is attached, and the aspiration procedure is repeated. After 2 aspiration attempts or when marrow flecks are recovered, the needle is removed.

Marrow samples collected in EDTA/isotonic saline solution and expelled into a Petri dish are prepared as follows. The Petri dish is tilted and/or rotated under a soft light so the marrow flecks can be seen and distinguished from fat droplets. Marrow flecks have a clear to slightly opaque, light gray appearance; fat droplets have a clear, glistening appearance. Marrow flecks may be slightly irregular in shape; fat droplets are spherical. Also, marrow flecks tend to be slightly larger than fat globules. Generally, marrow flecks are easily located if an adequate sample has been collected.

Flecks are transferred from the sample in the Petri dish to glass microscope slides by tilting the Petri dish, causing the sample to drain to one side of the dish. Some flecks cling to the bottom of the Petri dish, and the fluid portion of the sample drains away from them. These flecks are harvested with a microhematocrit capillary tube. One end of the capillary tube is touched to the side of the fleck. Often the fleck is partially aspirated into the capillary tube and can be transferred to the glass microscope slide. If the fleck does not partially aspirate into the capillary tube, the tube is advanced gently, forcing the fleck into it. The marrow fleck is then transferred onto the glass microscope slide by tapping the capillary tube end containing the fleck on the slide. In some

Figure 3. Smear preparation for bone marrow aspirates collected in EDTA/isotonic saline solution. A. A fleck, collected from the Petri dish containing the sample, is placed on a glass microscope slide. B. A microscope slide coverslip is placed over the fleck at a 45-degree angle to the slide. This spreads the fleck and accompanying fluid. C. The coverslip is slid horizontally and smoothly off the glass slide. D. Both the glass microscope slide preparation and coverslip preparation can be used. However, the coverslip preparation is usually hard to handle during staining and is often discarded. Multiple preparations can be made on a glass slide, and multiple slides can be prepared.

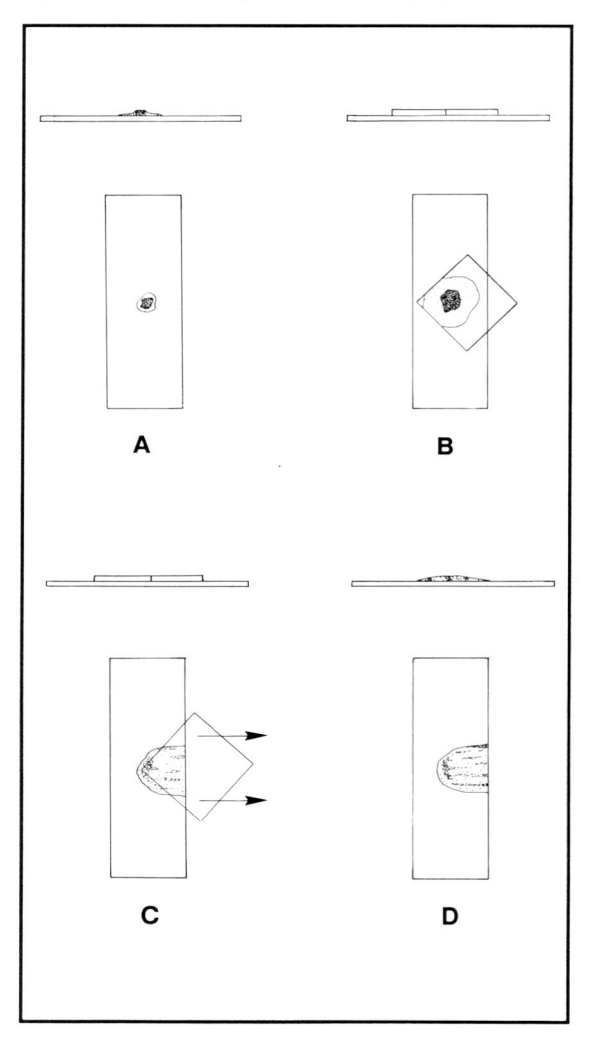

cases, it may be necessary to blow gently over the top of the capillary tube to dislodge the fleck. Any excessive fluid transferred can be removed by touching the fluid with a piece of absorbent paper or cloth.

After the fleck is transferred to the glass microscope slide, a 22 x 22-mm coverslip is placed over the fleck at a 45° angle to the glass microscope slide, allowing one corner of the coverslip to hang over the edge of the microscope slide (Fig 3). When the coverslip is placed over the fleck, the fleck spreads to about twice its previous size. Some smears should be made without any pressure other than that caused by the coverslip, and others should be made with sufficient gentle thumb pressure to cause the smears to spread to about twice the diameter caused by coverslip pressure alone. This ensures that some of the flecks are optimally spread.

Excessive pressure, causing rupture of cells, is the most common error in preparing cytologic smears of marrow flecks. When making smears from marrow samples in EDTA/isotonic saline solution, using another glass microscope slide instead of a coverslip to spread the fleck usually causes excessive pressure and results in rupture of nucleated cells.

Core Biopsy

Core biopsies can be collected with a Jamshidi infant (cats and small dogs) or pediatric (large dogs) marrow biopsy needle. The same procedure is used for collecting core biopsies as described for collecting marrow aspirate biopsies, except after the point of the needle has penetrated the cortex of the bone and entered the marrow cavity, the stylet is removed from the needle and the needle is advanced about 3 mm with a rotating motion. This cuts and collects a core of bone marrow. The needle is removed from the animal and the core of marrow is forced onto a glass microscope slide by passing the stylet through the barrel of the needle from the hub end.

Using the point of the needle, the core of marrow is gently rolled the length of the microscope slide. After making 1-2 slide preparations in this manner, the core of marrow is placed in a container filled with 10% formalin. If the cytologic preparations are to be sent to an outside laboratory, they should not be mailed with the formalin-filled container because formalin vapors alter the cells' staining qualities.

Collecting Marrow Samples from Dead Animals

Bone marrow samples occasionally are collected from dead animals. As mentioned earlier, if a complete evaluation of the marrow is expected, the samples must be collected and the cytologic preparations made immediately (within 30 minutes) after the animal's death. When collection and/or preparation are delayed, the preparations can be evaluated for cellularity, organisms, mast-cell infiltration, plasmacytosis, erythrophagocytosis and iron-containing pigments, but should not be evaluated for myeloid or lymphoid neoplasia. Delay in sample preparation can result in rupture of all the cells.

Though samples can be collected from most flat bones and the extremities of most long bones of dead animals, it is advisable to collect marrow samples from the same location(s) used in live animals (Fig 1). Remember, in adults, the central areas of long bones contain mostly fat. Access to the marrow can be gained by sawing the bone, cutting it with rongeurs, or fracturing it. If the bone is sawed, heat generated at the "saw line" can damage adjacent cells. Therefore, samples from sawed bones should be collected well away from the "saw line." Marrow is dug from between bony trabeculae, trying to avoid collecting bone spicules. The marrow is placed on a glass microscope slide at one end of the slide and gently rolled (by lifting upward with a needle or other instrument at the back of the sample) the length of the slide. Several slides are prepared from samples collected from several different areas of the bone marrow. The slides are air dried and stained as described below.

Staining Marrow Preparations

After fleck smears or core biopsy or necropsy imprints are made, they are air dried. The general Romanowsky-type staining procedures for staining blood smears are followed, except the stains and buffers are left in contact with the cells for a longer time. The extent to which the times must be lengthened depends on the thickness and cell density of the smears. Usually, staining times must be increased 2 times or more. Macroscopically, the marrow fleck streaks in the smear appear blue-purple to purple when the smear is properly stained.

Cells in Marrow

To evaluate cytologic preparations of bone marrow, one must be able to recognize the nor-

Figure 4. Bone marrow aspirate. A rubriblast (RB), rubricyte (R), metarubricyte (MR), myeloblast (MB), progranulocyte (PG), myelocyte (M), metamyelocyte (MM) and band cell (B) are indicated. (Wright's stain, original magnification 250X)

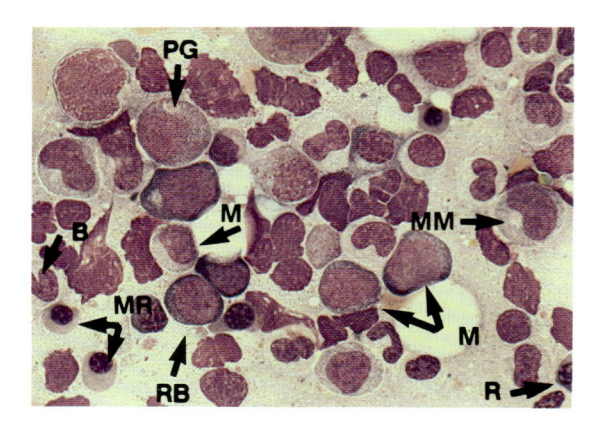

mal cells that occur in bone marrow, the neoplastic cells that have a propensity for infiltrating bone marrow, the organisms that can infect the marrow, and the processes (eg, erythrophagia) that occur in some pathologic conditions.

Erythroid Series

During proliferation and maturation, erythroid progenitor cells undergo 4-5 mitoses, producing 16-32 daughter cells. As they mature, erythroid cells decrease in size, their nuclei condense, and their cytoplasm changes from dark blue to red-orange. The general characteristics of the different cell stages of erythroid production are described below. Table 1 lists the different stages of erythroid development and provides an estimate of their relative proportions, a brief description of each stage, and a generalized schematic of the classic morphology of each stage.

Rubriblasts: The rubriblast is the most immature identifiable erythroid cell. Its nucleus is round, with a smooth nuclear border, a fine granular chromatin pattern, and 1-2 pale to medium blue nucleoli (Figs 4-6). Its cytoplasm is intensely basophilic and forms a narrow rim around the nucleus. The rubriblast has the highest nucleus:cytoplasm ratio of the erythrocyte series.

Prorubricytes: The next maturation stage of the erythroid series is the prorubricyte. Its nucleus is round, with a smooth nuclear border, and has a nuclear chromatin pattern slightly coarser than that of the rubriblast (Figs 5,6). Nucleoli usually are not visible in the prorubricyte stage. The cytoplasm is slightly less intensely blue and forms a thicker rim around the nucleus. The nucleus: cytoplasm ratio is less than that of the rubriblast, but greater than that of the rubricyte (the next stage of maturation). Mitosis continues through the prorubricyte stage.

Rubricytes: The next stage of erythroid maturation is the rubricyte. This stage is sometimes divided into the stages of basophilic and polychromatophilic rubricytes, or sometimes divided into the stages of basophilic, polychromatophilic and orthochromic rubricytes. The rubricyte and its nucleus are smaller than the prorubricyte and its nucleus. The rubricyte nucleus has an extremely coarse chromatin pattern that may resemble the spokes of a wheel (Figs 4-6). The cytoplasm is blue (basophilic) to bluish-red-orange (polychromic or polychromatophilic) to red-orange (orthochromic). The nucleus: cytoplasm ratio is less than that of prorubricytes but greater than that of metarubricytes (the next stage of maturation). Mitosis occurs in the early rubricyte stage but ceases by the latter rubricyte stages.

Metarubricytes: The next stage of erythroid development is the metarubricyte. Its nucleus is extremely pyknotic and appears black, without a distinguishable chromatin pattern (Figs 4,6). The cytoplasm of metarubricytes may be polychromatophilic or orthochromic.

Figure 5. Bone marrow aspirate from a cat with a bacterial bone marrow infection. *Salmonella* was cultured from the bone marrow. A rubriblast (RB), prorubricyte (PR), rubricyte (R), myeloblast (MB), early progranulocyte (PG), metamyelocyte (MM), band cell (B) and mature neutrophil (MN) are indicated. A macrophage (narrow arrow) containing bacteria and a large phagocytic vacuole, and numerous cells showing karyolysis (broad arrows) are also present. (Wright's stain, original magnification 250X)

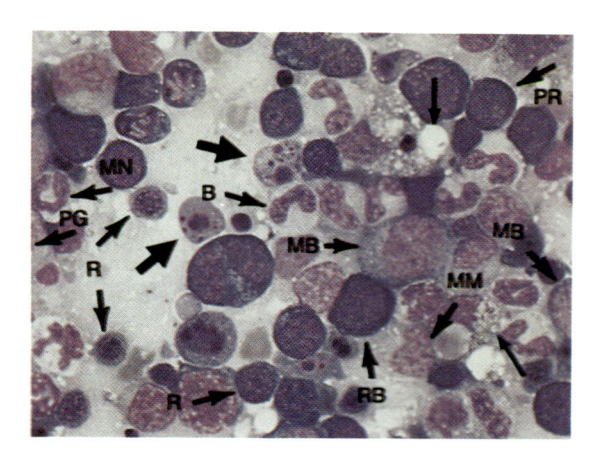

Polychromatophilic Erythrocytes: The next stage of development is the polychromatophilic erythrocyte. In blood smears stained with Romanowsky stains, polychromatophilic erythrocytes are nonnucleated, larger than mature erythrocytes (orthochromic erythrocytes), and bluish pink (polychromatophilic). Polychromatophilic erythrocytes stain as reticulocytes with supravital stains, such as new methylene blue.

Reticulocytes are nonnucleated erythrocytes that develop one or more granules or a network of granules when stained with supravital stains. More mature reticulocytes may be orthochromic (red-orange). As a result, all polychromatophilic cells are reticulocytes, but some reticulocytes are not polychromatophilic; instead, they are orthochromic.

The cytoplasm of some cells matures before the nucleus is extruded. These cells skip the polychromatophilic erythrocyte stage.

Mature Erythrocytes: The last stage of erythroid development is the mature erythrocyte. They stain red-orange (orthochromic) with Romanowsky stains. They do not stain with new methylene blue, nor do they form granules (reticulocyte formation) when stained with new methylene blue.

Granulocyte Series

The developmental stages, immature to mature, of the granulocyte series are: myeloblast, progranulocyte (promyelocyte), myelocyte, metamyelocyte, band cell and segmented granulocyte (mature neutrophil, eosinophil and basophil). The myeloblast, myelocyte and metamyelocyte stages of neutrophilic granulocytes cannot be differentiated reliably from monocytes. Table 2 lists the different stages of development of the granulocyte series, gives the relative proportions, and briefly describes the classic morphology of each stage.

Myeloblasts: The myeloblast is large and may be round or irregular in shape. It has a large nucleus, with a fine to finely stippled chromatin pattern and one or more visible nucleoli (Figs 4,5). The cytoplasm is blue to blue-gray and does not contain visible granules. The myeloblast has the highest nucleus:cytoplasm ratio of any of the granulocytic developmental stages. Mitosis occurs during the myeloblast stage.

Progranulocytes (Promyelocytes): The next stage of granulocyte development is the progranulocyte or promyelocyte. Often, the progranulocyte is slightly larger than the myeloblast. This increase in size is due to increased cytoplasm. The major differentiating feature of the progranulocyte is the presence of scattered small azurophilic (red-purple) primary granules throughout their cytoplasm (Figs 4,5). Primary granules are also called nonspecific granules. The nucleus is the same size to slightly smaller than the nucleus of the myeloblast. It has a lacy to coarse chromatin pattern and may contain visible nucleoli (but usually fewer and less prominent than the myeloblast) or nucleolar rings. Nucleolar rings are rings of densely staining chromatin that demark obscured nucleoli. The nucleus:cytoplasm ratio of the promyelocyte is less than that of the myeloblast. Mitosis occurs during the promyelocyte stage.

The presence of primary granules allows the progranulocyte to be recognized as a member of the granulocyte series and differentiates it from the monocyte series. Therefore, the progranulocyte can be more specifically identified than the myeloblast, neutrophil myelocyte and neutrophil metamyelocyte, which lack visible primary granules. As a result, the term progranulocyte, instead of promyelocyte, can be used to identify members of this developmental stage.

Myelocytes: The next developmental stage of the granulocyte series is the myelocyte. The disappearance of the primary granules (seen in the progranulocyte stage) aids differentiation of the myelocyte from the progranulocyte). Also, myelocytes are smaller than

Figure 6. Bone marrow aspirate from a cat with disseminated histoplasmosis. A rubriblast (RB), prorubricyte (PR), rubricyte (R), metarubricyte (MR), myelocyte (M), metamyelocyte (MM), band cell (B) and mature neutrophil (MN) are indicated. A macrophage containing several *Histoplasma* organisms is indicated by the broad arrow. (Wright's stain, original magnification 250X)

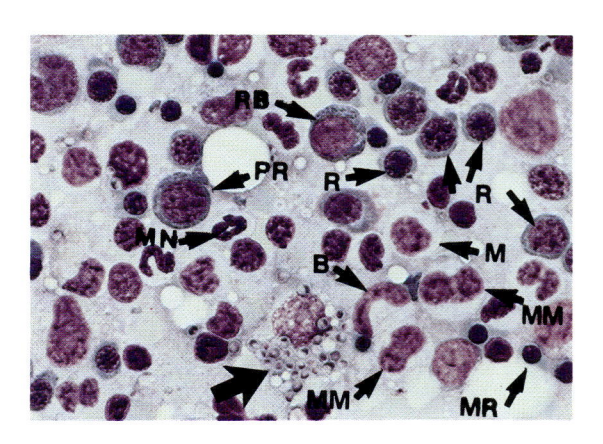

Figure 7. Bone marrow aspirate. *Top:* A promegakaryocyte with a small amount of basophilic cytoplasm and a nucleus that is polyploid but has not formed lobulations. (Wright's stain, original magnification 250X) *Bottom:* An immature (basophilic) megakaryocyte is on the right and a mature (eosinophilic) megakaryocyte at the left. (Wright's stain, original magnification 250X)

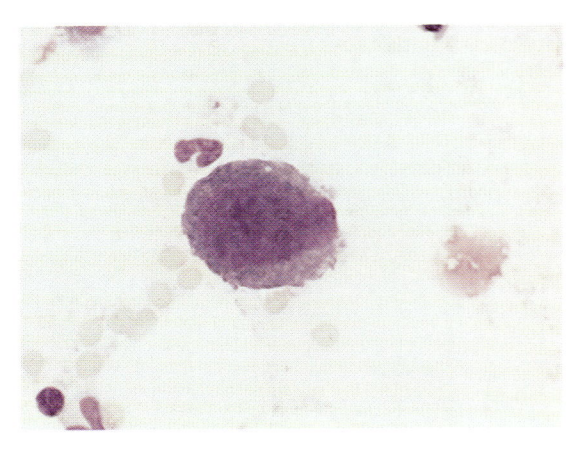

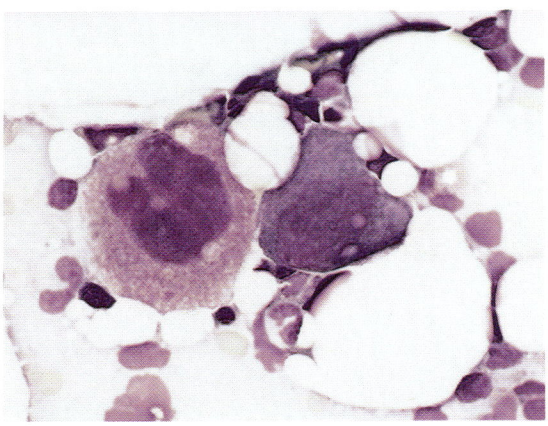

progranulocytes and their nuclear chromatin is more dense, giving a coarser pattern (Figs 4, 6). The nucleus is round to oval and nucleoli are not visible. The cytoplasm of the myelocyte is light blue to clear and contains secondary (specific) granules. These granules are poorly visualized in the neutrophil series but give the eosinophil and basophil their characteristic appearance.

The granules of feline eosinophils are rod shaped, while the granules of canine eosinophils are pleomorphic (but typically round) and variable in size. Feline basophils contain granules that are oval, tend to stain lavender, and fill the cytoplasm. The oval granules may appear round when viewed end-on. Some feline basophils also contain a few red-purple granules. Canine basophils contain a few to many round, variably sized, red-purple (metachromatic) granules. Mitosis can occur during this stage.

Metamyelocytes: The next stage of granulocyte development is the metamyelocyte. Its nucleus is classically described as kidney bean shaped. Generally, cells with nuclei having indentations extending less than 25% of the way into the nucleus are classified as myelocytes, whereas those with nuclei having indentations extending 25-75% of the way into the nucleus are classified metamyelocytes (Figs 4-6). The cytoplasmic characteristics of the metamyelocyte are similar to those of the myelocyte, with the neutrophil myelocyte cytoplasm being clear. This stage and subsequent stages do not undergo mitosis.

Band Cells: The next stage of granulocyte development is the band cell. It has a nucleus with a curved band or rod shape (Figs 4-6). Some chromatin clumps are present. The sides of the band cell nucleus are smooth and parallel. No area of the nucleus has a diameter less than one-half the diameter of any other area of the nucleus. Membrane irregularity and excessive narrowing of the nucleus warrant classifying of the cell as a mature neutrophil. The cytoplasmic characteristics of the band cell are similar to those of the metamyelocyte.

Segmented Granulocytes: The final stage of granulocyte development is the segmented granulocyte (mature neutrophil, eosinophil or basophil). Its nucleus is lobate or has areas of marked constriction (Figs 5, 6). The nuclear border is often irregular and large dense clumps of chromatin are present. Its cytoplas-

Figure 8. Bone marrow aspirate from a cat with lymphosarcoma. Numerous lymphoblasts are seen, along with 2 mitotic figures and a metarubricyte (upper left). (Wright's stain, original magnification 330X)

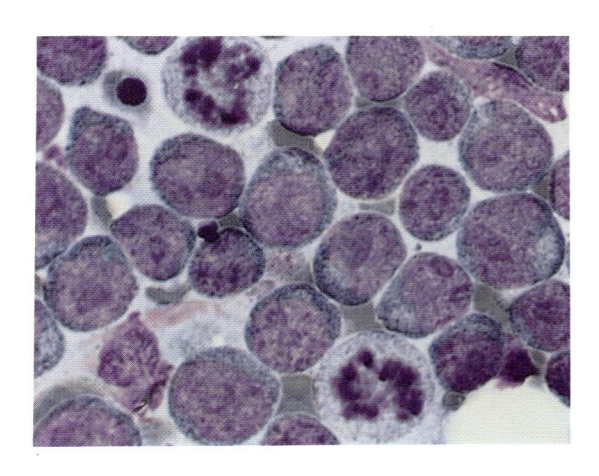

mic characteristics are similar to those of the myelocyte, metamyelocyte and band cell.

Monocyte Series

Cells of the monocyte series account for only a small percentage of the total marrow cells. As mentioned earlier, monoblasts cannot be differentiated from myeloblasts by light microscopy. Also, promonocytes are morphologically similar to neutrophilic myelocytes and metamyelocytes in bone marrow cytologic preparations stained with Romanowsky stains. Mature monocytes in bone marrow smears have the same appearance as monocytes in peripheral blood.

Thrombocyte (Megakaryocyte) Series

Megakaryoblasts: The most immature developmental stage of the megakaryocyte series recognizable by light microscopy is the megakaryoblast. However, it is not commonly identified in marrow aspirates because it usually occurs in small numbers and is difficult to differentiate from other blast cells.

Promegakaryocytes: The promegakaryocyte is the next recognizable stage. It has deep blue cytoplasm and contains 2-4 nuclei that may appear separate, but are linked by thin strands of nuclear material (Fig 7). Promegakaryocytes are much larger than WBC and RBC precursors.

Megakaryocytes: The megakaryocyte is the next developmental stage. Megakaryocytes are gigantic (50-200 μ in diameter). They contain >4 nuclei that are joined and form a lobulated mass (Fig 7). The larger the cell, the greater the nuclear ploidy (number). Megakaryocytes with deeply basophilic cytoplasm are less mature than those with light blue cytoplasm containing eosinophilic granules. Immature megakaryocytes are sometimes called basophilic megakaryocytes, while mature megakaryocytes are sometimes called eosinophilic or granular megakaryocytes. Bare nuclei of megakaryocytes may be seen in bone marrow cytologic preparations. They may represent nuclei of megakaryocytes that have shed their cytoplasm as platelets into the peripheral blood, or megakaryocytes whose cytoplasm has been torn from their nucleus during smear preparation.

Lymphocytes and Plasma Cells

The morphology of lymphoid cells and plasma cells has been described in Chapter 8. Briefly, mature (small) lymphocytes (Figs 1-5, Chapter 8, and Plate 1) are recognizably smaller than neutrophils, have a scanty amount of light to medium blue cytoplasm, and have an indented but otherwise round nucleus, with a dense smudged chromatin pattern without visible nucleoli. Prolymphocytes (Fig 5, Chapter 8) are about the same size as neutrophils. They have a little more medium to light blue cytoplasm than small lymphocytes. Their nuclei are round, other than an indentation in one area of the nucleus where the cytoplasm is most visible. The nuclear chromatin pattern appears smudged and nucleoli may be, but usually are not, visible. Lymphoblasts (Fig 8) are larger than neutrophils and have a small to moderate amount of light to dark blue cytoplasm. Their nuclei may be indented or irregular and have a fine reticular or lacy chromatin pattern. Multiple prominent nucleoli often are present.

Plasma cells are about the same size as or slightly larger than neutrophils. They have a round, eccentric nucleus and a moderate to abundant amount of deep blue cytoplasm. The Golgi apparatus can be recognized as a clear area in the cytoplasm adjacent to the nucleus where the cytoplasm is most abundant. Sometimes the cytoplasm contains round structures called Russell's bodies. These are areas of rough endoplasmic reticulum that are markedly dilated by immunoglobulin. Plasma cells packed with Russell's bodies are called Mott's cells (Fig 3, Chapter 8).

The bone marrow of normal dogs and cats usually contains <15% and <20%, respectively, lymphocytes and <2% (both dogs and cats) plasma cells.[3-5] Lymphocytes and plasma cells are not uniformly distributed throughout the bone marrow. Therefore, their proportions vary from area to area and fleck to fleck.

Macrophages

Usually <2% of the cells in normal canine and feline marrow are macrophages. Marrow macrophages are large, but not as large as early myeloid precursor cells (Figs 5,6). Their nuclei are usually eccentric and their cytoplasm is abundant and light blue staining, with indistinct boundaries. The cytoplasm is often vacuolated and may contain phagocytized material, such as pyknotic nuclear debris, WBCs, RBCs and/or their breakdown products, or organisms (*eg, Histoplasma capsulatum, Leishmania donovani*).

Osteoclasts and Osteoblasts

Osteoclasts and osteoblasts occasionally are encountered in bone marrow aspirates. Osteoclasts are giant multinucleated cells that phagocytize bone. They can be confused with megakaryocytes. Osteoclast nuclei are discernibly separate, whereas megakaryocyte nuclei are fused. The cytoplasm of osteoclasts stains blue and often contains azurophilic granular material. Osteoclasts are more common in aspirates from young animals than from old animals.

Osteoblasts are relatively large cells that somewhat resemble plasma cells (Fig 1, Chapter 11). They have eccentric nuclei and basophilic, sometimes foamy, cytoplasm. The Golgi apparatus may be visible as a clear area adjacent to the nucleus. Osteoblasts are larger and have less condensed nuclear chromatin than plasma cells. The osteoblast nucleus is round to oval, with a reticular chromatin pattern and 1-2 nucleoli. As with osteoclasts, they are more common in bone marrow aspirates from young growing animals than from older animals.

Miscellaneous Cells

Fat cells (adipocytes, lipocytes, Plate 8), endothelial cells (Plate 8), a few fibrocytes/fibroblasts (Plate 7), a few mast cells (Plate 2), unidentifiable blast cells, and free nuclei may be found in aspirates from normal animals. The free nuclei may be hematogones (small, round, condensed nuclei shed from metarubricytes) or basket cells (large free nuclei with dispersed lace-like chromatin from ruptured cells).

Organisms in Marrow

Though bacterial infections may involve bone marrow, the organisms usually sought on bone marrow cytologic preparations are *Histoplasma capsulatum* (Fig 6 and Plate 4), *Toxoplasma gondii* (Plate 5), *Leishmania donovani* (Plate 5) and *Ehrlichia* spp (Plate 6). By far, *Histoplasma capsulatum* is the most common organism identified in bone

Figure 9. Aspirates from 4 different bone marrows. A. Very hypocellular marrow. (Wright's stain, original magnification 25X) B. Normocellular marrow for an old dog, but mildly hypocellular marrow for a young dog. (Wright's stain, original magnification 25X) C. Mildly to moderately hypercellular marrow for an old dog, but normocellular marrow for a dog < 1 year old. (Wright's stain, original magnification 33X) D. Hypercellular marrow. (Wright's stain, original magnification 25X)

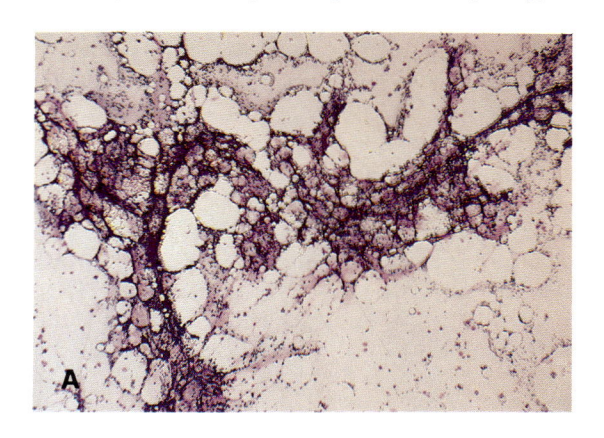

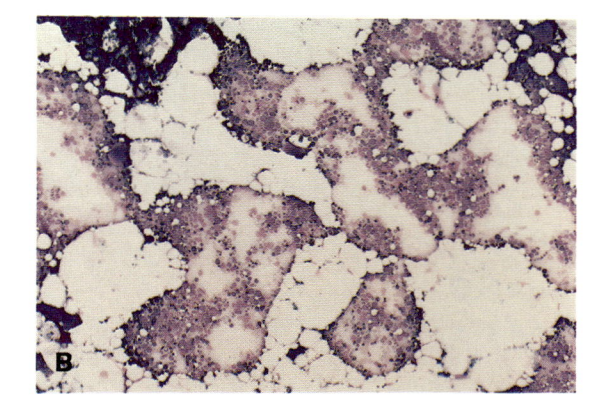

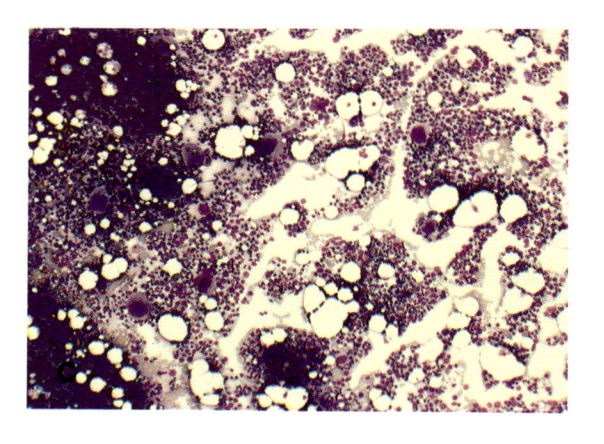

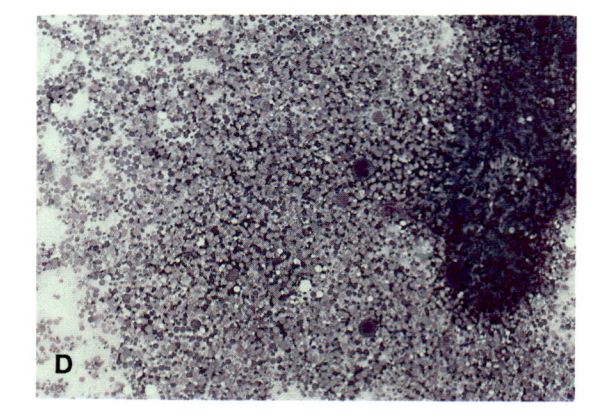

marrow cytologic preparations from dogs and cats. Systemic histoplasmosis often causes nonresponding anemia, thrombocytopenia and/or neutropenia. In a very high proportion of systemic histoplasmosis cases, the organism can be identified in bone marrow cytologic preparations.

Though *Ehrlichia* morulae can be found in the bone marrow of dogs during the early stages of ehrlichial infection, they seldom are identified during chronic ehrlichiosis. Because chronic ehrlichiosis is the most common stage in which clinical disease is recognized, bone marrow evaluation is seldom rewarding in diagnosis of clinical ehrlichiosis. Care must be taken not to mistake platelets overlying monocytes, macrophages and/or neutrophils for *Ehrlichia* morulae.

Bone Marrow Evaluation

Evaluation of bone marrow cytologic preparations must be made in light of available historical information, the animal's clinical signs, findings of physical examination, and the hematologic findings from a peripheral blood sample collected within hours of the bone marrow cytologic sample. For nonregenerative anemia, knowledge of the BUN level is important. Care should be taken not to overinterpret. When an interpretation cannot be made with certainty, the cytologic preparations, a concurrent blood smear, and hemogram results should be referred for interpretation.

Marrow Sample Evaluation

Bone marrow evaluation begins with aspiration. Easy collection of numerous flecks suggests normocellular or hypercellular marrow. On the other hand, if the marrow collection technique is adequate, difficult aspiration or failure to aspirate flecks from several sites suggests hypocellular, fibrotic or very densely packed marrow.

Aspirate samples containing only a few or no flecks and very little fat suggest fibrotic marrow. Those containing a few or no flecks and many fat globules suggest fatty hypoplastic marrow. Those containing many flecks suggest normocellular or hypercellular marrow. These subjective impressions should be confirmed by microscopic examination.

Core biopsies that yield red-gray marrow suggest normocellular or hypercellular marrow, while white or yellow-white marrow suggests hypocellular or fibrotic marrow. Core biopsies of fibrotic marrow may be recognizably firm.

There is some natural variation from fleck to fleck in cellularity and cell composition; therefore, several flecks should be evaluated. Macroscopically, hypercellular marrow tends to have large flecks that yield large, densely staining smears, while hypocellular marrow has small flecks that yield small smears with a reticular network of stain material outlining small to large unstained areas. Macroscopically, well-stained bone marrow preparations should be dark blue-purple. Reddish areas usually indicate clots.

Microscopic evaluation of bone marrow cytologic preparations should be methodical and thorough. Again, several flecks should be evaluated. The following order of examination can be used.

Adequacy of Preparation: At low magnification (4-10X objective) the smear is quickly scanned to ensure there are well-stained areas where flecks have been sufficiently spread (without excessive rupturing of cells) to form a cell monolayer with good cell morphology. If the flecks are insufficiently spread or excessive numbers of cells are ruptured, new preparations can be made if the sample was collected in EDTA. If the fleck smears are adequate but not sufficiently stained, they can be restained. If they are overstained, they can be destained in methanol and restained.

Evaluation of Marrow Cellularity

Bone marrow cellularity is estimated on low magnification (4-10X objective) by comparing the proportion of fat to cells in the fleck smear. Normal marrow cellularity varies, depending on the age of the animal (Fig 9). Marrow flecks of very young animals contain very little fat, while flecks from juvenile animals contain about 25% fat and 75% cells. Flecks from adult animals contain about 50% fat and 50% cells, and flecks from old animals contain about 75% fat and 25% cells. Cellularity also varies from fleck to fleck. Therefore, several flecks should be evaluated to form an estimate of overall marrow cellularity. Many interpretations made from bone marrow preparations hinge on marrow cellularity. For example, seldom can a diagnosis of neoplasia be made from hypocellular marrow flecks. Table 3 lists some diseases that affect bone marrow according to the marrow cellularity commonly seen during the disease.

Hypocellular marrow usually yields only a few flecks, or on some occasions, may not yield any flecks (dry tap). The flecks collected have a low cell:fat ratio (age must be considered). Hypocellular marrow can result from suppressive conditions (*eg*, feline leukemia virus marrow suppression), hypoplastic conditions (*eg*, renal insufficiency), infectious diseases (*eg*, parvovirus infection), toxic conditions (*eg*, estrogen toxicity), and idiopathic hypoplastic diseases. Other clinical, historical and/or clinicopathologic information often suggests the cause of hypocellular marrow.

Normocellular marrow usually yields many marrow flecks with a normal (considering the animal's age) cell:fat ratio. Normocellular marrow may be normal, or contain dysplastic and/or dyscrasic changes or organisms indicating pathologic changes. Dysplastic changes are alterations in cell morphology caused by a pathologic process. Dyscrasic changes are abnormal proportions of developmental stages of a cell series or abnormal proportions of different cell series. For example, excessive numbers of rubriblasts constitute a dyscrasia or dyscrasic change; whereas the presence of rubriblasts with abnormal cellular morphology, such as abundant cytoplasm, very coarse chromatin and eccentric nuclear location, is a dysplasia or dysplastic change. Also, normal cellular marrow preparations may contain organisms, macrophages demonstrating erythrophagocytosis, excessive numbers of mast cells, or metastatic tumor cells, such as metastatic carcinoma cells.

Hypercellular marrow usually yields an abundance of marrow flecks, but occasionally, tightly packed neoplastically hypercellular marrow may yield only a few or no flecks. Hypercellular marrow has an increased cell:fat ratio (the animal's age must be considered). Hypercellular marrow can be caused by erythroid hyperplasia, myeloid or granulocytic hyperplasia, myeloproliferative diseases, or infiltration of neoplastic cells, such as lymphosarcoma, plasma-cell tumors (multiple myelomas) and mast-cell tumors. The hemogram (including RBC morphology and thrombocyte count), clinical signs, historical information, and duration of the animal's illness help differentiate the causes of different types of hypercellular marrow.

Evaluation of the Megakaryocytic Series

The abundance and maturation of megakaryocytes are estimated on low magnification (4-10X objectives). Normally, each fleck contains several megakaryocytes. Less than 3 megakaryocytes per large fleck suggests megakaryocytic hypoplasia. The maximum number of megakaryocytes per fleck is not well established. However, >50 per large fleck generally suggests megakaryocytic hyperplasia. Usually, ≥50% of the megakaryocytes are mature (see description of megakaryocytic stages earlier in this chapter). When <50% of the megakaryocytes are mature, a regenerative response in the megakaryocytic series is suggested. If numerous promegakaryocytes (≤4 nuclei) are present, a maturation defect or early regenerative response is suggested.

Thrombocytopenia can be caused by platelet destruction (immune-mediated thrombocytopenia, etc), utilization (disseminated intravascular coagulation), sequestration (often in the spleen), or by suppression of platelet production (estrogen toxicity, etc). In thrombocytopenic animals, megakaryocytic hyperplasia indicates platelet destruction or utilization, whereas megakaryocytic hypoplasia indicates suppression of platelet production. Platelet sequestration usually is associated with normal megakaryopoiesis.

Bone marrow aspiration is seldom indicated in evaluation of patients with thrombocytosis, but it may be helpful in evaluation of patients with suspected polycythemia vera or megakaryocytic leukemia; both cause thrombocytosis but are very rare.

Figure 10. Bone marrow aspirate from a cat with megaloblastic change associated with FeLV infection. Numerous cells of the erythroid series are present. Most of the cells show megaloblastic changes, including increased cytoplasm, increased hemoglobin concentration and hence increased polychromatophilia of very immature erythroid cells, and excessively coarse chromatin patterns in immature erythroid cells. (Wright's stain, original magnification 250X)

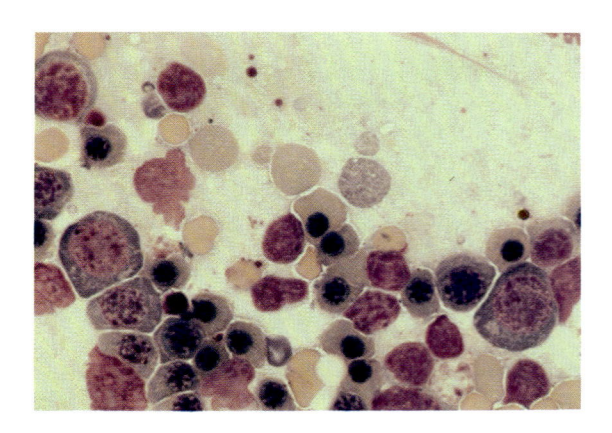

Table 1. The nucleated erythroid cell developmental stages and their relative percentage, description and schematic morphology.

Developmental Stage	Approximate Percentage of Classifiable Nucleated Erythroid Cells of Marrow* Dogs	Approximate Percentage of Classifiable Nucleated Erythroid Cells of Marrow* Cats	Description	Schematic of the Classic Morphology
Rubriblast	0.5	0.5	*Cell*: large; small to moderate amount of dark blue cytoplasm *Nucleus*: large; 1-2 nucleoli; dense granular chromatin	
Prorubricyte	2.0	3.5	*Cell*: medium to large; moderate amount of medium to dark blue cytoplasm *Nucleus*: medium to large; nucleoli usually not visible; coarse chromatin pattern	
Rubricyte	65	75	*Cell*: medium to small; small to moderate amount of medium blue (basophilic) to blue-pink (polychromatophilic) to orange (orthochromic) cytoplasm *Nucleus*: medium to small; no visible nucleoli; coarse clumped chromatin pattern with clear spaces	
Metarubricyte	32.5	21	*Cell*: small; small amount of blue-pink (polychromatophilic) to orange (orthochromic) cytoplasm *Nucleus*: small and pyknotic; no nucleoli visible; chromatin is densely clumped with few or no clear spaces	

* Broad variations may occur in normal animals due to the influence of such things as the subjectivity of cell classification and normal variation among individuals.

Evaluation of the Erythrocytic Series

The abundance, proportions and morphology of the erythrocytic series should be assessed using the 10X, 20X, 40X and 100X (oil immersion) objectives. Determination of the abundance of erythroid cells (erythroid hypoplasia/hyperplasia) requires consideration of the overall marrow cellularity and proportion of the marrow cells of the erythroid series. Table 1 gives the relative proportions of the different maturational stages of the erythroid series. The morphology of the erythroid cells can be evaluated for abnormalities, such as megaloblastic change, karyolysis, pyknosis of immature cells, and cytoplasmic and/or nuclear vacuolation. Megaloblastic changes include excessively coarse chromatin patterns, increased cytoplasm, macrocytic orthochromic erythrocytes, and increased hemoglobin content (causing polychromasia or orthochromia) in immature rubricytic cells (Fig 10). Megaloblastic change is most commonly seen in cats with FeLV-induced erythroid dysplasia. Karyolysis (Fig 5), pyknosis, and cytoplasmic and nuclear vacuolation can be caused by such conditions as marrow necrosis due to toxins (drugs, etc), infectious agents (bacterial or viral), and irradiation.

Nonregenerative anemia is a common indication for cytologic examination of bone marrow. Some causes of nonregenerative anemia in dogs and cats are given in Table 4. Associated bone marrow findings and procedures that can help differentiate the causes are also listed. Table 3 presents some causes of nonregenerative anemia according to the level of marrow cellularity with which they often are associated. Bone marrow cytologic examination seldom is of diagnostic value in evaluating polycythemic animals, but it may be helpful in evaluating patients with suspected polycythemia vera, an extremely rare neoplasia.

Evaluation of the Granulocytic Series

The abundance, proportions and morphology of the granulocytic series are assessed using the 10X, 20X, 40X and 100X (oil immersion) objectives. Normal proportions for the different granulocytic maturation stages are given in Table 2. To determine if there is an overall increase in the granulocytic series, marrow cellularity and the proportion of the marrow cells that are granulocytes must be considered. The presence of excessive numbers of one or more developmental stages, in comparison to the other developmental stages of the series, is referred to as dyscrasia. Dyscrasias can be caused by neoplasia, regenerative response and/or maturation arrest (with or without neoplasia). Some causes of abnormal morphology (dysplasia) are chemicals, nutritional imbalances (eg, folic acid/B_{12} deficiency), hereditary disorders (eg, macrocytosis of Poodles), neoplasia, feline leukemia virus infection, marrow necrosis, and marrow infection (eg, parvovirus infection).

Occasionally, bone marrow is examined to evaluate animals with persistent neutropenia. Some causes of persistent neutropenia are canine ehrlichiosis, feline leukemia virus suppression, myeloproliferative disease, lymphosarcoma, myelofibrosis (sclerosis), estrogen toxicity, marrow necrosis, histoplasmosis and cyclic hematopoiesis (cyclic neutropenia). These conditions, except cyclic hematopoiesis, also can cause severe nonregenerative anemia and/or thrombocytopenia. Cyclic hematopoiesis is associated with periodic marrow hypoplasia that is synchronous with the cycle of neutropenia. The bone marrow changes usually associated with these diseases, except cyclic hematopoiesis, and some procedures that may help diagnose them are given in Table 4. Table 3 lists some causes of neutropenia according to the level of marrow cellularity with which they usually are associated.

Bone marrow cytologic examination may aid in diagnosis of extreme neutrophilia and/or abnormal neutrophil morphology. However, leukemoid inflammatory responses (nonneoplastic extreme neutrophilia with or without an extreme left shift) can cause severe marrow dyscrasia. If a diagnosis of granulocytic leukemia cannot be made from the peripheral blood, it often cannot be made from bone marrow cytologic evaluation. Cytochemistry stains may be necessary to differentiate granulocytic neoplasia from a leukemoid response.

Evaluation of the Myeloid: Erythroid Ratio

The myeloid:erythroid (M:E) ratio is the ratio of myeloid cells to nucleated erythroid cells. Quantitative M:E ratios are determined by appropriately classifying 500 nucleated cells as myeloid or erythroid. This should be done using the 100X (oil immersion) objective. Cells should be classified from several fields of several different flecks. Harvey suggests 50% of the cells be classified from areas of the marrow flecks and 50% be classified from interfleck areas.[3] On the other hand, subjective

Table 2. The developmental stages of neutrophils and their relative percentage, description and schematic morphology.

Developmental Stage	Approximate Percentage of Classifiable Neutrophilic Granulocytes of Marrow* Dogs	Approximate Percentage of Classifiable Neutrophilic Granulocytes of Marrow* Cats	Description	Schematic of the Classic Morphology
Myeloblast	1	1	*Cytoplasm*: light to medium blue without granules *Nucleus*: round with prominent nucleoli *Chromatin pattern*: fine lacy	
Progranulocyte (promyelocyte)	3	3	*Cytoplasm*: light blue with scattered, small, red/purple (azurophilic) nonspecific (primary) granules *Nucleus*: round to oval; nucleoli indistinct or not visible *Chromatin pattern*: becoming coarse	
Myelocyte	12	10	*Cytoplasm*: nonspecific (primary) granules are no longer visible, so it is clear to slightly granular *Nucleus*: round to oval with slight indentation *Chromatin pattern*: coarse	
Metamyelocyte	19	20	*Cytoplasm*: clear to slightly granular *Nucleus*: kidney bean shaped *Chromatin pattern*: coarse with clumps	
Band neutrophil	26	29	*Cytoplasm*: clear to slightly granular *Nucleus*: curved rod or band shaped, with smooth borders *Chromatin pattern*: coarse with dense clumps	
Segmented neutrophil	38	35	*Cytoplasm*: clear to slightly granular *Nucleus*: marked indentations are present *Chromatin pattern*: coarse with dense clumps	

* Broad variations may occur in normal animals due to the influence of such things as the subjectivity of cell classification and normal variation among individuals.

Table 3. Some diseases that can cause nonregenerative anemia, neutropenia and/or thrombocytopenia in dogs and cats, classified by the overall marrow cellularity with which they can be associated.

Hypocellular Marrow	Normocellular Marrow	Hypercellular Marrow

FeLV suppression (cat) — A
Ehrlichiosis (dog) — A
Renal insufficiency — NA
Marrow necrosis — A, a
Radiation, cytotoxic drugs, etc — A, a
Myelofibrosis (sclerosis) — A, b
Aplastic anemias — NA, c
   Immune-mediated
   idiopathic
	FeLV suppression (cat) — A, d
	Ehrlichiosis (dog) — A, d
	Histoplasmosis — A, e
	Myeloproliferative disease — A, e
	Lymphosarcoma — A, e
		Histoplasmosis — A
		Ehrlichiosis (dog) — TP, f
		Myeloproliferative disease — A
		Lymphosarcoma — A
		Anemia of inflammatory
		   disease — (anemia of
		   chronic disease, etc) — NA

A — One to all of the marrow cell lines may be affected.
NA — Nonregenerative anemia
NP — Neutropenia
TP — Thrombocytopenia
a — Anemia may not be present in the acute phase.
b — Flecks, if any are collected, may appear small but hypercellular. This is because fibrous tissue has replaced most of the marrow elements, but a few pockets of hypercellular marrow may remain.
c — Rarely, thrombocytopenia and/or neutropenia may be present also.
d — Usually associated with hypocellular marrow.
e — Usually associated with hypercellular marrow.
f — Ehrlichiosis can be associated with hypercellular marrow, but when it is, it is usually in the acute to subacute phase of infection and is associated with thrombocytopenia alone; clinical signs are often inapparent.

Table 4. Some diseases that can cause severe nonregenerative anemia in dogs and cats. The prominent marrow features associated with the diseases and some procedures that can help diagnose the diseases are also listed.

Disease	Prominent Marrow Features	Helpful Diagnostic Procedures
Renal insufficiency	Erythroid hypoplasia	BUN and/or serum creatinine concentration
FeLV marrow suppression (cat)	Erythroid hypoplasia with or without maturation arrest and/or abnormal morphology (such as megaloblastic erythroid cells). Granulocytic hypoplasia may also be present.	Increased MCV on hemagram and/or the presence of megaloblastic erythrocytes in peripheral blood smears. FeLV serology and/or fluorescent antibody test for FeLV on bone marrow smears.
Ehrlichiosis (dog)	*Early*: Variable findings. *Late*: Erythroid hypoplasia, usually granulocytic hypoplasia, increased plasma cells.	*Ehrlichia* titer and/or response to therapy.
Estrogen toxicity	Erythroid, granulocytic and megakaryocytic hypoplasia.	History and physical examination.
Aplastic anemias Immune-mediated, idiopathic	Erythroid hypoplasia.	Rule out other diseases, response to androgens or immune suppressants.
Marrow necrosis Irradiation, cytotoxic drugs, etc	Erythroid, granulocytic and mega karyocytic hypoplasia with pink homogeneous strands of necrotic nuclear material. Early changes include cytoplasmic and nuclear vacuolation.	History, core biopsy.
Myelofibrosis (sclerosis)	Erythroid hypoplasia: Flecks are sparse, collected flecks may be normocellular or hypercellular.	Core biopsy.
Anemia of inflammatory disease (anemia of chronic disease, etc)	Erythroid hypoplasia and granulocytic hyperplasia, with increased marrow iron and plasma cells.	History, physical examination, clinical signs, marrow iron.
Histoplasmosis	Organisms present: Variable findings, but most commonly erythroid hypoplasia and granulocytic hyperplasia.	Refer slide for identification.
Nonerythroid neoplasia (lymphosarcoma, granulocytic leukemia, metastatic neoplasia)	Erythroid hypoplasia with marked increase in cells of the neoplastic cell line.	Cytochemistry to specifically identify the type of neoplasia.
Erythroid neoplasia	Increased erythroid cells often with a maturation arrest and/or abnormal morphology. May need to repeat aspirate to separate from early regenerative response.	Refer bone marrow cytologic sample and peripheral blood smear for interpretation.

M:E ratios are estimated from the proportions of myeloid and erythroid cells while evaluating the marrow cytologic preparations.

Accurate quantitative M:E ratios require classification of all myeloid and erythroid cells encountered in the fields viewed. This requires considerable experience and can be very frustrating. Though M:E ratios for normal dogs and cats usually are between 0.75:1 and 2.0:1, the range of M:E ratios for normal dogs and cats is very broad and can extend from 0.6:1 to 4.4:1.[2-8] Because of the difficulty in classifying some cells, the broad range of M:E ratios encountered in normal dogs and cats, and the ease with which most diagnostically significant changes in the M:E ratio can be perceived subjectively, quantitative M:E ratios usually are more masochistic than diagnostic. However, as Lewis and Rebar fluently state, "If business is slack...good luck! Certainly, there is no better way to learn hematopoietic

Table 5. Some causes of nonregenerative anemia and commonly associated bone marrow and peripheral blood findings.

Cellularity	Erythroid Series	Myeloid Series	M:E Ratio[a]	Other	Differential Diagnoses
↑	↑	↑	Variable	Neutropenia and/or thrombocytopenia may be present.	Neoplasia involving both leukocytes and erythrocytes (erythroleukemia).
↑	↑	↓	↓	Neutropenia and/or thrombocytopenia may be present.	Myeloproliferative disease in which erythrocytes predominate. Erythremic leukemia, reticuloendotheliosis, erythremic myelosis.
↑ or normal	↓	↑	↑	Without neutropenia.	Inflammation,[b] histoplasmosis or myeloproliferative disease in which leukocyte series predominate (eg, granulocytic leukemia, myelomonocytic leukemia).
↑ or normal	↓	↓	↑	With neutropenia.	Histoplasmosis or myeloproliferative disease in which leukocyte series predominate (eg, granulocytic leukemia, myelomonocytic leukemia).
↑ or normal ↓	↓	Variable	Variable	Neutropenia and/or thrombocytopenia may be present. Marked lymphoid infiltrate in bone marrow.	Lymphosarcoma.[c]
↓ or normal	↓	Normal	↑	Possible thrombocytopenia.	Ehrlichiosis, FeLV suppression, renal insufficiency, or aplastic anemias (immune-mediated or idiopathic).
↓	↓	↓	Variable	Depending on cause, neutropenia and thrombocytopenia may be present.	Ehrlichiosis, FeLV infection, marrow necrosis (irradiation, cytotoxic drugs, etc), myelofibrosis, estrogen toxicity, some aplastic anemias.

a — Remember, an increase or decrease in the M:E ratio indicates a shift of the M:E ratio out of the normal range, not just a shift from 1:1. Normal M:E ratio ranges vary between evaluators. A range of 0.75:1 to 2:1 often is used, but a broader range of 1:3 to 3:1 has been suggested.
b — Inflammation can cause anemia of inflammatory disease. Anemia due to inflammatory seldom, if ever, results in a PCV < 2/3 of the animal's normal PCV.
c — The marrow is usually hypercellular due to lymphoid infiltrate.

cell morphology."[9] In general, subjective evaluation of the proportions of myeloid and erythroid cells (subjective M:E ratio) is sufficient for diagnostic purposes, while quantitative ratios may be necessary in research studies.

The M:E ratio is interpreted in relation to marrow cellularity and peripheral blood (hemogram) values. Tables 5 and 6 give some causes of nonregenerative anemia and persistent chronic neutropenia, respectively, and some of the bone marrow findings, including M:E ratios, often associated with them.

Examination of Bone Marrow for Organisms

Bone marrow cytologic preparations can be examined for organisms, such as *Histoplasma capsulatum* (Fig 6 and Plate 4), *Leishmania donovani* (Plate 5), *Toxoplasma gondii* (Plate 5), and *Ehrlichia* spp (Plate 6), using the 40X and 100X (oil immersion) objectives. Usually, the areas of the smear adjacent to the fleck and the edges of the fleck are the most rewarding. These areas tend to contain a greater concentration of marrow macrophages than other areas. When organisms are suspected, a short

Table 6. Some causes of persistent chronic neutropenia and commonly associated bone marrow and peripheral blood findings.

Cellularity	Erythroid Series	Myeloid Series	M:E Ratio[a]	Other	Differential Diagnoses
↑	↑	↑	Variable	Erythroid and granulocytic abnormalities often are present in the peripheral blood. Nonregenerative anemia and thrombocytopenia usually are present.	Myeloproliferative disease involving myeloid and erythroid series (erythroleukemia).
↑	Normal or ↓	↑	↑	Usually a left shift in the peripheral blood. Nonregenerative anemia and thrombocytopenia usually are present.	Myeloproliferative disease in which the myeloid series predominates (eg, granulocytic and myelomonocytic leukemia).
↑ or normal	↓	↓	Variable	Marked lymphoid infiltrate in marrow. Nonregenerative anemia and thrombocytopenia usually are present.	Lymphosarcoma.[b]
↓	Normal	↓	↓	Thrombocytopenia may be present.	Ehrlichiosis, FeLV suppression.
↓	↓	↓	Variable	Nonregenerative anemia and thrombocytopenia are present.	Ehrlichiosis, FeLV suppression, marrow necrosis (irradiation, cytotoxic drugs, etc), estrogen toxicity, myelofibrosis.

a — Remember, an increase or decrease in the M:E ratio indicates a shift of the M:E ratio out of the normal range, not just a shift from 1:1. Normal M:E ratio ranges vary between evaluators. A range of 0.75:1 to 2:1 often is used, but a broader range of 1:3 to 3:1 has been suggested.
b — Lymphosarcoma with marrow infiltration causing neutropenia usually produces hypercellular marrow.

search should be performed. If they are not found quickly, the cytologic preparations should be sent to a consultant with more experience in identifying organisms and time to search for them. However, the examiner who has the time and enjoys bone marrow perusal should not be dissuaded from performing longer searches.

Examination for Erythrophagocytosis, Plasmacytosis, Iron-Containing Pigments, Neoplastic Cell Infiltration and Myelofibrosis

The marrow is examined for these conditions at all magnifications and their presence is confirmed on the higher magnifications (40X and 100X objectives).

Erythrophagocytosis is rarely seen in marrow samples from normal animals. When erythrophagocytosis is a prominent feature of the marrow sample, ineffective erythropoiesis and/or extravascular hemolysis is suggested. Ineffective erythropoiesis is the destruction of erythroid cells before they leave the marrow. Mild ineffective erythropoiesis may occur in some strongly regenerative anemias. However, marrow samples are seldom collected from animals with regenerative anemia.

In dogs and cats, usually <2% of nucleated marrow cells are plasma cells. When >3% are plasma cells, immune stimulation should be suspected. Sometimes, chronic immune stimulation results in development of Mott's cells (plasma cells stuffed with Russell's bodies). Marrow plasmacytosis usually is associated with myeloid hyperplasia. Plasmacytosis sometimes is associated with myeloid hypoplasia or a normal myeloid component in canine ehrlichiosis.

With multiple myeloma, there is usually an increase in the concentration of plasma cells throughout the marrow. However, a definitive diagnosis seldom can be made by bone marrow cytologic examination without aspiration of a focus of tumor proliferation. Tumor foci can be identified radiographically and aspirated. These foci yield sheets of plasma cells.

Evaluation of the marrow for iron pigments may require special stains, such as Prussian blue. Hemosiderin usually can be seen as blue-black particulate material in macrophages when iron stores are plentiful in dogs. However, recognizable iron pigments may not be present in Romanowsky-stained marrow preparations from normal cats. Recognizable marrow iron associated with low serum iron and ferritin levels can result from anemia of inflammatory disease. Depleted marrow iron stores associated with low serum iron and ferritin levels is associated with iron deficiency.

Cytologically, mast cells are easily recognized in bone marrow smears. A few mast cells may be present normally; however, when mast cells are abundant, infiltration by mast-cell neoplasia should be considered.

Lymphoid neoplasia often infiltrates bone marrow (Fig 8). Marrow preparations from normal dogs and cats can contain up to 15% and 20%, respectively, lymphoid cells, most of which are small lymphocytes.[3-5] Lymphoblasts can be difficult to differentiate from other blasts in the bone marrow. When ≥ 20% of the nucleated cells in marrow can be definitely recognized as lymphoblasts, lymphoid neoplasia is likely. Often, by the time the animal shows sufficient clinical signs to merit bone marrow examination, neoplastic lymphoid cells have completely, or almost completely, replaced the marrow elements. The hallmark of this situation is that recognizable granulocytes are sparse.

Occasionally, such neoplasms as carcinomas may metastasize to bone marrow. These usually are not encountered in bone marrow aspirations unless the site of metastasis has been radiographically located and the aspirate is taken from that area.

Myelofibrosis is the displacement of normal marrow elements (myelophthisis) by fibrous tissue. Usually, a few pockets of marrow persist within the fibrous tissue. These pockets of marrow undergo compensatory hyperplasia. Aspiration usually does not yield any marrow flecks, but occasionally a few small flecks may be recovered. These flecks usually contain very little fat and therefore appear hypercellular.

References

1. Davenport et al: Platelet disorders in the dog and cat, Part II: diagnosis and management. *Comp Cont Ed Pract Vet* 4:788-796, 1982.

2. Hoff et al: An appraisal of bone marrow biopsy in assessment of sick dogs. *Can J Comp Med* 49:34-42, 1985.

3. Harvey: Canine bone marrow: Normal hematopoiesis, biopsy techniques and cell identification and evaluation. *Comp Cont Ed Pract Vet* 6:909-926, 1984.

4. Schalm: The histology of mammalian bone marrow. *Feline Pract* 10(3):48-51, 1980.

5. Perman: Bone marrow evaluation in dogs and cats. *Proc 55th Ann Mtg AAHA*, 1988. pp 99-100.

6. Jain: *Schalm's Veterinary Hematology.* 4th ed. Lea & Febiger, Philadelphia, 1986. pp 126-139.

7. Duncan and Prasse: Clinical examination of bone marrow. *Vet Clin No Am* 6:597-609, 1976.

8. Seybold *et al*: The clinical pathology laboratory: Examination of bone marrow. *VM/SAC* 75:1517-1521, 1980.

9. Lewis and Rebar: *Bone Marrow Evaluation in Veterinary Practice.* Ralston Purina, St. Louis, 1979.

10

Synovial Fluid

B. W. Parry

The nature, chemical constituents and function of synovial fluid are well reviewed elsewhere.[1] Basically, synovial fluid is a dialysate of plasma. Hence, concentrations of electrolytes and nonelectrolytes (such as glucose and urea) are similar to those in blood, plasma or serum. It has a relatively low total protein concentration. Most of the proteins in synovial fluid that are derived from plasma are the lower-molecular-weight proteins. It is essentially without fibrinogen and most other clotting factors, and therefore does not clot, even *in vitro*.

The plasma dialysate is modified by type-B cells of the synovial membrane, principally by addition of hyaluronate. The latter glycosaminoglycan forms protein complexes that result in the fluid's characteristic high viscosity ("stickiness"). This viscosity depends on the length, structure and interactions of these hyaluronic acid polysaccharide chains. Longer, more polymerized and interactive molecules result in higher viscosity. These complexes are referred to as synovial mucin.

Normal synovial fluid has a low cellularity, with virtually no RBC and only small numbers of nucleated cells, mainly nonphagocytic mononuclear cells.

The principal functions of synovial fluid are nutritive support, lubrication and "cushioning" of the articular cartilage, which has no blood vessels, lymphatics or nerves.

Evaluation of synovial fluid is a valuable adjunct to assessment of many lameness cases. It can be readily performed with a minimum of equipment, in a fairly short time. In addition to cytologic evaluation, the fluid should be assessed for volume obtained, color, turbidity, viscosity, mucin (hyaluronic acid) quality/concentration, and protein concentration. Based on these findings, the arthropathy can usually be categorized as degenerative or inflammatory in origin. With further tests, including clinical examination, clinical pathologic testing and radiography, these categories can be further subdivided (see below).

There is a paucity of published data on synovial fluid analysis in cats. Sample volumes anticipated from normal and abnormal joints are obviously less than for most dogs. For other values and for clinical interpretation of findings, direct extrapolation from dogs is probably satisfactory. Unless otherwise stated, this chapter pertains to dogs.

Collection

Restraint

The animal must be restrained adequately to allow controlled manipulation and immobilization of the joint. This allows insertion of a needle directly into the joint space without causing damage to surrounding or adjacent structures, especially blood vessels, nerves, synovial membrane and articular surfaces. Consequently, the clinician must gauge the method of restraint most appropriate for each animal. This may vary from manual restraint, possibly with tranquilization and local anesthesia, to general anesthesia. When the animal's tractability is in doubt, it is best to opt for tranquilization or anesthesia if possible. This will probably result in easier and faster sample collection and help minimize blood contamination.

Asepsis

Routine aseptic technique should be followed. Normal joint spaces are sterile.

Equipment

Sterile disposable 2- to 5-ml syringes and 1-inch, 20- to 22-ga hypodermic needles are recommended in most cases. If the joint space to be tapped is small (*eg,* carpus of small dogs or cats), a 25-ga spinal needle may be preferable, since its shorter bevel is more likely to enter the articulation properly.

Approaches for Arthrocentesis

Approaches to the more commonly sampled joints are detailed below. Arthrocentesis from most of these joints is most readily achieved with the animal in lateral recumbency and the affected limb uppermost.[2] Exceptions are the carpal joints, where sternal recumbency may be preferred, and the hip joint, where a ventral approach may be preferred (hence necessitating dorsal recumbency).

Palpation of affected joint(s) during manual flexion and extension may help identify the space to be entered. In all cases the needle should be advanced gently toward and through the joint capsule to avoid damaging the articular cartilage. If the needle encounters bone before entering the joint, it should be withdrawn slightly and redirected.

Once the needle is inside the joint space, the volume of fluid obtained depends on the particular joint and the disorder. Ordinarily, some synovial fluid is fairly readily collected from the stifle joint, but it is difficult to obtain from the carpal and tarsal joints. Obviously, when joint spaces are swollen, fluid is more easily aspirated. The plunger of the syringe should be released before the needle is removed from the joint space. This minimizes blood contamination of the sample as the needle is withdrawn.

Radiocarpal Joint: The carpus is flexed and the needle is inserted from the cranial aspect, between the radius and the radiocarpal bone.

Intercarpal Joint: The carpus is flexed and the needle is inserted from the cranial aspect, between the radiocarpal bone and the second and third carpal bones. This joint space is connected with that of the carpometacarpal joint. The latter is difficult to tap *per se.*

Elbow Joint: The elbow is flexed slightly and the needle is inserted from the caudolateral aspect of the joint, such that it is caudal and medial to the lateral condyle of the humerus and slightly dorsal to the olecranon tuberosity of the ulna. The needle will pass through the anconeus muscle and the tendon of insertion of the triceps muscle.

Shoulder Joint: The shoulder is slightly flexed and the needle is inserted just medial and ventral to the acromion process of the humerus. It is advanced obliquely ventrocaudad to pass through the biceps brachii muscle and medial to the deltoideus muscle.

Tarsal Joint: The needle can be inserted from the craniolateral or craniomedial aspect. It should pass beside the flexor tendons.

Stifle Joint: Arthrocentesis of the stifle joint can be from either side of the straight patellar ligament, since both joint spaces are connected. The stifle is flexed to extend the joint capsule, while applying digital pressure over the capsule on one side of the patellar ligament. This causes protrusion of the capsule on the opposite side. The needle is advanced through the latter area in an obliquely distal direction, toward the intercondylar space of the tibia. Abduction of the limb may improve joint access.

Hip Joint: A lateral or ventral approach can be used. For the former, the femur is abducted and rotated craniad (usually by grasping the stifle). This maneuver widens the joint space and tenses the capsule. The needle is inserted cranial to the greater trochanter of the femur and advanced caudoventrad toward the joint. Care must be taken to avoid the circumflex femoral artery, which crosses the joint capsule, and the sciatic nerve, which is caudal to the joint.

For the ventral approach, the animal is placed in dorsal recumbency, with both femurs gently abducted until they are perpendicular to the midline. The ventral aspect of the acetabular fossa is located just caudal to the origin of the pectineus muscle at the ileopectineal eminence of the pelvis. The needle is advanced craniad at a 45-degree angle, through the joint capsule and ligamentum teres into the joint space.

Sample Handling and Test Priorities

Normal synovial fluid does not clot. However, with blood contamination, intraarticular hemorrhage, or protein exudation in various inflammatory diseases, samples may clot unless processed immediately or added to an anticoagulant. EDTA is preferred for cytologic examination, whereas heparin is recommended for the mucin clot test. Either anticoagulant is suitable for other routine tests.

Laboratory tests performed on a sample mainly depend on the volume of fluid collected. When only a few drops are obtained, volume, color and turbidity should be noted at the time of collection (while the sample is in the syringe). Viscosity is then assessed as the sample is expelled onto a glass slide. Direct smears are immediately made for subsequent cytologic examination and subjective assessment of cellularity (see below). See Chapter 1 for a discussion of slide preparation techniques. When larger volumes of fluid are collected, a total nucleated cell count, mucin clot test and total protein estimation (in order of priority) can be added to the above procedures.

When sufficient fluid is collected to allow cell counting, various types of smears can subsequently be made in accordance with the sample's cellularity. If the nucleated cell count is <500/μl, cytologic examination is enhanced by centrifugation of the sample to concentrate cells. About 5 minutes at 1500 rpm is satisfactory. The supernatant is decanted and saved for a mucin clot test (see below). Sedimented cells are gently resuspended in a small amount (about 0.5 ml) of supernatant. Smears are made from this suspension, as outlined in Chapter 1. Fluids with nucleated cell counts >5000/μl can be smeared directly onto slides. Fluids with counts of 500-5000/μl are usually more easily evaluated if sediment smears are prepared. Obviously, when only a small volume of fluid is collected, direct smears at any cell count are preferable to no smears.

Cells in sediment smears and direct smears of fluid with high (normal) viscosity may not spread out well on slides, especially in the thicker areas of the smear. This makes cell identification difficult. This problem can be overcome by mixing equal amounts of synovial fluid and hyaluronidase (solution of 150 IU/ml) together for at least 10 minutes.[3] The fluid is then quite watery, facilitating good cell morphology.

Cytocentrifuges are now available for concentration of low-cellularity fluids directly onto a small area of a glass slide. Samples with good to fair viscosity must be pretreated with hyaluronidase (as above), otherwise the synovial fluid mucin clogs the cytocentrifuge filter paper, interfering with slide preparation. These machines are too expensive for the average practitioner to justify purchase.

Slides can be stained with any Romanowsky-type stain for routine cytologic evaluation. Staining with new methylene blue demonstrates any fibrin strands in the smear (causing clumping and uneven distribution of cells). However, this is rarely done. (See Chapter 1 for a discussion of stains and staining techniques.)

It is advisable to make synovial fluid smears soon after collection. Delays of several hours, particularly at warm temperatures, can result in artificial vacuolation of macrophages, and pyknosis and karyorrhexis of all nucleated cells.

Microbiologic evaluation of samples collected aseptically can be undertaken if cytologic and clinical findings suggest an infectious agent may be present.

Laboratory Analysis and Reference Values

Volume

The approximate volume of fluid collected should be recorded. In normal animals this varies from joint to joint.[4] In one study of 70 arthrocenteses from 70 normal canine joints (carpi, elbows, shoulders, hocks and hips), the volumes collected ranged from 0.01 to 1.0 ml.[4] In other less extensive studies, volumes were 0.2-1.0 ml (17 samples from stifle, shoulder or carpal joints) and 0.03-0.25 ml (about 20 stifle joints.)[3,5]

Clinical experience is an extremely valuable guide to detecting an articular effusion. This judgment is based on the degree of joint capsule distension, ease of fluid collection, and volume readily obtained. The aim of arthrocentesis for synovial fluid analysis is not to drain the joint space. Hence, all fluid present is not necessarily removed. In contrast, treatment of some disorders, such as septic arthritides, may include synovial lavage with joint drainage.

Color and Turbidity

Normal synovial fluid is transparent and colorless to yellow. Abnormal samples, which have increased cellularity, exhibit variable discoloration and increased turbidity.

If the fluid is blood tinged, hemarthrosis must be distinguished from iatrogenic contamination at collection. In cases of hemarthrosis, the sample is uniformly bloody throughout the collection period. If the fluid was initially free of blood, with subsequent admixture during the collection procedure, contamination should be suspected. When the volume of fluid collected is sufficiently large, centrifugation of an aliquot is helpful. Recent

Figure 1. Direct smear of synovial fluid from a dog with acute suppurative arthritis. Note the markedly increased cell count and linear arrangement of cells. The latter, referred to as "windrowing," suggests normal viscosity. (Wright's stain 160X) (From Parry, in Pratt: *Laboratory Procedures for Veterinary Technicians*. 2nd ed. American Veterinary Publications, Goleta, CA, 1992.)

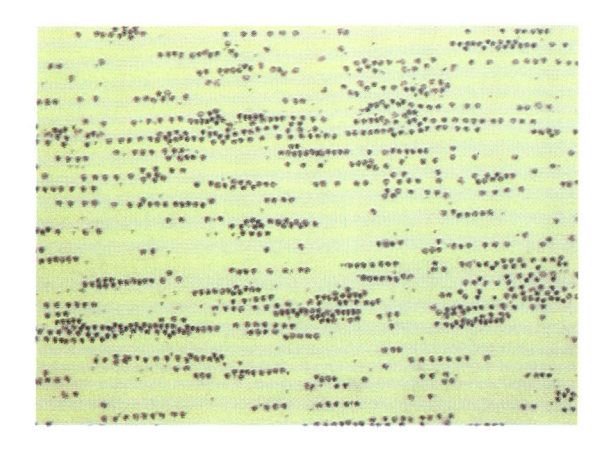

hemorrhage is associated with a sediment of RBC and a clear to straw-yellow supernatant, whereas chronic hemorrhage is associated with yellow discoloration of the supernatant (because of hemoglobin breakdown products). Cytologic differences between acute and chronic hemorrhage are discussed below under Acute Hemarthrosis.

Viscosity

Normal synovial fluid is very viscous because of its high concentration of hyaluronic acid. Viscosity can be measured using a viscometer; however, this is rarely done in small animal practice. Instead it is usually assessed subjectively. When slowly expressed from a needle attached to a syringe held horizontally, normal synovial fluid forms a long "strand" (usually >2.5 cm) before separating from the needle. Alternatively, when a drop of fluid is placed between thumb and forefinger, a similar strand bridges the 2 digits as they are moved apart. Viscosity is usually recorded as normal, decreased or markedly decreased.

Viscosity is easily assessed at the time of collection. However, if it must be evaluated after the sample is added to an anticoagulant, heparin is probably preferable to EDTA for sample preservation. EDTA tends to degrade hyaluronic acid and might therefore decrease the sample's viscosity.[1]

Viscosity can also be subjectively assessed when cytologically evaluating direct or sediment smears. Such smears of fluids with high (normal) viscosity tend to have cells aligned in a linear fashion, sometimes referred to as "windrowing" (Fig 1). In contrast, synovial fluid samples with decreased viscosity have cells more randomly arranged on the smear (Fig 2).

Mucin Quality and Concentration

If sufficient sample remains after the above tests, the quality and quantity of synovial fluid mucin (and hence hyaluronic acid) may be assessed using a mucin clot test. EDTA interferes with the mucin clot test by degrading hyaluronic acid.[1] Hence, if anticoagulant must be used to prevent sample coagulation before the test can be run, use of heparin is recommended.

Following centrifugation (see above), undiluted synovial fluid supernatant is added to 2-5% glacial acetic acid at a ratio of about 1:4. This causes mucin to agglutinate (clot). The test can be performed in test tubes when sufficient fluid is collected or on glass slides when only a drop is available for this test (Fig 3). The mixture is gently agitated and the nature of the clot observed.

The following subjective classifications are commonly used: good (normal), when there is a compact ropey clot in a clear solution; fair (slightly decreased), when there is a soft clot in a slightly turbid solution; poor, when there is a friable clot in a cloudy solution; and very poor, when there is no actual clot, just some

Figure 2. Sediment smear of synovial fluid from a dog with degenerative arthropathy. Note the normal (low) cell count and random distribution of cells. The latter suggests decreased viscosity. (May-Grünwald-Giemsa stain, 200X)

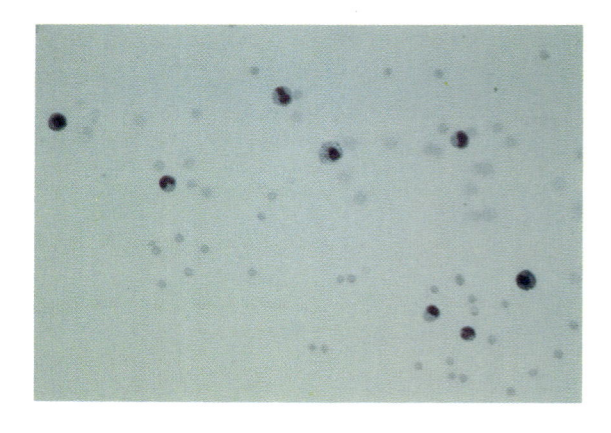

Figure 3. Mucin clot tests. Reading from left to right, these tests were graded as good (normal), good, fair, poor and poor.

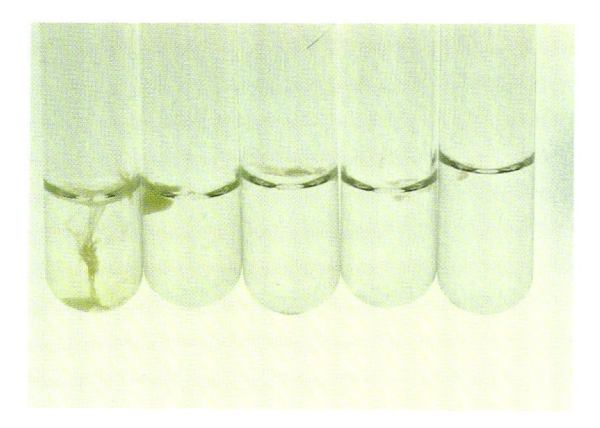

large flecks in a very turbid solution. If clot quality is initially debatable, it can be reassessed after about 1 hour at room temperature. When the solutions are gently shaken during assessment, good clots remain ropey, while poor clots fragment. Assessment is enhanced by reading the test against a dark background.

Hyaluronic acid concentration can be measured directly;[6] however, this is rarely performed on clinical cases in dogs and cats.

Total Cell Counts

Nucleated cell counts in normal synovial fluid vary from one joint to another in the same animal.[3] However, no surveys have been done to show that these differences are statistically significant or that they should be of concern when interpreting clinical results. Most studies have been on stifle samples. Various reference ranges have been reported (Table 1). As a generalization from these studies, most normal joints have nucleated cell counts $<3000/\mu l$.

Nucleated cell counts are usually performed using a microscope and hemacytometer, similar to other cell counts. The sample may be counted undiluted if the cell count is low, as in nonturbid specimens. However, if the sample is turbid and the anticipated cell count is high-normal to increased, the specimen should be diluted. A WBC diluting pipette and physiologic saline are suitable for this purpose. The Unopette system (Becton Dickinson) can also be used, provided the diluent selected is not acetic acid. The latter is often used as a diluent for WBC counts in blood samples but cannot be used on synovial fluid because it causes the sample's mucin to clot, invalidating results.

Recently, manual nucleated cell counts were compared to electronic particle counter-derived values.[9] Samples from 19 normal canine stifles were evaluated. The mean ±SD hemacytometer value was 848 ±533/μl, while the electronic particle counter value was 1008 ±405/μl. Analysis of their data by paired t test reveals that these results were not significantly different ($P>0.05$). Hemacytometer results may be more accurate at low counts. However, provided the "background count" of an electronic particle counter is very low (arbitrarily $<60/\mu l$), even at low cell counts the electronic particle counter method (when available) would be preferable to the hemacytometer, since results are more readily and quickly obtained. Further, any difference in values between the 2 techniques is not diagnostically (clinically) important.

One study of heparin-preserved human synovial fluid samples from rheumatoid arthritis patients with abnormally high nucleated cell counts showed that these laboratory cell counts were increased by in-vitro addition of hyaluronidase to the specimen before dilution in a pipette.[10] Hyaluronidase pretreatment counts averaged 2.5 times greater than values obtained on untreated samples. Without hyaluronidase pretreatment, samples tended to stick to the walls of the diluting pipette stems. Similar studies have not been conducted in

Table 1. Reference ranges for synovial fluid total nucleated cell counts in dogs.

Range ($/\mu l$)	Joints Sampled
33-2495[3]	12 joints: stifle, shoulder, carpus
0-2900[4]	55 joints: hip, stifle, hock, elbow, shoulder, carpus
700-4400[5]	20 stifles
327-1450[7]	14 stifles
50-2725[8]	58 stifles
209-2070[9]	19 stifles

dogs and cats. Since EDTA reportedly decreases synovial fluid mucin quality (and probably therefore viscosity), counts on fluid samples collected into EDTA may not be increased by hyaluronidase. Such pretreatment of samples for cell counts in dogs and cats has not been recommended in previous papers.[1,4,5,9]

Red blood cell counts are not usually performed on synovial fluid. Normal samples contain very few RBC. However, minor blood contamination at collection is not uncommon. One study reported normal RBC counts of 0-320,000/µl, with a mean of 12,150/µl.[4] The author indicated that blood contamination was noted when some samples were collected. The RBC counts can be performed manually at the same time nucleated cells are enumerated.

Cytologic Examination

When only a few drops of fluid are collected, cytology reports should include subjective assessments of the amount of blood present, total nucleated cell count, and sample viscosity. When a cell count and mucin clot test have been performed, these subjective assessments should still be made for corroboration of results. However, it is not as important to actually record subjective findings unless they were at variance with test results.

Normal synovial fluid contains very few RBC. Increased RBC numbers may result from hemorrhage at collection and/or hemorrhage associated with trauma to, or inflammation of, the joint capsule. Differentiation of these causes is discussed later.

With practice, the cellularity of synovial fluid direct smears can be reliably and uniformly estimated. The body of the smear of normal specimens contains about 2 cells/field at 400X magnification. It is usually sufficient to categorize samples as having normal (Fig 2), slightly increased, moderately increased or markedly increased (Fig 1) cellularity. Obviously, such assessment is impractical and unnecessary on sediment and cytocentrifuge-prepared smears. Actual cell counts should be available in these situations.

Because of the high viscosity of normal synovial fluid, cells of direct and centrifuged sediment smears tend to line up in rows (windrowing, Fig 1). This characteristic arrangement of cells can therefore be used to comment on sample viscosity when insufficient volume is collected for viscosity and mucin clot tests. At very low cell counts, windrowing may not be apparent even though viscosity is normal.

Smears of both normal and abnormal synovial fluid often have an eosinophilic granular proteinaceous background (Fig 10). This is a normal finding and must not be confused with bacteria.

Nucleated cells should be classified as neutrophils, eosinophils, lymphocytes or large mononuclear cells. The last group encompasses mononuclear cells with phagocytic potential without attempting to determine their origin. These cells could be derived from blood monocytes, tissues macrophages or synovial membrane cells (clasmatocytes).[1] Their origin has little practical importance as far as clinical diagnosis and therapy are concerned. The proportion of large mononuclear cells that are vacuolated and/or phagocytic of debris, cells or microorganisms is more important and should be recorded, together with assessment of the degree of vacuolation or phagocytic activity. The latter is reported as mild, moderate or marked. Overall cell morphology should also be noted, with comments on the degree of karyolysis, pyknosis and/or karyorrhexis. Finally, other cells, such as chrondrocytes, osteoblasts, osteoclasts and lupus erythematosus (LE) cells, which are not present in normal samples, and any microorganisms should also be noted.

Results of synovial fluid differential cell counts are usually reported as percentage values. Though absolute numbers of individual cell types are not actually calculated, results must be interpreted taking into account the sample's total nucleated cell count or subjectively assessed cellularity.

Reports of synovial fluid differential cell counts are quite variable in their reference values;[3-5,7,8] however, the following generalizations are appropriate. Neutrophils, when present, are in small numbers and represent ≤12% (frequently ≤5%) of nucleated cells.[3-5,7] Eosinophils are absent.[3-5,7,8] Lymphocyte values can be quite variable. One study (of 64 samples) reported values of 0-100%, with a mean of 44%.[4] Another study (of 19 samples) reported a range of 3-28%, with a mean of 11%.[3] Average lymphocyte percentages in other studies were between these 2 mean values.[5,7,8] Large mononuclear cells account for the remainder of nucleated cells in samples from normal joints, ranging from 64-97% in one study, to 60-92% in another study.[3,7]

As noted earlier, slides should be made as soon as possible after the sample is collected. Delayed processing can lead to increased numbers of markedly vacuolated large mononuclear cells and nuclear degeneration.[3] In samples from normal joints that were processed immediately by direct smear, the percentage of large mononuclear cells that were markedly vacuolated was about 9%.[3] Pretreatment of samples with hyaluronidase to improve cytologic morphology before direct smears or cytocentrifugation smears were made also increased the percentage of large mononuclear cells that were markedly vacuolated (from about 9% to about 14-18%).[3]

Total Protein Concentration

Synovial fluid usually has a low total protein concentration. This can be measured by refractometry or biochemical assay. Comparatively few studies have reported baseline values for total protein concentration. This probably reflects the relatively low priority given to this value. Other tests (mentioned above) are usually run in preference, and sample volume is usually insufficient to allow protein measurement as well. One study of 15 normal stifle, shoulder and carpal joints reported reference total protein concentrations of 1.8-4.8 g/dl, measured by refractometer.[3]

Normal synovial fluid is essentially free of fibrinogen and other clotting factors, and therefore does not clot *in vitro*. However, if samples are left undisturbed for several hours, they may gel. The latter phenomenon is referred to as thixotropism. It is distinguishable from clotting in that normal fluidity is restored simply by gently shaking the sample. If a specimen does clot after collection, this indicates hemorrhage and/or protein exudation into the joint space. The latter usually results from inflammation, which would be evident from increased sample cellularity.

Other Tests

The small volume of fluid obtained from dogs and cats precludes consideration of additional tests in almost all cases. Such tests are reviewed elsewhere and include assays for glucose, urea, electrolytes, enzymes, pH and aldehyde groups.[1,3,11]

Ancillary Tests

Various other procedures are extremely useful when evaluating dogs and cats with lameness or arthropathies. These include:

- Full case history and complete physical examination.[12-16]
- Biochemical assays and urinalysis, especially when a multisystemic disease is suspected (*eg*, systemic lupus erythematosus).[12-14,16]
- Radiography.[12-16]
- Arthroscopy.[13,17]
- Synovial membrane biopsy.[2]
- Microbiologic testing.[13,14]

Detailed consideration of their contribution to case workup is beyond the scope of this chapter. The above references will serve as an introduction to these topics for the interested reader.

Synovial Fluid Changes in Diseased Joints

Synovial fluid has a limited number of ways in which it can respond in disease. Consequently, 2 main categories have formed the basis of various classification schemes: degenerative arthropathies (also referred to as noninflammatory and nonpurulent by some authors) and inflammatory arthropathies.[1,12-14,18] Table 2 summarizes the characteristics and causes of these categories of response, and suggests acute hemarthrosis as a separate classification.

All fluids do not fall neatly into 1 of the above categories. This is especially true of longer-standing problems, which tend to develop characteristics of other categories, thus making classification and interpretation more difficult. For example, resolving hemarthrosis has a concurrent secondary chronic to chronic-active inflammatory response, while a long-standing purulent arthropathy may have low-grade but significant hemorrhage and erythrophagocytosis. Further, degenerative arthropathy can become secondarily infected, while septic arthritis can result in secondary degenerative joint disease.

The remainder of this chapter discusses the categories of Table 2 in more detail.

Acute Hemarthrosis

True hemarthrosis must be distinguished from accidental blood contamination of samples at collection and from hemorrhage associated with various causes of nonpurulent and (especially) purulent effusions.

Chapter 10

Figure 4. Direct smear of synovial fluid from a dog. Note the platelet clump, indicating recent hemorrhage. In this case, hemorrhage was due to iatrogenic contamination. May-Grünwald-Giemsa stain, 500X.

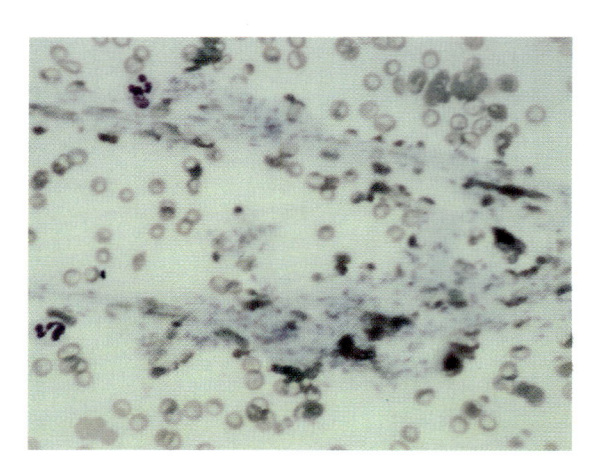

Figure 5. Synovial fluid from a dog with degenerative arthropathy. Note the erythrophagocytic macrophage, which indicates concurrent chronic hemorrhage (*ie*, not iatrogenic contamination). May-Grünwald-Giemsa stain, 1250X.

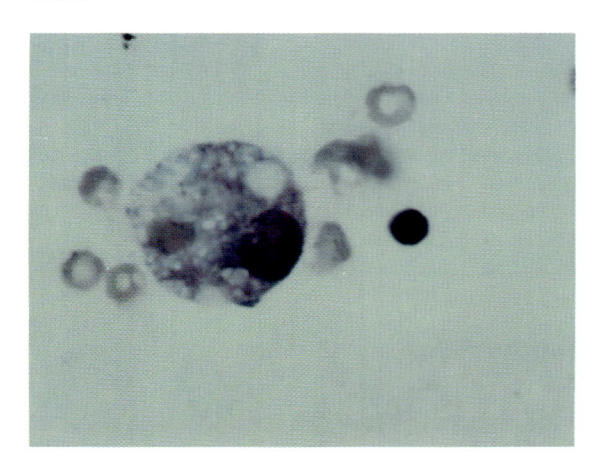

Table 2. Characteristics and major causes of 3 main categories of synovial fluid responses to articular injury.[1,4,13-17]

Category	Color	Turbidity	Viscosity	Mucin Clot Test	Nucleated Cell Numbers Total	Nucleated Cell Numbers Differential	Causes
Acute hemarthrosis	Bloody	Increased proportionally with amount of hemorrhage	Decreased mildly to markedly	Fair to poor	Probably increased	Mo: Normal to increased PMN: Increased[a]	Coagulopathy, especially Factor deficiency, such as Hemophilia A; severe acute trauma
Degenerative arthropathy	Usually normal	Usually normal	Usually normal to mildly decreased	Usually normal; sometimes poor	Normal to slightly increased	Mo: Normal to slightly increased[b] PMN: Usually normal (often absent, sometimes increased)	Hydrarthrosis; degenerative joint disease; traumatic joint disease; neoplasia
Inflammatory arthropathy	Variable (yellow to off-white; muddy brown if also bloody)	Increased proportionally with amount of inflammation and hemorrhage	Variable; usually mildly to markedly decreased	Variable; fair to very poor	Increased (usually markedly)	Mo: Normal to increased[b] PMN: Increased	Infections; immune-mediated arthropathies; nonimmune-mediated inflammation (See Table 3)

Key:
Mo = Large mononuclear cells   PMN = Neutrophils
a - Differential may actually be similar to peripheral blood; possibly with platelets present.
b - With increased phagocytic activity.

In acute hemarthrosis, arthrocentesis yields bloody fluid from the time the sample first flows through the needle. Turbidity is directly proportional to, and the viscosity and mucin clot test tend to be inversely proportional to, the amount of hemorrhage present. Hemarthrosis elicits an inflammatory response. Within hours, erythrophagocytosis is evident and the neutrophil count is mildly increased. In longer-standing cases the fluid may have a xanthochromic supernatant. Lameness caused by hemarthrosis is usually acute in onset. There may or may not be a history of trauma to the joint. Recurrent hemarthrosis has been described in dogs with hemophilia A, and eventually resulted in chronic degenerative joint disease.[19] Thus, cytologically, chronic recurrent hemarthrosis may resemble nonpurulent arthropathies.

In cases of iatrogenic hemorrhage at collection, the synovial fluid usually is not bloody at the beginning of arthrocentesis. Thus the practitioner often notes admixture of blood at some stage during the procedure, frequently toward the end of collection. Blood contamination can be minimized by releasing the negative pressure on the syringe before withdrawing the needle from the joint space. Cytologically, often only a small amount of blood is present without erythrophagocytosis. Platelets may also be observed with recent hemorrhage (including blood contamination) (Fig 4).

Figure 6. Synovial fluid from a dog with degenerative arthropathy, showing 5 mononuclear cells, 1 lymphocyte and 4 macrophage-type cells. The latter cells exhibit absent to moderate phagocytic activity. (May-Grünwald-Giemsa stain, 1250X)

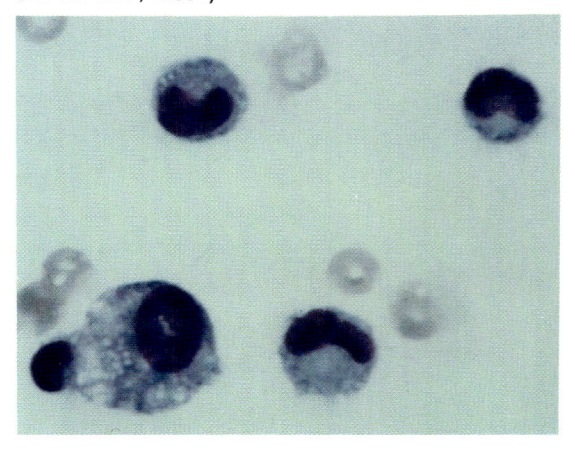

Hemorrhage associated with degenerative and inflammatory arthropathies is usually mild when compared to that in true hemarthrosis. Cytologically, erythrophagocytosis is usually apparent, together with changes characteristic of the underlying cause (Fig 5).

Degenerative Arthropathies

This category of disease usually results from trauma to a joint and/or degenerative changes of the articular surfaces. The latter may be idiopathic but is most often caused by acute or chronic trauma, which may result from accidental injury, congenital or acquired anatomic disorders that impose abnormal stresses on articular surfaces, metabolic and nutritional abnormalities, and neoplasia.[12-15] Diseases that may cause degenerative arthropathies include osteoarthritis (also called osteoarthrosis or "degenerative joint disease"), osteochondritis dissecans, elbow dysplasia, avascular necrosis of the femoral head, hip dysplasia, chronic patellar dislocations, and joint instabilities due to ligament damage (eg, rupture of the cranial cruciate ligament).[12-15]

General synovial fluid changes are outlined in Table 2. Cytologic findings may be abnormal before radiographic changes are readily apparent.[17] The volume of fluid present may vary from slightly to markedly increased.

Cytologic examination of the effusion may reveal a number of changes.[1,4,13-15,17] The total nucleated cell count is usually normal to slightly increased, with a marked predominance of large mononuclear cells, >10% of which are moderately to markedly vacuolated or phagocytic (Figs 6,7). Neutrophils are usually normal in number or absent, though in some cases their number may be somewhat increased. The total protein concentration is usually normal to slightly increased, and the fluid usually does not clot. Hemorrhage is usually minimal or absent. However, there may be superimposed acute bouts of mild inflammation and hemorrhage associated with capsular trauma. This causes a transient increase in neutrophil and RBC numbers. If damage to articular cartilage is severe enough, osteoclasts and chondrocytes may be seen in the sample (Fig 8). In equine synovial fluid samples, cytologic classification of cartilage fragments has been used to estimate the depth of articular damage.[20] This approach has not been reported for dogs and cats.

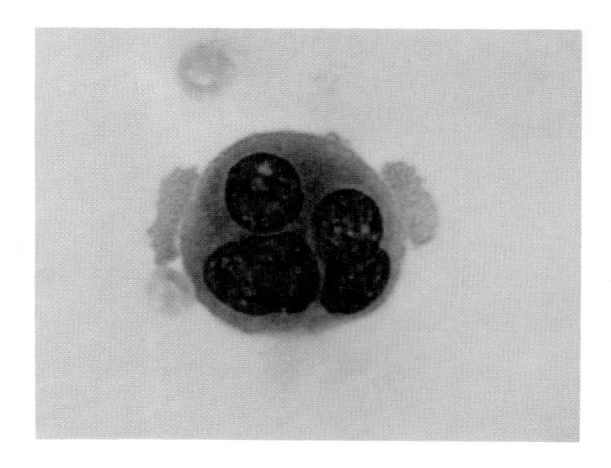

Figure 7. Synovial fluid from a dog with degenerative arthropathy. Note the leukophagocytic macrophage, indicating chronic inflammation. (May-Grünwald-Giemsa stain, 1250X)

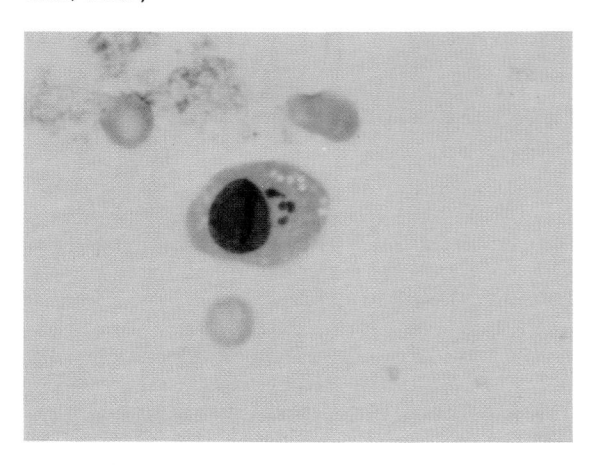

Neoplasia involving joint spaces is very rare.[13] Tumors can arise within joints, invade or erode joints from adjacent tissues, or metastasize to joints. Tumors that may affect the joints include synoviomas (synovial-cell tumors), chondrosarcomas, osteosarcomas, fibrosarcomas, bronchial carcinomas and lymphosarcomas.[13,14] Diagnosis is usually by the radiographic and clinical appearance, and biopsy of the lesion or mass. Cytologic examination of such biopsies is described in other chapters throughout this textbook. Synovial fluid changes *per se* are poorly described. The fluid could conceivably have characteristics of a degenerative or an inflammatory arthropathy. Neoplastic cells might be evident in these fluids. However, limited experience with synovial-cell tumors is discouraging in this regard, in that neoplastic cells were not evident in the synovial fluid of any of 3 such cases.[21]

Inflammatory Arthropathies

There are numerous causes of inflammatory arthropathies. Basically they can be divided into 2 groups: infectious and noninfectious (Table 3). Both are usually associated with an effusive exudate showing a moderate to marked increase in neutrophil numbers and variable increase in large mononuclear cell numbers, many of which are often vacuolated and/or phagocytic of debris. Concurrent, relatively mild hemorrhagic diapedesis is common. Other findings are listed in Table 2.

Essentially, the greater the inflammatory reaction, the more discolored and turbid the fluid, and the poorer the viscosity. Mucin clot test results often parallel sample viscosity. The total protein concentration is increased and the sample readily clots. Fibrin strands often cause clumping of inflammatory cells in the smear. If not apparent on a routinely stained smear, fibrin strands may be demonstrated by staining with new methylene blue (Fig 9).

Infectious Arthritides

Infectious arthritides in dogs and cats are uncommon, but when they occur they are usually of bacterial origin.[13,15] Associated lameness is characteristically nonshifting and involves 1 or more joints. As a generalization, most infectious arthritides in mature animals are monoarticular and probably result from puncture wounds. Polyarticular infectious arthritides, though less common, may occur following hematogenous spread of organisms, as in navel ill in neonates and bacterial endocarditis in more mature animals. Clinical signs characteristic of such diseases should be apparent on physical examination. In contrast, noninfectious inflammatory arthropathies are seldom truly monoarticular. Though only 1 joint may be clinically involved at any one time, arthrocentesis of several joints often reveals the polyarticular nature of these disorders.

Synovial fluid changes are outlined above. Cell morphology is variable. Most neutrophils are usually intact; however, karyolysis or pyknosis and karyorrhexis may be evident. Karyolytic degeneration of cells suggests that a joint

Figure 8. Synovial fluid from a dog with degenerative arthropathy. Note the osteoclast, which indicates articular cartilage erosion to subchondral bone. (May-Grünwald-Giemsa stain, 1250X)

Figure 9. Synovial fluid from a dog with degenerative arthropathy. Note the large clump of fibrin with enmeshed cells. This is more often seen in inflammatory arthropathies. (May-Grünwald-Giemsa stain, 500X)

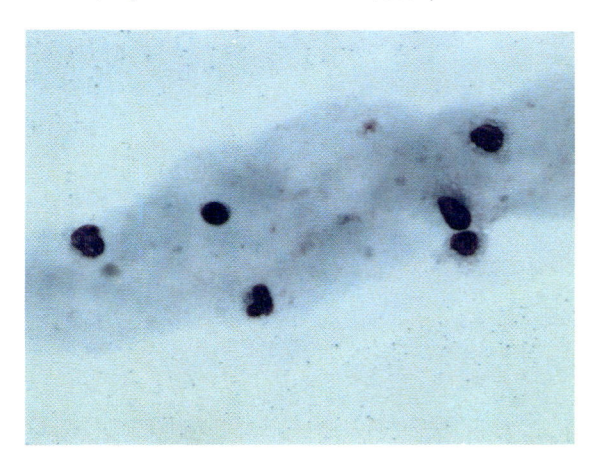

is septic. However, this change is not common, and organisms are frequently not observed in synovial fluid smears. When septic arthritis is a possibility, joint fluid and, if possible, a biopsy of synovial membrane should be cultured. Organisms commonly involved include coliforms, *Corynebacterium*, *Erysipelothrix*, *Pasteurella*, *Salmonella*, staphylococci and streptococci.[15] Failure to isolate organisms on culture does not necessarily exclude a bacterial cause.

Mycoplasmal arthritis is rare in dogs and cats.[13,15] The inflammatory reaction is purulent, typically with good cell morphology. Organisms may be observed on Romanowsky-stained smears or on mycoplasmal culture.

Fungal arthritides caused by *Blastomyces dermatitidis*, *Coccidioides immitis*, *Cryptococcus neoformans* and *Sporothrix schenckii* have been reported rarely in dogs.[13] Synovial fluid changes were not included in the original reports. Presumably, the organisms might be visible in synovial fluid of such cases.

Protozoal arthritides have been reported in dogs. *Leishmania donovani* has been demonstrated in macrophages in synovial fluid of a few dogs with visceral leishmaniasis.[22] Based on microscopic examination of synovial fluid smears, nucleated cell count and cell distribution were considered normal. Based on cytologic examination of tissue aspirates, other tissues, namely lymph node and bone marrow, were also infected by the protozoan, as is more usually the case (see Chapter 2).

Polyarthritis has recently been associated with *Ehrlichia* infections in dogs from Missouri, Tennessee and Oklahoma.[23-25] The species of *Ehrlichia* involved has not been definitively determined but it is serologically more closely related to *E canis* than *E equi*. Synovial fluid samples have markedly increased cellularity, most of which is attributable to neutrophils (60-80% of nucleated cells). *Ehrlichia* morulae are present in only about 1-2% of neutrophils in synovial fluid and sometimes in 1-2% of neutrophils in peripheral blood (Fig 10).

Viral arthritis has not been convincingly demonstrated in dogs or cats.[13,15] Feline calicivirus infection has been associated with lameness in kittens. However, synovial fluid changes in experimental infections were minimal. Synovial fluid macrophage numbers were subjectively increased to a moderate degree, and some exhibited leukophagocytosis.[26]

Noninfectious Inflammatory Arthropathies

The noninfectious inflammatory arthropathies are a heterogeneous group of diseases from clinical, clinicopathologic (especially with respect to hematologic and biochemical findings) and radiographic viewpoints.[12,13,15,16,18,27-32] Diagnostically they can be subgrouped into immune-mediated and nonimmune-mediated causes.[14] Further subclassification varies among authors; one approach is outlined in Table 3. Differential diagnosis of these diseases is achieved by various

Figure 10. Synovial fluid from a dog with ehrlichial polyarthritis. Note the *Ehrlichia* morula in neutrophil and normal granular, eosinophilic proteinaceous background. (Wright's stain, 1250X) (Courtesy of Dr. R.L. Cowell, Oklahoma State University)

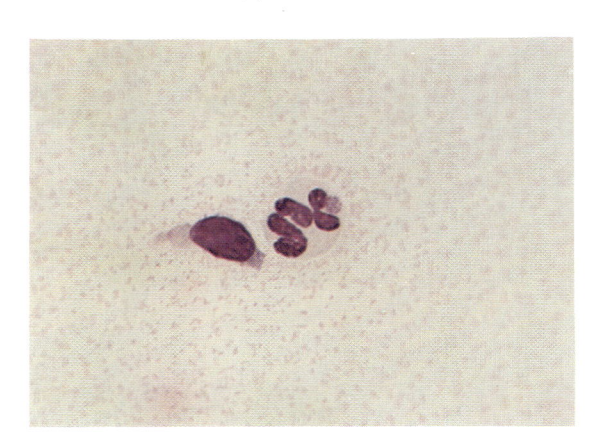

Table 3. Subclassifications of noninfectious inflammatory arthropathies and their more important diagnostic features.

Category	Subgroups[a]	Salient Features
Immune-mediated	**Erosive Arthritides**	*Radiography*: characteristic erosive arthropathy.
	Rheumatoid arthritis (dog)[12,16,18,25,27]	Probably RF positive; usually negative on LE prep and ANA titer.
	Polyarthritis of Greyhounds[16]	Characteristic breed.
	Chronic progressive polyarthritis (cat)[16]	A variant form of chronic progressive polyarthritis, less common.
	Proliferative Arthritis	*Radiography*: Periosteal osseous proliferation, leading to ankylosis (especially carpi and tarsi).
	Chronic progressive polyarthritis (cat)[16]	Associated with feline syncytial virus and often FeLV infections.
	Nonerosive Arthritis[b]	*Radiography*: Not as in erosive arthritides or proliferative arthritis.
	Systemic lupus erythematosus[18,29,30]	Positive LE prep and ANA titer; by definition, it is a multisystemic disease.[c]
	Polyarthritis/polymyositis syndrome[31]	Negative LE prep and ANA titer. Muscle soreness; biopsy shows polymyositis. CPK activity normal to increased.
	Idiopathic polyarthritis[18,32]	Not as in SLE or polyarthritis/polymyositis. Probably an "immune-complex" arthropathy (synovitis).
	Type I: "Uncomplicated"	No evidence for Types II, III or IV.
	Type II: Concurrent infection elsewhere in the body	Especially infections involving the respiratory and urinary systems. Arthritis associated with RMSF may fit into this classification.
	Type III: Concurrent gastrointestinal disease	For example: Gastroenteritis, ulcerative colitis and unspecified diarrhea.
	Type IV: Concurrent neoplasia elsewhere in the body	Associated with various malignancies; remote from affected joints.
	Drug-associated	Decribed in Doberman pinschers and Weimaraners on repeated courses of sulfa-trimethoprim preparations.[34-36] May have other tissues involved also.
Nonimmune-mediated	**Crystal-induced**	Very uncommon in dogs and cats.[14]
	Chronic hemarthrosis	Especially hemophilia A.[19]

Key:
a - Styled from references 13 and 14.
b - Polyarthritis nodosa is in this group[14] and is probably best categorized as a type-1 idiopathic polyarthritis
c - Investigate immune-mediated: hemolytic anemia, leukopenia, thrombocytopenia, dermatitis, glomerulonephritis, polymyositis and pleuritis.
RF = Rheumatoid factor   LE prep = Lupus erythematosus cell preparation
ANA = Antinuclear antibody   RMSF = Rocky Mountain spotted fever.

Figure 11. Synovial fluid from a dog with systemic lupus erythematosus and resultant immune-mediated polyarthritis. Note the LE cell. (Wright's stain, 1650X) (Courtesy of Dr. R.L. Cowell, Oklahoma State University.)

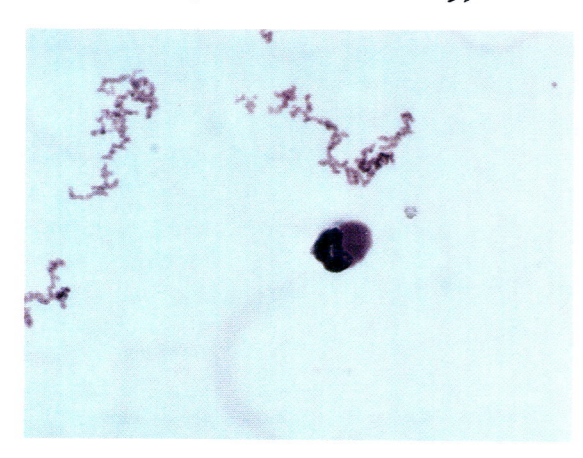

clinicopathologic tests and radiography (Table 3).

As a generalization, lameness from noninfectious inflammatory arthropathies is polyarticular and frequently of a shifting nature. The clinical picture was compared to that in infectious arthritides above.

Synovial fluid changes in this group of diseases are fairly uniform and usually indistinguishable from each other. They may also be difficult to distinguish from septic arthropathies in some cases, unless cytologic and microbiologic examinations establish the latter diagnosis.

Nucleated cell counts in noninfectious inflammatory arthropathies tend to be markedly increased.[18,27-32] Neutrophils are usually the predominant cell type, ranging from about 40% to 100% of nucleated cells (average 80%). The remaining cells are large and small mononuclear cells.

Three noninfectious inflammatory arthropathies may be distinguishable cytologically.

Systemic Lupus Erythematosus: Lupus erythematosus (LE) cells may be seen in synovial fluid of some dogs with systemic lupus erythematosus (SLE) (Fig 11).[37] They are diagnostic for the disease when present; however, they must not be confused with leukophagocytic macrophages (Fig 7) or neutrophils containing particulate nucleic acid (Fig 12). The latter have been referred to as ragocytes.[37] However, the term ragocyte is more correctly used to refer to neutrophils with numerous small dark intracytoplasmic granules observed on unstained wet preparations, not on stained smears.[1] These granules are phagocytosed immunoglobulins and complement. To avoid confusion, it is simpler to describe the neutrophils' contents observed on a stained smear and avoid attaching a noncontributory and possibly misleading name.

Canine Plasmacytic-Lymphocytic Synovitis:[14] This condition may be a variant of rheumatoid arthritis; however, it is minimally erosive and proliferative and thus does not fit neatly into any of the subgroups listed in Table 3. Cytologic examination reveals a moderate to marked increase in cell numbers (5000-20,000/μl), with 10-40% neutrophils. Most of the remaining cells are lymphoid cells.

Idiopathic Eosinophilic Polyarthritis: A case of eosinophilic polyarthritis was described in a Great Dane bitch.[38] Synovial fluid total cell counts were mildly increased (3800-5300/μl), with 20-52% eosinophils, 5-48% neutrophils, 20-75% mononuclear cells, and markedly increased phagocytic activity. No cause was discovered; however, the dog responded to treatment with antiinflammatory drugs. The pathogenesis was postulated to be immune-mediated.

Charts 1 and 2 present algorithms of diagnostic approaches to interpretation of synovial fluid examination.

Figure 12. Synovial fluid from a dog with immune-mediated polyarthritis. Note the neutrophil containing phagocytosed material, probably nucleic acid. This material must be distinguished from bacteria. This dog was negative on an LE preparation, positive on antinuclear antibody assay and rheumatoid factor assay. Culture of synovial membrane and fluid was unproductive. Stain precipitate is present in the right of the photograph. (May-Grünwald-Giemsa stain, 1250X)

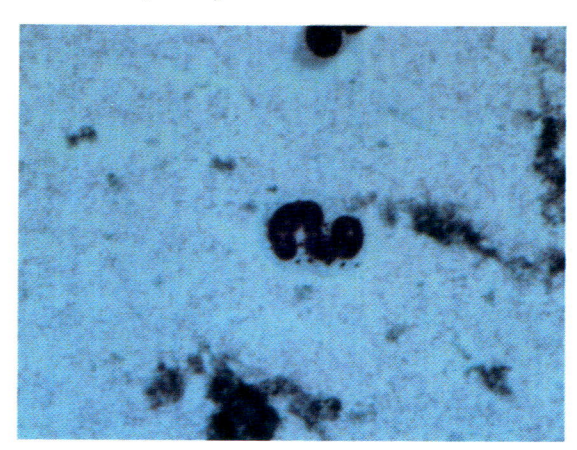

Chapter 10

Chart 1. Initial diagnostic plan for evaluation of synovial fluid. Is the sample bloody? Hemorrhage into synovial fluid may be a primary problem or secondary to degenerative or inflammatory arthropathies.

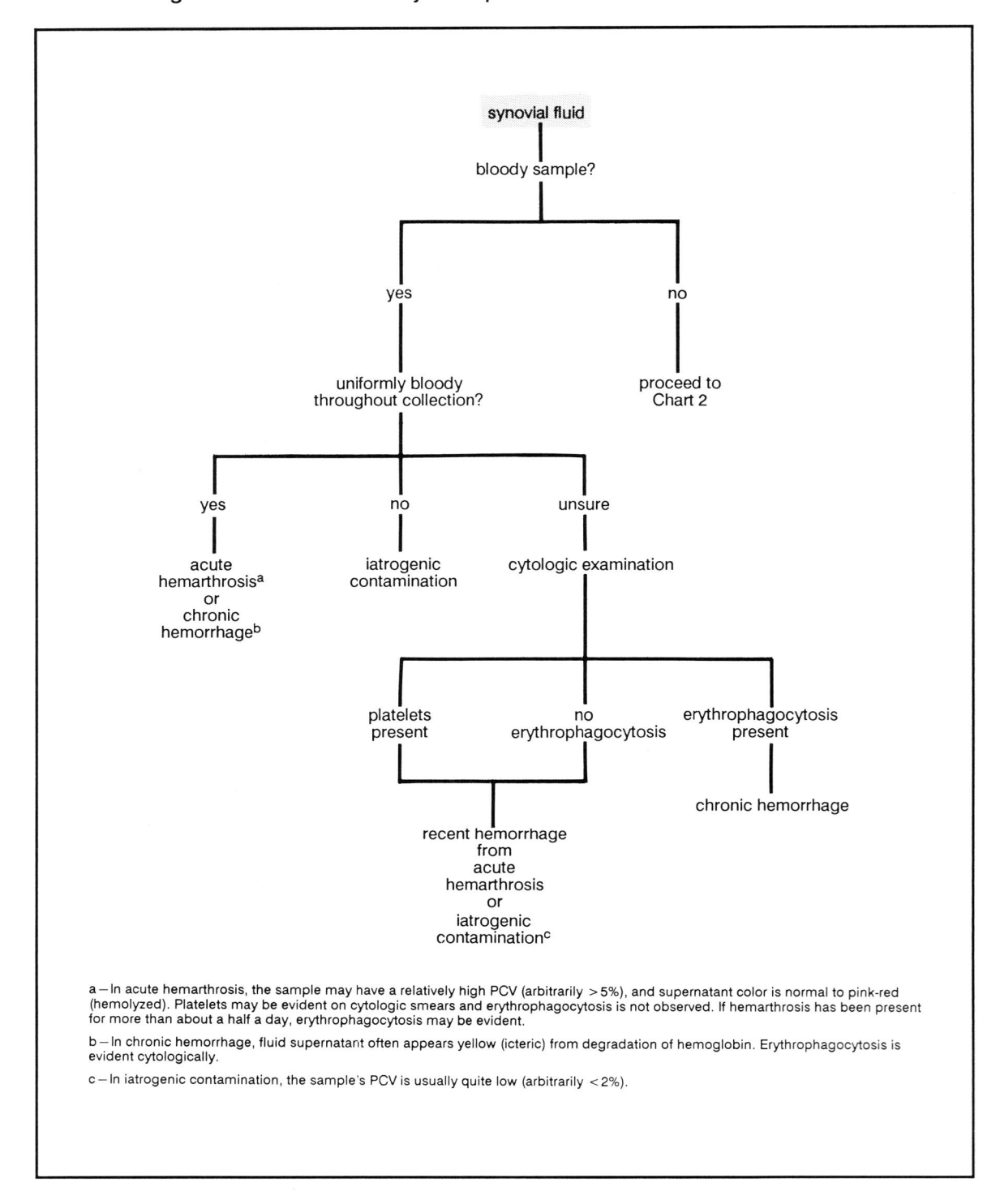

```
                        synovial fluid
                             │
                       bloody sample?
                      ┌──────┴──────┐
                     yes             no
                      │              │
              uniformly bloody   proceed to
          throughout collection?   Chart 2
              ┌───────┼───────┐
             yes      no    unsure
              │       │       │
           acute  iatrogenic  cytologic
        hemarthrosisᵃ contamination examination
             or                     │
          chronic          ┌────────┼────────┐
         hemorrhageᵇ   platelets   no     erythrophagocytosis
                       present  erythrophagocytosis  present
                           └─────────┬─────────┘        │
                                     │           chronic hemorrhage
                              recent hemorrhage
                                   from
                                  acute
                               hemarthrosis
                                    or
                               iatrogenic
                              contaminationᶜ
```

a — In acute hemarthrosis, the sample may have a relatively high PCV (arbitrarily >5%), and supernatant color is normal to pink-red (hemolyzed). Platelets may be evident on cytologic smears and erythrophagocytosis is not observed. If hemarthrosis has been present for more than about a half a day, erythrophagocytosis may be evident.

b — In chronic hemorrhage, fluid supernatant often appears yellow (icteric) from degradation of hemoglobin. Erythrophagocytosis is evident cytologically.

c — In iatrogenic contamination, the sample's PCV is usually quite low (arbitrarily <2%).

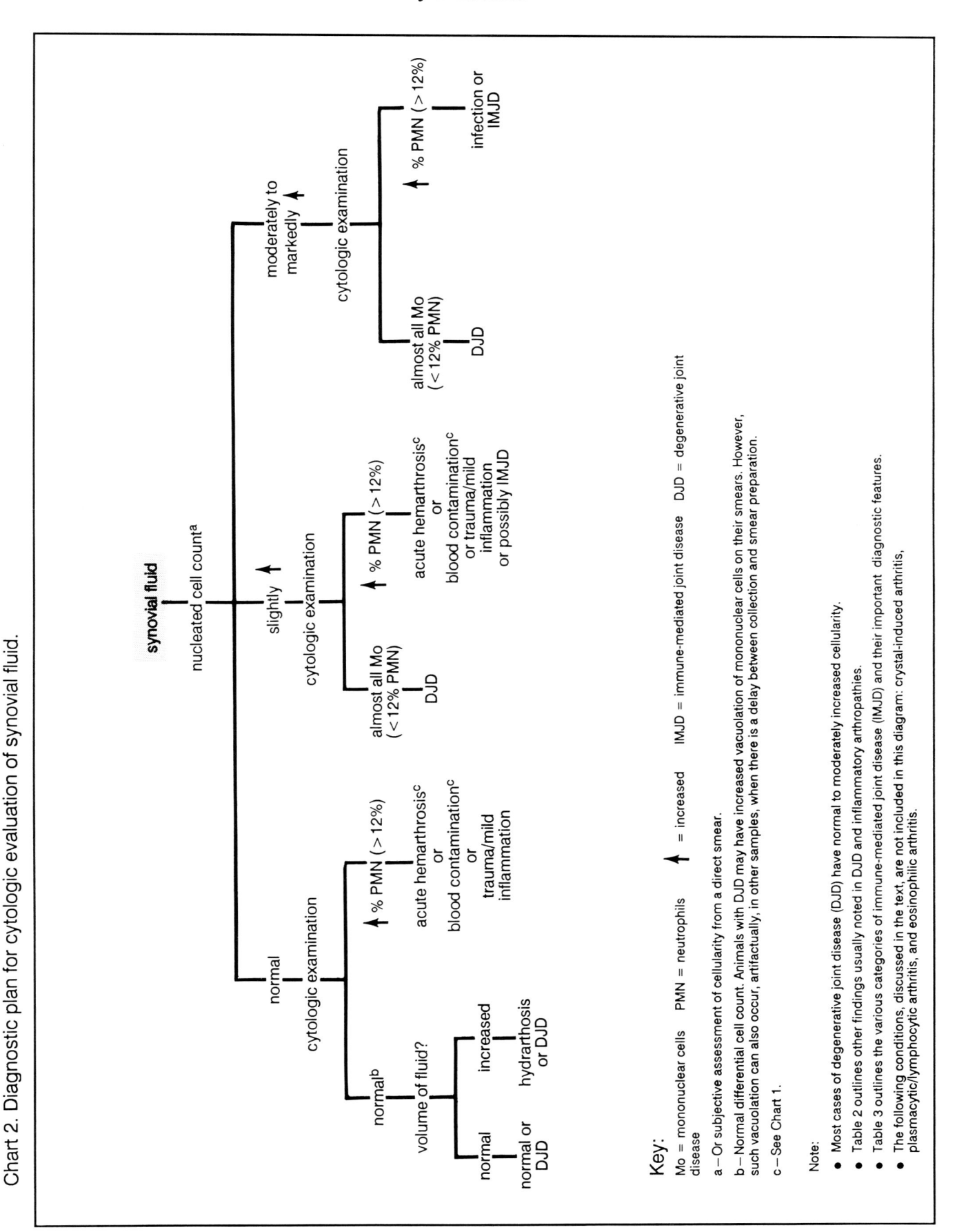

Chart 2. Diagnostic plan for cytologic evaluation of synovial fluid.

synovial fluid
→ nucleated cell count[a]

normal → cytologic examination
- volume of fluid?[b]
  - normal → normal or DJD
  - increased → hydrarthosis or DJD
- ↑ % PMN (>12%) → acute hemarthrosis[c] or blood contamination[c] or trauma/mild inflammation

slightly ↑ → cytologic examination
- almost all Mo (<12% PMN) → DJD
- ↑ % PMN (>12%) → acute hemarthrosis[c] or blood contamination[c] or trauma/mild inflammation or possibly IMJD

moderately to markedly ↑ → cytologic examination
- almost all Mo (<12% PMN) → DJD
- ↑ % PMN (>12%) → infection or IMJD

Key:
Mo = mononuclear cells   PMN = neutrophils   ↑ = increased   IMJD = immune-mediated joint disease   DJD = degenerative joint disease

a – Or subjective assessment of cellularity from a direct smear.
b – Normal differential cell count. Animals with DJD may have increased vacuolation of mononuclear cells on their smears. However, such vacuolation can also occur, artifactually, in other samples, when there is a delay between collection and smear preparation.
c – See Chart 1.

Note:
- Most cases of degenerative joint disease (DJD) have normal to moderately increased cellularity.
- Table 2 outlines other findings usually noted in DJD and inflammatory arthropathies.
- Table 3 outlines the various categories of immune-mediated joint disease (IMJD) and their important diagnostic features.
- The following conditions, discussed in the text, are not included in this diagram: crystal-induced arthritis, plasmacytic/lymphocytic arthritis, and eosinophilic arthritis.

References

1. Perman, in Kaneko: *Clinical Biochemistry of Domestic Animals*. 3rd ed. Academic Press, Orlando, FL, 1980. pp 749-783.

2. Hardy and Wallace: Arthrocentesis and synovial membrane biopsy. *Vet Clin No Am* 4:449-462, 1974.

3. Fernandez et al: Synovial fluid analysis: preparation of smears for cytologic examination of canine synovial fluid. *JAAHA* 19:727-734, 1983.

4. Sawyer: Synovial fluid analysis of canine joints. *JAVMA* 143:609-612, 1963.

5. Atilola et al: Intra-articular tissue response to analytical grade metrizamide in dogs. *Am J Vet Res* 45:2651-2657, 1984.

6. Rowley et al: Quantitation of hyaluronic acid in equine synovia. *Am J Vet Res* 43:1096-1099, 1982.

7. Warren et al: The significance of cellular variations occurring in normal synovial fluid. *Am J Path* 11:953-968, 1935.

8. McCarty et al: Crystal-induced inflammation in canine joints: An experimental model with quantitation of the host response. *J Exp Med* 124:99-114, 1966.

9. Atilola et al: A comparison of manual and electronic counting for total nucleated cell counts on synovial fluid from canine stifle joints. *Can J Vet Res* 50:282-284, 1986.

10. Palmer: Total leukocyte enumeration in pathologic synovial fluid. *Am J Clin Path* 49:812-814, 1968.

11. Maldonado et al: Synovial aldehyde groups in equine joint disease. *Equine Vet J* 15:168-169, 1983.

12. McKeown and Archibald, in Catcott: *Canine Medicine*. 4th ed. American Veterinary Publications, Santa Barbara, 1979. pp 533-678.

13. Bennett, in Chandler et al: *Canine Medicine and Therapeutics*. 2nd ed. Blackwell, Oxford, 1984. pp 167-205.

14. Pedersen et al, in Ettinger: *Textbook of Veterinary Internal Medicine*. 2nd ed. Saunders, Philadelphia, 1983. pp 2187-2235.

15. Arnoczky and Lipowitz, in Slatter: *Textbook of Small Animal Surgery*. Saunders, Philadelphia, 1985. pp 2295-2302.

16. Lipowitz, in Slatter: *Textbook of Small Animal Surgery*. Saunders, Philadelphia, 1985. pp 2302-2311.

17. Lewis et al: A comparison of diagnostic methods used in the evaluation of early degenerative joint disease in the dog. *JAAHA* 23:305-315, 1987.

18. Pedersen et al: Noninfectious canine arthritis: the inflammatory, nonerosive arthritides. *JAVMA* 169:304-310, 1976.

19. Hall: *Blood Coagulation and Its Disorders in the Dog*. Bailliere Tindall, London, 1972. pp 34-53.

20. Tew and Hackett. Identification of cartilage wear fragments in synovial fluid from equine joints. *Arthr Rheum* 24:1419-1424, 1981.

21. Cowell, Oklahoma State University, and Parry, University of Melbourne: Unpublished data, 1988.

22. Yamaguchi et al: *Leishmania donovani* in the synovial fluid of a dog with visceral leishmaniasis. *JAAHA* 19:723-726, 1983.

23. Stockham et al: Canine granulocytic ehrlichiosis in dogs from central Missouri: a possible cause of polyarthritis. *Vet Med Rev* 6:3-5, 1985.

24. Bellah et al: *Ehrlichia canis*-related polyarthritis in a dog. *JAVMA* 189:922-923, 1986.

25. Cowell et al: Canine ehrlichiosis and polyarthritis in 3 dogs. Manuscript in preparation, 1989.

26. Pedersen et al: A transient febrile "limping" syndrome of kittens caused by two different strains of feline calicivirus. *Feline Pract* 13(1):26-35, 1983.

27. Pedersen et al: Non-infectious canine arthritis: Rheumatoid arthritis. *JAVMA* 169:295-303, 1976.

28. Bennett: Immune-based erosive joint disease of the dog. 1. Clinical, radiological and laboratory investigations. *J Small Anim Pract* 28:779-797, 1987.

29. Bennett: Immune-based non-erosive inflammatory joint disease of the dog. 1. Canine systemic lupus erythematosus. *J Small Anim Pract* 28:871-889, 1987.

30. Grindem and Johnson: Systemic lupus erythematosus: Literature review and report of 42 new canine cases. *JAAHA* 19:489-503, 1983.

31. Bennett and Kelly: Immune-based non-erosive inflammatory joint disease of the dog. 2. Polyarthritis/polymyositis syndrome. *J Small Anim Pract* 28:891-908, 1987.

32. Bennett: Immune-based non-erosive inflammatory joint disease of the dog. 3. Canine idiopathic polyarthritis. *J Small Anim Pract* 28:909-928, 1987.

33. Greene and Philip, in Greene: *Clinical Microbiology and Infectious Diseases of the Dog and Cat*. Saunders, Philadelphia, 1984. pp 562-575.

34. Werner and Bright: Drug-induced immune hypersensitivity disorders in two dogs treated with trimethoprim sulfadiazine: Case reports and drug challenge studies. *JAAHA* 19:783-790, 1983.

35. Harvey: Possible sulphadiazine-trimethoprim induced polyarthritis. *Vet Record* 120:537, 1987.

36. Whur: Possible trimethoprim-sulphonamide induced polyarthritis. *Vet Record* 121:91, 1987.

37. Miller et al: Synovial fluid analysis in canine arthritis. *JAAHA* 10:392-398, 1974.

38. Christopher and Wallace: Synovial fluid eosinophilia: a case report in a dog and review of the literature. *Vet Clin Path* 15(2):25-31, 1986.

11

The Musculoskeletal System

E.A. Mahaffey

Though cytologic techniques have not been used extensively in evaluating diseases of the musculoskeletal system, they can be valuable aids in the diagnosis of certain important diseases affecting this system. One perhaps would suspect that muscle, being a soft tissue, would be a more productive tissue for cytologic examination than bone. In fact, the opposite is true. Diseases of bone yield diagnostic cytology specimens more commonly than do diseases of muscle. Reasons for this difference are several:

Inflammatory and neoplastic lesions lend themselves to cytologic diagnosis, while degenerative diseases do not. There are relatively few clinically important inflammatory and neoplastic diseases of muscle in comparison to those affecting bone.

Aspirates and imprints of muscle tissue typically yield only blood. Striated muscle cells do not exfoliate readily, and inflammatory diseases of muscle, when they occur, are often characterized by modest infiltration of inflammatory cells.

Though healthy bone tissue is difficult to sample and contains few cells and abundant matrix, both inflammatory and neoplastic bone diseases are often acccompanied by bone lysis and increased cellularity. Both lytic and proliferative bone lesions are often easily aspirated.

Sample Collection

Collection of material from bone lesions for cytologic examination can be complicated by the hardness of cortical bone. Lesions with a major soft tissue component can be aspirated by techniques similar to those applicable to any soft tissue mass (see Chapter 1). Even heavily mineralized masses often can be aspirated with a fine needle by careful palpation and exploration of the lesion's surface with a needle. Radiographs may reveal portions of the lesion that are less heavily mineralized and more likely to produce useful aspirates.

Some lesions in which cortical bone remains intact will not yield to fine-needle aspiration. In such instances, the best way to obtain diagnostic material is to use a trephine to obtain a core biopsy specimen. Imprints can be made for cytologic evaluation before fixing the specimen in formalin for histologic processing.

Cytologic specimens from skeletal muscle lesions can be collected by methods similar to those used for dermal and subcutaneous masses. These techniques are described in Chapter 1.

Cytologic Findings

Inflammatory Diseases

Inflammatory lesions of the skeleton are important causes of disease in domestic animals, and cytologic exmination can be valuable in identifying certain of these lesions. Cytologic specimens from inflammatory lesions of bone are generally similar to exudates from other organs. Neutrophils typically predominate in specimens from animals with osteomyelitis, though epithelioid cells (activated macrophages) and multinucleate giant cells are a significant component of some exudates. The appearance of epithelioid cells and multinucleate giant cells in cytologic preparations is described in Chapter 1.

Inflammatory lesions accompanied by new bone proliferation may yield cytologic specimens also containing small numbers of os-

Figure 1. Neutrophils, a macrophage, and cells interpreted as osteoblasts from an animal with osteomyelitis.

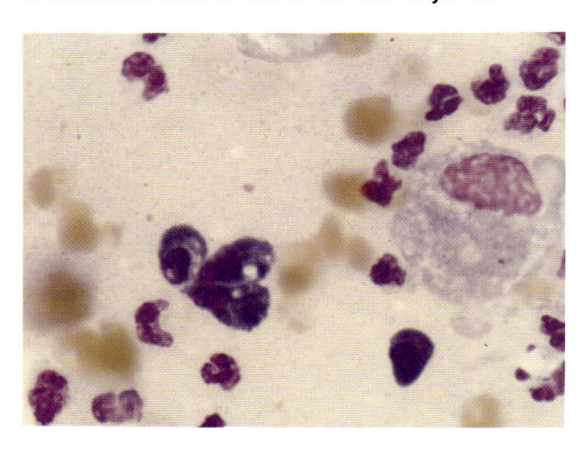

teoblasts (Fig 1). Those cells are typically ovoid to plump and fusiform, with round to ovoid eccentric nuclei and dark-blue cytoplasm. They differ from neoplastic osteoblasts in that they are smaller and more uniform, and lack nuclear manifestations of malignancy (see Chapter 1).

Osteoclasts may also be found in small numbers in specimens from inflammatory lesions. These cells resemble multinucleate giant cells and arise from precursor cells of the monocyte/macrophage cell line. They are very large and irregularly shaped, with variable numbers (typically 6-10) of uniform round nuclei arranged randomly in the cell and abundant light-blue cytoplasm.

Some specific infectious agents causing osteomyelitis may be identified in cytologic preparations. *Actinomyces* spp (Plate 3), a common cause of mandibular osteomyelitis in ruminants, occasionally cause osteomylelitis in dogs. These organisms appear as branching filamentous rods that cannot be distinguished from *Nocardia* on Romanowsky-stained slides. Neutrophils predominate in aspirates from actinomycotic lesions as well as in aspirates from other types of bacterial osteomyelitis. Bacterial cocci (Plate 3) in such aspirates indicate infection by *Staphylococcus* or *Streptococcus*, while bipolar rods (Plate 3) are typical of infection by Gram-negative organisms.

Osteomyelitis is also a relatively common manifestation of coccidioidomycosis (Plate 5), and the organisms may be detected in exudate. The exudate in coccidioidomycosis typically is more mixed than that of bacterial infections. The exudate from *Coccidioides immitis* infections contains a much larger component of activated macrophages and multinucleate giant cells. Other fungal organisms, including *Blastomyces dermatitidis* (Plate 4) and *Histoplasma capsulatum* (Plate 4), may produce osteomyelitis with a similar exudate.

Neoplastic Diseases

Neoplasms of bone are relatively common in domestic animals, and cytologic examination is useful in establishing the diagnosis in some of these diseases. As with interpretation of histologic sections of bone, evaluation of cytologic specimens from bone requires knowledge of the clinical and radiographic features of a specific lesion. Cytologic examination is probably more useful in distinguishing inflammatory bone disease from neoplasia than in identifying specific bone tumors; however, osteosarcomas and chondrosarcomas have characteristic cytologic features that can aid in diagnosing those tumors.

Osteosarcoma: Aspirates of osteosarcomas are often more highly cellular than aspirates of soft tissue sarcomas. Cells may occur singly or in clusters. One characteristic feature that may be evident on low-power examination of the slide is islands of osteoid surrounded by tumor cells (Fig 2).[1,2] Osteoid (Fig 2) appears as somewhat fibrillar bright-pink material on Wright's-stained slides. These structures are not found in most aspirates from osteosarcomas; however, when found, their presence provides strong evidence that a tumor is of bone origin.

Figure 2. Osteoblasts bordering an island of pink-staining osteoid from an osteosarcoma.

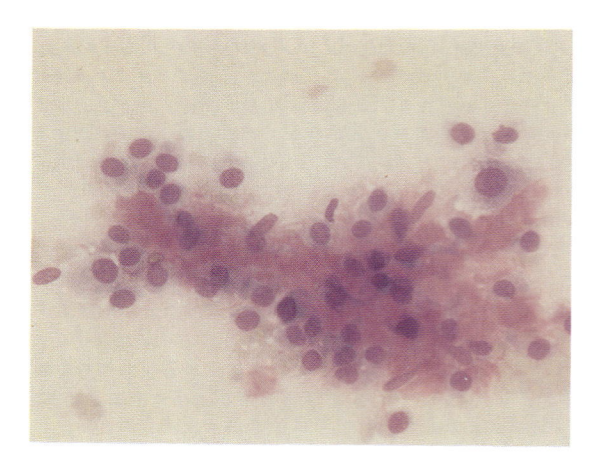

Individual tumor cells vary from round to plump and spindle-shaped, and often vary greatly in size (Fig 3). They often have many of the classic cytologic features of neoplasia, such as karyomegaly, anisokaryosis, large nucleoli and multiple nucleoli differing in size (see Chapter 1 for further discussion). Cytoplasm is typically dark blue and may contain several clear vacuoles (Fig 3). Some cells from most osteosarcomas contain scattered pink cytoplasmic granules (Fig 4). These granules are not specific for osteosarcomas; similar granules may also occur in cells from chondrosarcomas and, less commonly, from fibrosaracomas. Small numbers of inflammatory cells and nonneoplastic osteoblasts and osteoclasts similar to those described above in the section on inflammation may also be found in aspirates from osteosarcomas.

Chondrosarcoma: These tumors are the second most common sarcomas of bone. The ribs, turbinates and pelvis are the most common sites for chondrosarcomas of dogs, while the scapulae, vertebrae and ribs are more common sites in cats.[3] One useful cytologic feature of chondrosarcomas that may be evident on low-power examination of aspirates is lakes of bright pink, smooth or slightly granular material in which cells may be embedded (Fig 5). This material is the intercellular matrix of cartilage, sometimes called "chondroid."[2] Though this material suggests the possibility of cartilagenous origin of a tumor, it is not a consistent finding in aspirates of chondrosarcomas.

Individual chondroblasts from chondrosarcomas have cytologic features similar to those

Figure 3. Aspirate of an osteosarcoma showing marked variation in cell size and shape.

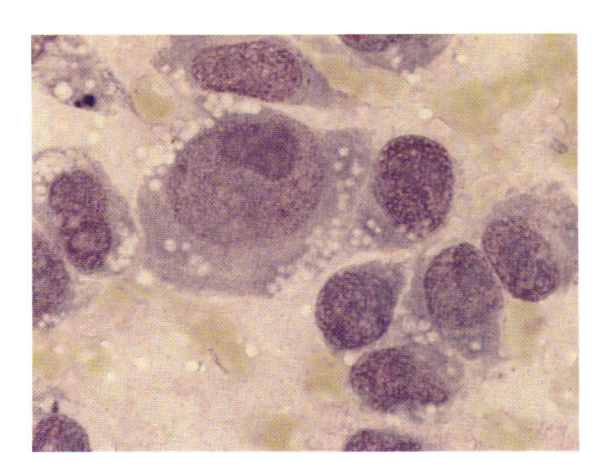

Figure 4. Cell from an osteosarcoma with vacuolated cytoplasm and fine pink cytoplasmic granules.

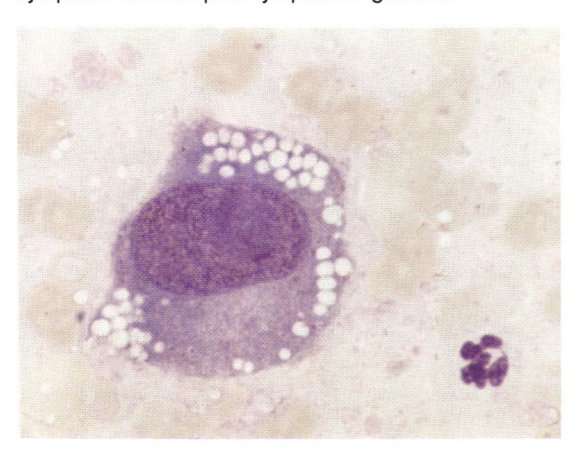

of osteosarcoma cells. They vary from round to fusiform, with large nuclei and dark-blue cytoplasm (Fig 6). Anisokaryosis is prominent, and multinucleate tumor cells may be found. Cytoplasm often contains several small clear vacuoles, and occasional cells may contain fine pink cytoplasmic granules similar to those seen in cells from osteosarcomas. If the tumor is causing bone lysis, osteoclasts may also be found in cytologic specimens. Even though it is not always possible to distinguish chondrosarcomas from osteosarcomas in cytologic specimens, characterization of the lesion as neoplastic is often clinically important.

Other Bone Neoplasms: Among other neoplasms arising with some frequency in bone are fibrosarcomas and hemangiosarcomas. Cytologic features of these tumors are similar to those of the same tumors when they occur in soft tissues. Metastatic tumors may also be manifested clinically as bone tumors; carcinomas exhibit this behavior most commonly (Plate 6). See Chapters 1 and 2 for a further discussion of carcinomas. The cytologic features of metastatic neoplastic cells are similar to those of the soft tissue tumors from which they originated.

Most hematopoietic neoplasms involving bone marrow are not manifested clinically as bone tumors. One major exception is the plasma-cell myeloma (Fig 7), which may show radiographic manifestations of bone lysis. Aspirates of lytic lesions may yield sheets of neoplastic plasma cells. Bone marrow aspirates from nonlytic areas often yield increased numbers of plasma cells, but do not

Chapter 11

Figure 5. Low-power view of an aspirate from a chondrosarcoma showing tumor cells surrounded by pink matrix material resembling mucus.

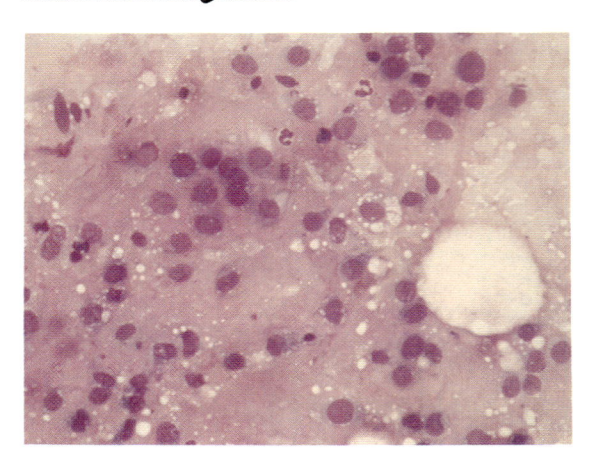

Figure 7. Sheet of neoplastic plasma cells from a lytic bone lesion in a dog with plasma-cell myeloma. (Courtesy of Dr. R.L. Cowell, Oklahoma State University)

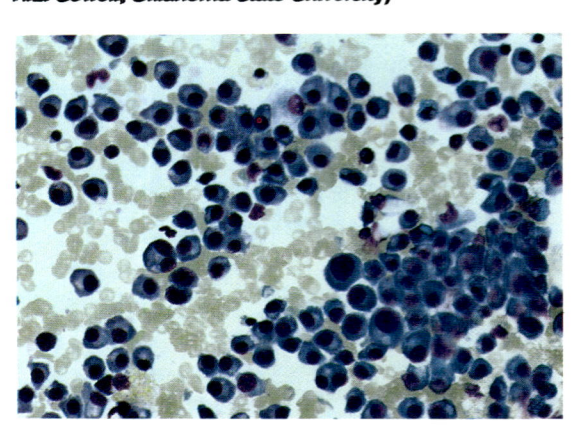

provide sufficient evidence for definitive diagnosis of plasma-cell myeloma.

Skeletal Muscle Tumors: Primary skeletal muscle tumors, rhabdomyomas and rhabdomyosarcomas, occur rarely. The cytologic features of one feline subcutaneous rhabdomyosarcoma have been described.[4] An aspirate from that tumor consisted of a pleomorphic population of connective tissue cells, including unusual multinucleate forms with long cytoplasmic projections. Among the more common tumors that appear to originate in skeletal muscle are lipomas, fibrosarcomas and malignant fibrous histiocytomas. While most of these tumors probably arise in the subcutis, they may infiltrate underlying muscle so extensively that they appear as muscle tumors on presentation. Their cytologic features are described in Chapter 2.

Figure 6. Aspirate of a chondrosarcoma with pleomorphic connective tissue cells including one cell in mitosis.

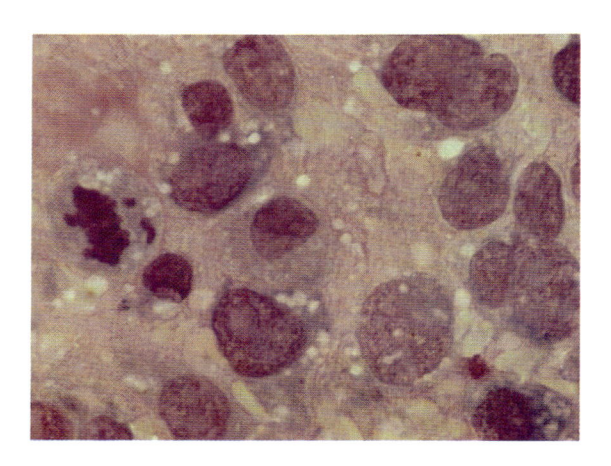

References

1. Rebar: *Handbook of Veterinary Cytology.* Ralston Purina, St Louis, 1978. pp 37-50.

2. Willems, in Linsk and Franzen: *Clinical Aspiration Cytology.* Lippincott, New York, 1983. pp 349-359.

3. Pool, in Moulton: *Tumors in Domestic Animals.* Univ Calif Press, Berkeley, 1978. pp 89-149.

4. Perman *et al*: *Cytology of the Dog and Cat.* American Animal Hospital Association, Denver, CO, 1979. pp 92-93.

12

Cerebrospinal Fluid

D. Brobst and G. Bryan

Diseases of the central nervous system (CNS) are often a diagnostic problem for the clinician. Careful, systematic physical and neurologic examination of the patient and elucidation of the history are necessary and useful, but may be inadequate for accurate diagnosis and prognosis. The clinician generally finds that other procedures and techniques must be employed to identify the etiology of CNS disorders.

Neurologic examination may reveal brain or spinal cord disease. A logical means of determining the cause of the disease is to evaluate the cerebrospinal fluid (CSF) filling the spaces within and around the CNS. Alterations in CSF composition often occur in CNS disease, especially if the involved area is in contact with the CSF spaces.

Lesions involving the CNS do not consistently or uniformly cause changes in the CSF. Alterations of CSF probably depend more on the location and extent of the CNS lesion than on cellular abnormalities. Thus, disease of the meninges produces greater alterations in CSF than do most diseases of CNS parenchymal tissue. Septic meningitis may cause suppuration within the CSF; inflammatory cells may be numerous (several thousand/μl), and levels of exudative protein markedly increased. In contrast, viral diseases affecting the CNS, such as canine distemper, usually cause only a mild increase in nucleated cell numbers in CSF.

Dogs with tumors of the brain and spinal cord or fungal, protozoal or rickettsial disease involving CNS tissue may or may not show CSF abnormalities. Consequently, laboratory findings must be interpreted in light of the clinical abnormalities and the duration and severity of clinical signs.

To interpret CSF changes reflecting diseases involving the CNS, one must be familiar with normal CSF physiology and factors determining CSF composition. Chart 1 presents an algorithm for examining CSF.

Formation and Circulation of CSF

Cerebrospinal fluid is an ionic solution with a low protein content. It is produced largely by secretory activity of the vascular choroid plexus cells, ependymal lining cells of the ventricles, and probably to a lesser extent by capillary endothelial cells of the brain.[1] Concentrations of Na, Cl and Mg are greater in CSF than in plasma, while concentrations of glucose and K are lower in CSF.[2] The osmolality of CSF is 6-7 mOsm/kg greater than that of plasma. The secretory process of the choroid plexus involves active movement of Na from blood to CSF via adenosine triphosphatase (ATPase) of the Na-K pump located on the surface of choroidal cells.[2] Some K exchange occurs via this pump and, in addition, Cl and HCO_3 may accompany Na secretion. The presence of an active chloride pump has been postulated in choroidal cells. In cats, furosemide, a chloride inhibitor, inhibits CSF formation.[3,4]

Cerebrospinal fluid production in anesthetized cats is about 20 μl/minute.[5] In hypothermia, decreased flow of blood to the brain and choroid plexus may decrease CSF formation. The CSF circulates from the ventricles of the brain into the subarachnoid space, where it bathes the surfaces of the brain and spinal cord both internally (within the central canal) and externally. The CSF is important in regulation of intracranial pressure.[6] Turnover is quite rapid and most animals replace CSF over a period of about 4 hours.[7] Its absorption occurs primarily via the arachnoid villi located in cerebral veins or venous sinuses around the brain. Veins and lymphatics located around the spinal nerve roots also resorb CSF. Cerebrospinal fluid also may enter the brain parenchyma through ependymal cells.[4] The rate of formation of CSF is independent of pressure, while the rate of resorption depends on the pressure gradient between CSF and venous blood in the dural sinuses.[8]

Functions of CSF

The CSF completely covers the CNS, forming an aqueous solution in which brain and spinal cord are suspended. In addition to protecting the CNS, CSF helps supply nutrients to the CNS and remove metabolic waste products from the CNS. The CSF also reflects changes in peripheral blood to chemosensitive receptor areas of the brain, which in turn alter respiration to aid in maintaining acid-base balance.[7]

At least 2 barriers can be identified between the capillary blood supply to the CNS and the interstitial fluid about neuronal cells. The first of these, the blood-CSF barrier, protects the CNS from a variety of substances. This barrier, consisting of capillary endothelial cells joined by tight junctions, represents a significant obstacle, even to free diffusion of ions. Penicillin does not pass through layers of the choroid plexus. Passage of materials through the blood-CSF barrier is determined to a great extent by their lipid solubility.[4]

Table 1. CSF evaluation in dogs and cats with CNS disease.

CNS Disease	Species	RBC/μl	Nucleated Cells/μl	Neutrophil (%)	Mononuclear (%)	Total Protein (mg/dl)	Albumin (mg/dl)	IgG (mg/dl)
Bacterial meningitis[6]	Dog	0	2332	80	20	220	—	—
Blastomycosis[6]	Cat	127	39	8	92	162	—	—
Extradural lymphosarcoma[6]	Cat	2019	20	50	50	65	—	—
Diskospondylitis with extradural fibrosis[6]	Dog	4	9	0	100	101	—	—
Focal granulomatous meningoencephalomyelitis[17]	Dog	50	750	1	99	251	1.4	31.8
Normal values[4,6,18]	Dogs, Cats	0	<8	<10	>90	<48	4.4-7.6	0.5-2.4

A second barrier, the CSF-brain barrier permits some materials to be transported from the CSF into the interstitial fluid of the brain and spinal cord. Ependymal cells lining the ventricles of the brain and the cerebral aqueduct provide a component of this barrier. In chemosensitive regions of the brain, openings in this membrane may provide virtually free communication between CSF and brain interstitial fluid.[7]

In systemic acid-base derangements the pH of CSF changes to a lesser degree than that of blood. The remarkable constancy of CSF pH, and probably brain extracellular fluid pH, in the presence of systemic acid-base disorders is believed due partly to PCO_2-dependent intracellular synthesis of HCO_3 by the choroid plexus.[9,10]

CSF Collection and Processing

Collection

Cerebrospinal fluid evaluation can be an important diagnostic procedure in dogs and cats with CNS disease. However, there are contraindications for its use. Collection of CSF is contraindicated after trauma because collection may be dangerous and you already have an etiologic diagnosis. Collection also may be hazardous in conditions causing increased intracranial pressure, such as cerebral edema, hydrocephalus and intracranial hemorrhage. Sudden release of this pressure at the time of CSF collection can result in tentorial or foramen magnum herniation.[6]

Cerebrospinal fluid usually is removed from dogs and cats at the cisterna magna at the atlanto-occipital articulation. With the patient under general anesthesia, the atlanto-occipital area is surgically prepared. For the right-handed individual, the animal is placed in right lateral recumbency and the atlanto-occipital joint is flexed by an assistant and maintained at a right angle to the long axis of the neck. The nose should be elevated so that the head is parallel to the top of the table. This position separates the occipital condyles from the atlas and increases the area for puncture.

An imaginary line is drawn across the neck between the cranial borders of the wings of the atlas. A second line is drawn from the occipital crest to the dorsal border of the axis. The puncture is made in the middle of the animal's neck at the intersection of these lines. A 20- to 22-ga, 1 1/2- to 3-inch spinal needle with stylet is passed through the skin and fascia perpendicular to the dorsal midline of the neck. When the needle is in the cisterna magna, the stylet is withdrawn and CSF normally drips from the needle hub. A syringe can also be used to aspirate CSF.[6] Aspiration should be done slowly, changing syringes with every ml withdrawn.

A more difficult method of collection is by subarachnoid puncture at the lumbar cisterna.[2] Because CSF flows down the spinal subarachnoid space and central canal, thoracolumbar spinal cord lesions may cause changes in CSF from the lumbar cistern, while fluid collected simultaneously from the cisterna magna cistern is normal. For this reason, the lumbar space is often used for CSF collection when a solitary thoracolumbar spinal cord lesion is suspected.[6]

Measurement of CSF pressure is not routinely done. However, the procedure is not difficult in animals weighing >6-7 kg. The CSF pressure appears to have a wide range of normal values. These variations may relate to the depth of anesthesia during measurements and the size of the animal. Normal CSF pressure is 50-180 mm H_2O. Many animals with neurologic disease have normal CSF pressure.

In performing CSF aspiration in some animals, an intervertebral vein may be entered and blood obtained. If there is only slight contamination of the aspirate with blood, permitting CSF to flow through the hub of the needle for a few seconds may render a clear sample.

For most CSF evaluation procedures, 1-3 ml are usually adequate. Indeed, it may be dangerous to remove >4-5 ml of fluid from dogs. In cats, no more than 0.5-1 ml of fluid should be removed at any one time, as they are susceptible to meningeal hemorrhage when too much fluid is removed. Cerebrospinal fluid collection from kittens should be done cautiously, with no more than 0.33 ml collected.

Processing

The specimen should be placed in EDTA anticoagulant at the same concentration as used for blood samples.[13] Refrigeration at 4 C also aids cell preservation. Samples of CSF are generally examined as soon as possible after collection. Because cells in CSF sometimes degenerate rapidly, cell counts and cytologic examination should be performed within 30 minutes of collection.[4,11] Cells in some CSF samples, however, remain well preserved, even when cell counts and cytologic examination are done 24 hours or more after collection.[12]

Chapter 12

Examination of CSF

Examination of CSF should include physical, cytologic and biochemical evaluations. Total and differential cell counts and quantitative protein determinations should be done routinely on all specimens. Microbiologic cultures of CSF should be done if a septic process is suspected. Enzyme activity in CSF may also reflect CNS disease. The glucose concentration in CSF, however, is not considered a sensitive indicator of CNS disease.

Physical Examination

Color: Normal CSF is clear and colorless. If the sample is red or yellow, it should be centrifuged and the supernatant examined visually. A bright-red discoloration is caused by contamination with blood as a result of a traumatic tap. When centrifuged, such specimens characteristically have a clear supernatant. In contrast, red to brown to yellow CSF samples are more characteristic of old hemorrhage resulting from intracranial lesions. Yellow (xanthochromic) CSF is usually attributed to disintegration of RBC within the subarachnoid space, with subsequent formation of bilirubin.

Turbidity: The CSF becomes turbid when the total cell count exceeds 300-500 cells/μl. Total red and nucleated cell counts and differential counts should be done to determine the nature of the increased nucleated cell count or pleocytosis.

Coagulation: Normal CSF does not coagulate. Coagulation may occur if damage to barrier membranes permits fibrinogen to enter the CSF or if CSF collection results in hemorrhage.

Cell Counts

Cell counts of CSF can be determined either on fluid that is undiluted or diluted. To determine the cell count of undiluted fluid, use a capillary pipette to place CSF on one chamber of a hemacytometer with a Neubauer ruling. Count the cells in all 9 squares. The number of cells is multiplied by 1.1 to determine the total cell count/μl.[6,11]

When the volume of CSF is small, it is appropriate to perform cell counts using undiluted fluid. Differentiation of RBC and nucleated cells can also be done directly on CSF in the counting chamber, using the high-dry objective of the microscope. Nucleated cells are larger than RBC, and have a granular appearance.

Dilution of CSF is done by drawing commercially prepared Rosenthal's diluting fluid into a WBC diluting pipette up to the "1" mark and filling to the "11" mark with CSF. Mix thoroughly and discard 2 or 3 drops. Fill each side of the hemacytometer and wait 2 minutes for the cells to settle. Count all the cells within the entire ruled areas on both sides of the counting chamber and multiply by 0.6 to obtain the number of cells/μl.[6,11]

The diluting fluid contains acetic acid, which lyses RBC, and sometimes a stain that aids in identification of cells. Normal CSF of dogs and cats is free of RBC and contains <8 nucleated cells/μl. In normal dogs, the nucleated cell count of cisternal fluid is slightly greater (1.04-1.86 cells/μl) than in lumbar CSF (0.22-0.88 cells/μl).[14] Perhaps there are fewer cells entering the lumbar CSF or there is a greater rate of cell lysis in lumbar CSF.

In dogs with a normal peripheral blood WBC count, CSF samples contaminated with blood (>500 RBC/μl) have an increase in nucleated cell count by at least 1 cell/μl and in total protein by at least 0.5 mg/dl.[14]

Cytologic Examination

When the nucleated cell count is above normal, it is important to differentiate the types of cells present. The types of cells present in CSF can provide additional information that may aid in determining the nature of the CNS disorder. Cells can be differentiated by centrifugation and by a cytocentrifuge technique.

Centrifugation: When the total cell count is <500/μl, centrifuge the sample at 1000/rpm for 5 minutes. After centrifugation, aspirate off the supernatant, add 1 drop of homologous serum to the sediment, and make a smear of the sediment. Air dry the smear and stain with Wright's stain as done for blood smears. Count and differentiate the nucleated cells. Note if microorganisms or other abnormalities are present.

Cytocentrifuge Technique: Most professional laboratories prefer the cytocentrifuge procedure for preparation of cells. This method requires only small amounts of fluid and causes little cell damage. Using this technique, 2 drops of CSF are placed in the centrifuge funnel and centrifuged 3-4 minutes at 1500 rpm. The slides are stained with Wright's stain.

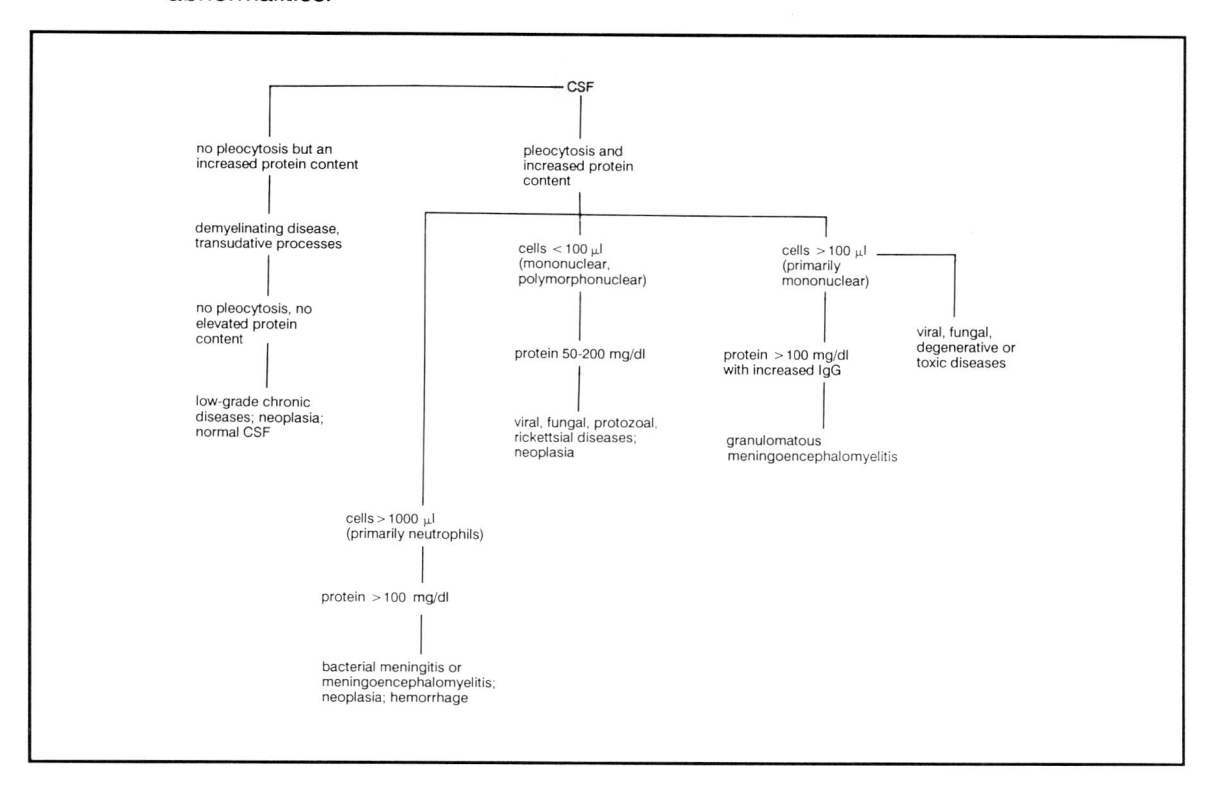

Chart 1. An algorithm for differential diagnosis of various diseases and lesions causing CSF abnormalities.

```
                                    CSF
        ┌───────────────────────────┼─────────────────────────────┐
  no pleocytosis but an       pleocytosis and
  increased protein content   increased protein
        │                     content
  demyelinating disease,              ┌─────────────────────┬──────────────────┐
  transudative processes         cells <100 μl         cells >100 μl
                                 (mononuclear,         (primarily
  no pleocytosis, no             polymorphonuclear)    mononuclear)
  elevated protein                    │                     │              viral, fungal,
  content                                                                  degenerative or
        │                        protein 50-200 mg/dl  protein >100 mg/dl   toxic diseases
  low-grade chronic                   │                with increased IgG
  diseases; neoplasia;           viral, fungal, protozoal,   │
  normal CSF                     rickettsial diseases;  granulomatous
                                 neoplasia             meningoencephalomyelitis

                             cells >1000 μl
                             (primarily neutrophils)
                                    │
                             protein >100 mg/dl
                                    │
                             bacterial meningitis or
                             meningoencephalomyelitis;
                             neoplasia; hemorrhage
```

Normal Cytologic Findings

Since the origin of cells in CSF is uncertain cells are classified according to their morphologic appearance as it relates to the nomenclature used in histopathology and hematology: lymphocytes, monocytes, neutrophils, eosinophils and plasma cells. Most cells in CSF are small lymphocytes, though a few monocytes may be observed. Nucleated cells resembling monocytes but with phagocytic vacuoles are macrophages. Neutrophils are not normally found in CSF unless the tap is traumatic. They should not constitute >10% of the total cells (Table 1). It should be remembered that increased numbers of apparently normal cells are a sign of abnormality.

Abnormal Cytologic Findings

Nucleated cell counts and cytologic findings of CSF examination can be difficult to fit into classifications conforming to specific diseases. All classifications appear to overlap. Pleocytosis of CSF indicates abnormality, but CNS disease may exist in which there is no pleocytosis, and the cells present are normal. A classification of abnormal cytologic characteristics follows:

Neutrophilic Pleocytosis: Observation of neutrophils usually indicates pyogenic or bacterial infection, an abscess, bacterial encephalitis or meningitis. However, neutrophils may occur in noninfectious inflammatory conditions. With these findings, one should attempt to identify bacteria, and the fluid should be cultured. Though other cells may be present, neutrophil numbers are often >1000/μl.

Interpreting results of CSF analysis can be confusing. For example, a predominance of polymorphonuclear cells is expected in bacterial infections, but mononuclear cells might predominate in the later stages of the disease.[15,16] Sequential CSF analysis over time may lessen this confusion. Protein concentrations in the CSF of dogs with suppurative meningoencephalitis may be as high as 220 mg/dl (Table 1).

Pleocytosis of Mixed Cell Types: Most CNS lesions rarely cause exfoliation of pure cell types into the CSF. The CSF of dogs with mycotic and protozoal encephalitides have varied pleocytosis, consisting of neutrophils, mononuclear cells or eosinophils.[17] An increase in total cell numbers, with primarily lymphocytic cells, may be a sign of viral infection. Total nucleated cell counts of CSF from dogs with distemper were reported to be <60 cells/μl.[16] These cells were 80% lymphocytes, 10% macrophages and 10% other cells. Polymorphonuclear cells, however, have been reported to predominate in the early stages of viral meningitis.

Nucleated cells in the CSF of dogs with granulomatous meningoencephalomyelitis are primarily of the mononuclear type, with lymphocytes predominating and fewer monocytes (Fig 1). However, nucleated cell differential counts have varied from 98% lymphocytes and 2% monocytes to 7% lymphocytes, 42% monocytes and 51% neutrophils.[17]

Metrizamide, an iodinated a contrast agent used for myelography, may cause histiocytic meningitis with CSF pleocytosis within 1 day after its use.[18] In such cases, cells in the CSF comprise a mixture of large monocytoid cells, though neutrophils may be present. Some of the monocytoid cells resemble macrophages and have intracytoplasmic material, presumably phagocytosed contrast medium.

In dogs and cats with noninflammatory conditions involving the CNS, pleocytosis is rarely observed. In dogs with spinal trauma, a slight increase in cell numbers may develop.[19] Dogs with congenital malformations (hydrocephalus, spinal dysraphism) generally have normal CSF.[19] Dogs with cerebral infarcts may have increased numbers of RBC in the CSF. Erythrophagocytosis by macrophages is a diagnostic feature.[19] The CSF may also be xanthochromic.

Pleocytosis with Neoplastic Cells: Primary tumors involving the CNS include astrocytomas, ependymomas, meningiomas, oligodendrogliomas and choroid plexus papillomas. In a study of 53 dogs with these types of brain tumors, nearly 40% of CSF samples had a normal or only slightly increased nucleated cell count, increased protein content and increased CSF pressure.[20] Nucleated cells consisted predominantly of mononuclear cells. Neutrophils predominated in dogs with meningiomas and increased cell counts. This abnormality correlated with necrosis or neutrophil infiltration of the tumors. None of these 53 dogs had neoplastic cells in the CSF; the neoplasia was diagnosed histopathologically.

Though neoplastic cells are difficult to identify in CSF, they may be present when the meninges are infiltrated. Malignant cells generally manifest variability in cell size and shape. Their nucleus may appear large relative to the amount of cytoplasm present. In dogs with CNS lymphosarcoma, CSF cytologic features were considered truly diagnostic because large numbers of lymphoblastic cells were readily recognized in the CSF sample.[19] Metastatic carcinoma cells tend to form aggregates and may show evidence of differentiation, such as gland formation.[15] Dogs with brain or spinal cord tumors may or may not have increased numbers of CSF cells. In some with pleocytosis, the cells are due to secondary effects of the tumor, rather than the tumor cells alone.

Proteins in CSF

Quantitation of CSF total protein and specific proteins is used to detect increased permeability of the blood-CSF barrier and increased synthesis of protein within the CNS. Because CSF is partly an ultrafiltrate of plasma, low-molecular-weight proteins, such as albumin, normally predominate.[4]

Normal CSF Proteins: The total protein concentration of normal CSF in dogs and cats is <48 mg/dl. The total protein content of

Figure 1. A CSF smear from a dog with granulomatous meningoencephalomyelitis. To the left a segmented neutrophil and larger monocyte are easily identified. The nuclear membrane of the neutrophil is lobated and its cytoplasm is pink. Monocytes of the CSF, like those of blood, are larger than neutrophils. Monocyte nuclei are extremely variable in shape; at times nuclear folds can be detected. Adjacent to these cells and on the far right are RBC. The pink-staining RBC are smaller than nucleated cells. In the middle of the photograph are monocytes and a smaller lymphocyte.

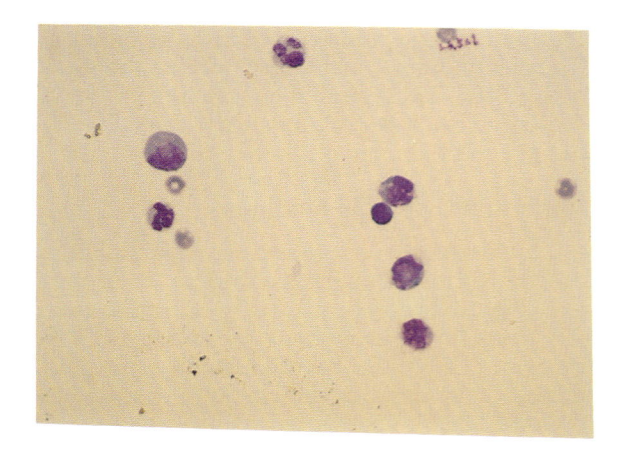

lumbar CSF in dogs is 26.6-30.7 mg/dl and the mean total protein content of cisternal CSF is 12.3-15.6 mg/dl.[14] The normal lumbar CSF protein level in cats is 40.6-47.4 mg/dl, while the normal cisternal CSF protein level is 9.4-44.6 mg/dl.[21] This higher protein content of lumbar CSF in dogs and cats may be due to sluggish spinal fluid circulation, leading to local protein accumulation.

Normal CSF should be relatively free of globulins. A rough approximation of globulin levels in CSF can be made using the Pandy test. Pandy reagent is prepared by adding 10 g of phenol crystals to 100 ml of distilled water.[6] About 1-2 drops of CSF are added to 1 ml of Pandy reagent. Normal CSF produces only faint turbidity. With abnormally large amounts of globulins, the solution becomes cloudy. Urinary protein reagent strips may be used to grossly detect protein. An elevated protein level would usually be represented on reagent strips as $\geq$ 100 mg/dl.[22]

Spectrophotometric procedures are required for accurate protein quantitation. In contrast to cell evaluation, protein quantitation need not be done immediately. Fluid may be frozen and submitted to a laboratory for evaluation. The Coomassie brilliant-blue technique and turbidimetric procedures have been used for total protein assay. In spectrophotometric measurement of CSF protein levels using Coomassie blue reagent, the linearity of the assay procedure is better than that of the turbidimetric procedure.[23]

Abnormal CSF Proteins: The permeability of blood-brain barrier to plasma proteins is markedly increased by bacterial meningitis and somewhat less altered by viral meningitis or encephalitis. Entrance of plasma proteins into the CSF may also result from high intracranial pressure due to a brain tumor or intracerebral hemorrhage. Metrizamide, the contrast agent used for myelography, causes histocytic meningitis in dogs, increasing the entrance of plasma proteins into the CSF.[18] The effect of these disease processes is that specific protein concentrations in the CSF increasingly resemble those characteristic of serum.

Quantitation of protein fractions in both serum and CSF may be necessary to differentiate leakage of plasma proteins across the blood-CSF barrier from increased synthesis of immunoglobulins (IgG) within the CNS. Intrathecal administration of metrizamide to dogs results in increased total CSF protein and IgG levels. The increased CSF IgG concentration might result from increased secretion of IgG by CNS tissue into the CSF or from increased leakage of serum constituents across the blood-CSF barrier.

Correlation between CSF albumin and CSF globulin concentrations indicates a blood-CSF barrier dysfunction with both albumin and globulin entering CSF with equal facility, but at a greater-than-normal rate. The high correlation between CSF albumin and IgG concentrations in metrizamide-treated dogs supports the likelihood of plasma origin of CSF albumin and IgG.[18] In contrast, dogs with focal granulomatous meningoencephalomyelitis had low serum IgG concentrations, high CSF concentrations of IgG, and normal concentrations of CSF albumin.[24] The increased CSF IgG level was considered a result of local CNS IgG production and not leakage across the blood-CSF barrier (Chart 1).

Electrophoresis of canine CSF from dogs with canine distemper encephalomyelitis revealed decreased albumin values. In contrast, gamma globulin values in CSF were elevated. This may indicate most of the gamma globulin was of intrathecal origin, with minimal blood-brain barrier disturbances.[25]

Electrophoresis of CSF from dogs with CNS neoplasms showed elevated albumin values accompanied by a spike in the alpha and beta globulin zones. These findings indicated transudation of plasma protein through an altered blood-brain barrier. This was believed to result from increased endothelial cell permeability. The degree of increased permeability depends on tumor location and cell type. Tumors in the ventricular system or highly malignant tumors are more likely to alter the blood-brain barrier and cause transudation of plasma proteins than are noninvasive tumors.[20,25]

The pathologic mechanisms altering CSF protein levels are complex; it should be remembered, however, that CSF protein content may increase without a concomitant increase in cell numbers.

Enzymes in CSF

Activity of several different enzymes has been measured in CSF to determine if the CNS or its protective barriers have been damaged. One source of abnormal amounts of enzyme in CSF may be diffusion across the blood-CSF barrier. A second source of CSF enzyme activity is from altered CNS tissue by diffusion across the brain-CSF barrier. Abnormally large numbers of cellular elements in CSF may also enhance some types of enzyme activity.[4,8]

Lactate Dehydrogenase: Activity of serum and CSF lactate dehydrogenase (LDH) and its isoenzymes has been measured in normal Beagles.[26] The LDH activity in serum was 10 times that in CSF. Most of the CSF activity was from LDH_1 and LDH_2, whereas most of the serum LDH activity was from LDH_4 and LDH_5. Therefore, some CSF LDH activity may come from brain tissue, and the blood-CSF barrier may effectively segregate CSF LDH from serum LDH. Simultaneous measurement of serum and CSF LDH activity and LDH isoenzyme profiles may thus help establish the nature of CNS disease.

Creatine Kinase: Increased CSF creatine kinase (CK) activity has been reported in a wide variety of neurologic disorders. In dogs with neurologic disease, the concentrations of CK in CSF and serum were diagnostically nonspecific, though elevated CK concentrations in CSF were associated with a guarded to poor prognosis.[27] Normal CSF CK concentrations had a mean value of 3.1 IU/L, with a high of 6.0 IU/L. The prognosis was guarded when the CSF CK level was 7-19 IU/L and poor when the CSF CK level was >20 IU/L. Concentrations of CK in CSF did not correlate significantly with serum CK values. Elevated CSF CK levels appear to be a nonspecific but sensitive index of CNS disease.

Glucose in CSF

The concentration of glucose in CSF is about 60-70% of the blood glucose level. Glucose enters the CSF by active transport and passive diffusion. Because of this relationship between blood and CSF glucose levels, the blood glucose concentration should be determined simultaneously with the CSF glucose concentration. Determining the glucose concentration in CSF is not useful in diagnosing a specific cause of CNS disease. Decreased CSF glucose concentrations may be due to increased utilization of glucose by microorganisms, WBC or CNS cells. Also there may be impaired transport of glucose from plasma to the CSF.

References

1. Nattie: Ionic mechanisms of cerebrospinal fluid acid-base regulation. *J App Physiol* 54:3-12, 1983.

2. Wright: Evaluation of cerebrospinal fluid in the dog. *Vet Record* 103:48-51, 1978.

3. Abbot *et al*: Chloride transport and potential across the blood-CSF barrier. *Brain Res* 29:185-193, 1971.

4. Coles, in Kaneko: *Clinical Biochemistry of Domestic Animals.* 3rd ed. Academic Press, Orlando, FL, 1980. pp 719-748.

5. Snodgrass and Lorenzo: Temperature and cerebrospinal fluid production rate. *Am J Physiol* 222:1524-1572, 1972.

6. Kornegay: Cerebrospinal fluid collection, examination, and interpretation in dogs and cats. *Comp Cont Ed Pract Vet* 3:85-90, 1981.

7. Molony and Jacobson, in Kokko and Tannen: *Fluids and Electrolytes.* Saunders, Philadelphia, 1986. pp 305-381.

8. Kjeldsberg and Kreig, in Henry: *Clinical Diagnosis and Management by Laboratory Methods.* 17th ed. Saunders, Philadelphia, 1984. pp 459-492.

9. Siesjo: The regulation of cerebrospinal fluid pH. *Kidney Intl* 1:360-374, 1972.

10. Bledsoe and Hornbein, in Hornbein: *Regulation of Breathing, Part I.* Marcel Dekker, New York, 1981. pp 347-428.

11. Coles: *Veterinary Clinical Pathology.* 4th ed. Saunders, Philadelphia, 1980. pp 267-278.

12. Cowell, RL, Oklahoma St Univ: Personal communication, 1987.

13. Doxey: *Clinical Pathology and Diagnostic Procedures.* 2nd ed. Bailliere Tindall, London, 1983. p 277.

14. Bailey and Higgens: Comparison of total white blood cell count and total protein content of lumbar and cisternal cerebrospinal fluid of healthy dogs. *Am J Vet Res* 46:1162-1165, 1985.

15. Shah: Cytology of cerebrospinal fluid. *Am J Med Technology* 48:829-831, 1982.

16. Sarfaty *et al*: Differential diagnosis of granu-lomatous meningoencephalomyelitis, distemper, and suppurative meningoencephalitis in the dog. *JAVMA* 188:387-392, 1986.

17. Bailey and Higgens: Characteristics of cerebrospinal fluid associated with canine granulomatous meningoencephalomyelitis: a retrospective study. *JAVMA* 188:418-421, 1986.

18. Johnson *et al*: Transient leakage across the blood cerebrospinal fluid barrier after intrathecal metrizamide administration to dogs. *Am J Vet Res* 46:1303-1308, 1985.

19. Vandevelde *et al*: Cerebrospinal fluid cytology in canine neurologic disease. *Am J Vet Res* 38:1827-1832, 1977.

20. Bailey and Higgens: Characteristics of cisternal cerebrospinal fluid associated with primary brain tumors in the dog: a retrospective study. *JAVMA* 188:414-417, 1986.

21. Hochwald *et al*: Exchange of proteins between blood and spinal subarachnoid fluid. *Am J Physiol* 217:348-353, 1969.

22. Duncan and Prasse: *Veterinary Laboratory Medicine, Clinical Pathology.* 2nd ed. Iowa State Univ Press, Ames, 1986. p 210.

23. Gaad: Protein estimation in spinal fluid using Coomassie blue reagent. *Med Lab Sciences* 38:61-63, 1981.

24. Murtaugh *et al*: Focal granulomatous meningoencephalomyelitis in a pup. *JAVMA* 187:835-836, 1985.

25. Sorjonen: Total protein, albumin quota, and electrophoretic patterns in cerebrospinal fluid of dogs with central nervous system disorders. *Am J Vet Res* 48:301-305, 1987.

26. Heavner *et al*: Lactate dehydrogenase isoenzymes in blood and cerebrospinal fluid from healthy Beagles. *Am J Vet Res* 47:1771-1775, 1986.

27. Indrieri *et al*: Critical evaluation of creatine phosphokinase in cerebrospinal fluid of dogs with neurologic disease. *Am J Vet Res* 41:1299-1303, 1980.

13

Abdominal and Thoracic Fluid

R.L. Cowell, R.D. Tyler and J.H. Meinkoth

Abdominal and thoracic viscera are bathed in and lubricated by a small amount of fluid. This fluid is essentially an ultrafiltrate of blood. The amount of lubricating fluid in the cavity is determined by the amount of fluid entering the cavity minus the amount exiting the cavity. Therefore, the amount of fluid increases when more fluid enters the cavity than is removed from it. Along with thoracic and abdominal effusions, ectopic sources of fluid, such as rupture of the urinary bladder, are discussed in this chapter.

Most effusions are not noticed by pet owners until they become severe. Dogs and cats with pathologic thoracic effusions often show dyspnea. With severe pleural effusion, a crouched, sternal recumbent position, with elbows abducted away from the chest, is characteristic. Extension of the head and neck, with open-mouth breathing and forceful abdominal respiration, may be present.[1] With milder effusions, lethargy and lack of stamina may be the only clinical signs. Animals, especially cats, with mildly to moderately severe effusions, often adapt by decreasing their activity and thus conceal their illness until it is severe. Dogs and cats with abdominal effusions may be presented for treatment of lethargy, weakness and abdominal distension. Owners may mistake the abdominal distension for weight gain (fat), gas or ingesta.

An increased amount of fluid in the abdominal or thoracic cavity is not a disease in itself but rather an indication of a pathologic process in the fluid production and/or removal system, or an accumulation from an ectopic source. Fluid analysis, including cytologic evaluation and classification, is a quick, easy, inexpensive and relatively safe way to obtain useful information for diagnosis, prognosis and treatment of diseases resulting in abdominal and/or thoracic fluid accumulations.

Collection Techniques

Thoracentesis

Pleural effusions are typically abundant and bilateral but may be mild, unilateral and/or compartmentalized. Radiographs help determine the extent and location of the effusion. If the effusion is compartmentalized, radiographs can help establish the fluid's location and guide thoracentesis. If the fluid is not compartmentalized, thoracentesis is done ventrad, at the seventh or eighth intercostal space.[1,2]

The animal is restrained in sternal recumbency or standing. The site of needle insertion is clipped and scrubbed, and an antiseptic is applied. Tranquilization and/or local anesthesia are generally not necessary for collecting a small sample for analysis, but may be needed if a large amount of fluid must be drained from the chest. An 18- to 20-ga, over-the-needle catheter (or other needle catheter unit) is preferred. The catheter unit allows the needle to be withdrawn after the catheter is introduced into the thoracic cavity, decreasing the chance of injury to intrathoracic organs.

The needle catheter unit should be inserted next to the cranial surface of the rib to minimize the risk of lacerating the vessels on the rib's caudal border. As long as the needle and/or catheter is below the fluid line, air will not be aspirated into the thoracic cavity. If only a single syringe of fluid is to be collected, the syringe may be attached to the catheter, the fluid aspirated, and the catheter withdrawn with syringe attached. However, if the syringe is to be repeatedly filled, a 3-way stopcock should be attached. Draining large quantities of fluid with a syringe may be difficult, especially if the fluid is viscid, full of debris and/or fibrin clots, or compartmentalization has occurred; placement of a chest tube may be necessary in such cases.[2]

A sample of the effusion should be collected in an EDTA (lavender top) tube to be used for a total nucleated cell count, total protein determination, and cytologic examination. Another sample should be collected in a serum (red top) tube if any biochemical analyses (eg, cholesterol, triglyceride) are to be performed.

Abdominocentesis

Many techniques have been described for collecting abdominal fluid from dogs and cats. Some of those techniques are discussed below, and some of their advantages and disadvantages are compared in Table 1.

The ventral midline of the abdomen, 1-2 cm caudal to the umbilicus, is the usual site of needle insertion. This site avoids the falciform fat, which can readily block the needle barrel. The urinary bladder is emptied to help avoid accidental cystocentesis. The site of needle insertion is clipped and scrubbed, and an antiseptic is applied. Neither local nor general anesthesia is usually needed, but the animal must be adequately restrained.

With the animal standing or in lateral recumbency, a ventral midline puncture is made using a 1-inch, 20-ga needle or an over-the-needle 20-ga, 1 1/4-inch plastic catheter. If a previous surgical incision is present, the needle should be inserted at least 1.5 cm away from the site to avoid abdominal viscera that may have adhered to the abdominal wall in the area of the scar. Open-needle abdominocentesis is reportedly more sensitive than aspiration via syringe; therefore, a syringe is usually not attached.[3]

The fluid is collected into an EDTA (lavender top) tube for cytologic examination, total protein determination, and total nucleated cell count. A serum (red top) tube of fluid also is collected if any biochemical tests (eg, creatinine) are to be performed. If a syringe is attached, only mild negative pressure should be applied because it is easy to aspirate omentum or other abdominal contents against the needle opening and inhibit fluid collection. To enhance fluid collection, abdominal compression may be applied when an over-the-needle catheter is used and the stylet has been removed, leaving only the catheter in the abdominal cavity. Though the catheter may kink, sufficient fluid can usually be collected for analysis.

If the above technique fails to yield fluid, passing a closed-ended multiply fenestrated polyethylene 3 1/2-Fr tom cat catheter (Sherwood Medical, St. Louis, MO) through a 14-ga, 2.5-inch around-the-needle Teflon catheter (Abbott, N. Chicago, IL) may be helpful.[3]

Placing a peritoneal dialysis catheter in the caudal portion of the abdomen is reportedly the most sensitive method of fluid collection.[4] The ventral midline area is clipped and prepped for catheter insertion 1-2 cm caudal to the umbilicus. The patient is placed in dorsal recumbency and the site of insertion is infiltrated with 1% lidocaine with epinephrine. A small skin incision is made and the catheter/trocar is inserted into the caudal abdomen and the stylet removed. One must be careful during insertion not to let the stylet damage abdominal organs.

Inserting the catheter by making a small (0.5- to 2-cm) incision 1-2 cm caudal to the umbilicus, being sure to tie off any bleeders to avoid blood contamination, spreading the loose subcutaneous fat, incising the linea alba, and inserting the catheter (without the trocar) into the caudal abdomen may be beneficial, especially in small patients.[5]

A syringe is attached and mild negative pressure is applied. If fluid cannot be aspirated, warm normal saline is infused (20 ml/kg body weight) while gently massaging the abdomen to aid fluid dispersion. When the fluid has been infused, the bottle is placed on the floor and vented, and the fluid is recollected via gravity drainage.[4]

Slide Preparation and Staining

Preparation of the sample for cytologic evaluation depends on the character and quantity of the fluid, the type of stain to be used, and whether the cytologic evaluation will be performed in-hospital or sent to a consultant.

The character of the fluid (turbid or clear) usually indicates the process(es) that may be occurring and the probable nucleated cell concentration. Clear, colorless fluids are usually transudates and of low cellularity. While fluids of low cellularity are the most difficult to prepare, diagnostic-quality smears can be made

Abdominal and Thoracic Fluid

Table 1. Some advantages and disadvantages of 4 different methods of collecting peritoneal fluid.

Technique	Advantages	Disadvantages
20-gauge needle	• Quick and easy • Inexpensive • Requires minimal equipment	• Risk of lacerating abdominal organs • Less successful if only small amount of fluid present • Needle easily occluded by omentum, fat, etc
Over-the-needle catheter	• Quick and easy • Inexpensive • Relatively safe • Less chance of lacerating abdominal viscera	• Catheter may kink • Less successful if only small amount of fluid present • Catheter easily occluded by omentum, fat, etc
Tom cat catheter passed through over-the-needle catheter	• Quick and easy • Relatively safe • Allows for use of multiple-opening collection catheter • Less chance of lacerating abdominal viscera than needle technique • More successful in sample collection than needle or over-the-needle catheter techniques if only small amount of fluid present	• May require local anesthesia • More expensive than needle or over-the-needle catheter technique
Peritoneal dialysis catheter	• Appears to be the best method of fluid collection when only small amount of fluid is present • May be used for abdominal lavage • Allows for use of multiple-opening collection catheter • Less chance of lacerating abdominal viscera	• More expensive than other methods • Requires more equipment • More time consuming • More discomfort to patient • Requires minor surgery • Requires at least local anesthetic • If catheter/stylet unit forced into abdomen, stylet may damage abdominal organs

from most low-cellularity fluids by using sediment smear or line smear techniques. Amber, clear to mildly opaque fluids are often modified transudates of low to moderate cellularity. However, moderate to markedly opaque fluids are usually exudates of moderately high to very high cellularity. Slide preparation techniques for various types of fluids are briefly presented below. Chapter 1 contains a detailed discussion and illustrations.

Sediment smears should be made on all nonturbid fluid specimens. This is done by centrifuging the fluid for 5 minutes at 165-360 G. This can be achieved in a centrifuge with a radial arm length of 14.6 cm by centrifuging the fluid at 1000-1500 rpm. After centrifugation, nearly all of the supernatant is poured off, leaving only about 0.5 ml of fluid with the pellet in the bottom of the test tube. The supernatant may be used for refractometric total protein determination and, if the supernatant was not collected from an EDTA tube, other chemical analyses. The pellet is then resuspended in the remaining 0.5 ml of fluid by gentle agitation, a drop of the suspension is placed on a glass slide, and a routine pull smear or squash prep is made (see Chapter 1, Figs 3,6). The smear is air dried and then stained with any hematologic stain.[6]

If it is not possible to centrifuge the fluid, line smears should be made from fresh, well-mixed fluid. Also, line smears are useful when making smears from the sediment of very low-cellularity fluids. Line smears are made by placing a drop of fluid on a glass slide and starting to make a pull smear. Instead of continuing until the fluid makes a feathered edge, go only a short distance, stop, and lift the pull slide directly up. Cells concentrate in the fluid following the pull slide, creating a line of increased cellularity where the pull slide is lifted (Chapter 1, Fig 7).[6]

Opaque fluids may need only a direct smear, as high cell concentrations are likely present. Direct smears may be made by making either pull smears or squash preps on well-mixed, uncentrifuged fluid.[6]

When submitting samples to an outside laboratory for cytologic examination, it is best to request instructions for sample preparation from the person who will be examining the preparations. However, the following instructions generally suffice unless the cytologist wishes to use Papanicolaou-type stains, in which case the sample must be wet fixed. Include some stained and unstained premade, air-dried slides, prepared as described above, along with an EDTA tube of the fluid. If premade, air-dried slides are not submitted and the fluid is delayed, the cellular constituents will become hypersegmented and pyknotic, and cell morphology will be difficult if not impossible to evaluate. Even if the cells in the EDTA tube have become pyknotic, a total nucleated cell count and refractometric total protein determination can be performed.[6]

Many acceptable stains are available. Diff-Quik (Harleco, Gibbstown, NJ) is one of the easiest to use, stains cellular elements well, and has little precipitate to confuse with bacteria. Some other commonly used hematologic stains are Wright's stain and new methylene blue. Gram's stain and acid-fast procedures may be used to classify bacteria but are much less sensitive than hematologic stains for finding bacteria. Also, care must be given to procedure when performing a Gram's stain because the cellular elements, proteins and other constituents in septic fluids can affect the staining.[6]

Laboratory Data

Cell Counts and Counting Techniques

A total nucleated cell count (TNCC), which is a count of all nucleated cells present in the fluid, may be done by automated or manual methods. The automated cell counters may count debris, so only relatively clear fluids should be used. The Unopette (Becton Dickinson, Rutherford, NJ) procedure is a good in-house method, and is performed the same as for peripheral blood leukocyte counts. Cell clumping, cell fragmentation, and noncellular debris can cause counting errors with both the automated and manual techniques.[6,7]

Red blood cell (RBC) counts offer little if any additional information over visual assessment and a PCV measurement on the effusion. Therefore, RBC counts are seldom performed unless the TNCC is done on an automated instrument that automatically counts RBCs. Noting the presence of RBCs in effusions is important because they indicate blood contamination of the fluid during collection, hemorrhage into the cavity, or increased capillary permeability with diapedesis of RBCs into the cavity.[6]

Total Protein Measurement and Techniques

Peritoneal or pleural fluid protein concentration is used, with the TNCC, to classify effusions (transudates, modified transudates, exudates) and to estimate the severity of inflammation. The total protein (TP) content may be determined biochemically or estimated by refractometry. In most practices TP is estimated by refractometry. If the fluid is opaque, it is best to determine the refractive index of the supernatant after centrifuging the fluid. Otherwise, refraction of light by suspended particles may result in an erroneously high TP reading.[6] Lipemic fluids often do not separate sufficiently to allow TP to be estimated by refractometry or chemical methods.

Microbiologic Cultures

Not all effusions need to be cultured (*eg*, true transudates). If cytologic evaluation of the fluid suggests infection, the fluid should be cultured for both aerobic and anaerobic bacteria. Fluid samples for aerobic and anaerobic cultures can be collected into a syringe, taking care to exclude air from the sample. The needle should be capped and the syringe containing

Abdominal and Thoracic Fluid

Figure 1. Some nondegenerate neutrophils and RBCs. The dark-staining, tightly clumped nuclear chromatin characterizes the nondegenerate neutrophil. Some hypersegmentation (age-related change) is present. (Wright's stain, original magnification 100X)

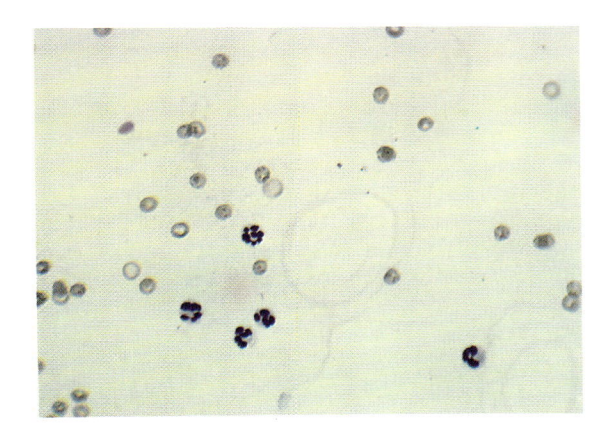

the sample taken immediately to the laboratory for culture. For optimal results or if a delay is anticipated, the fluid should be placed in a transport system that supports both aerobic and anaerobic bacteria.[6] Chapter 1 contains a further discussion of culturing.

Cells Seen in Effusions

Neutrophils

Neutrophils are present to some degree in most effusions and tend to predominate in effusions associated with inflammation. Cytologically, there are 2 general classifications of neutrophils: degenerate and nondegenerate. When evaluating neutrophil morphology, only neutrophils in the area of the slide corresponding to the monolayer of a blood slide should be evaluated. Neutrophils close to the feathered edge may appear degenerate due to mechanical stresses of smear preparation.

Degenerate neutrophils are neutrophils that have undergone hydropic degeneration (Fig 5 and Plate 1). This is a local change generally occurring due to bacterial toxins altering cell membrane permeability. This allows water to diffuse into the cell and through the nuclear pores, causing the nucleus to swell, fill more of the cytoplasm, and stain homogeneously eosinophilic. This swollen, loose, homogeneous eosinophilic nuclear chromatin pattern characterizes the degenerate neutrophil. Though all cell types are exposed to the same toxin, degenerative change is evaluated only in neutrophils.

Nondegenerate neutrophils are those with tightly clumped, basophilic nuclear chromatin, like peripheral blood neutrophils (Fig 1 and Plate 1). Some to many of the neutrophils may be hypersegmented. Hypersegmentation is an aging change; the nuclear chromatin eventually breaks into round, tightly clumped spheres (pyknosis). These aged neutrophils often are seen phagocytized by macrophages (cytophagia). The presence of nondegenerate neutrophils suggests the fluid is not septic. However, bacteria that are not strong toxin producers, such as the Actinomycetes family, may be associated with nondegenerate neutrophils. Also, nonbacterial infectious agents (eg, *Ehrlichia*, *Toxoplasma*, various fungi) may be associated with nondegenerate neutrophils.

Effusions may also contain toxic neutrophils. However, toxic changes (eg, Dohle bodies, toxic granulation, diffuse cytoplasmic basophilia, foamy cytoplasm) develop in the bone marrow and in response to inflammation. Therefore, toxic neutrophils in the peripheral blood migrate into the body cavity and are observed in effusions of the cavity.[6] While foamy cytoplasm is considered a toxic change, cytoplasmic vacuolation may be seen in neutrophils of peritoneal/thoracic fluid smears due to age-related change or EDTA-induced artifact.

Mesothelial/Macrophage-Type Cells

Mesothelial cells line the pleural, peritoneal and visceral surfaces and are present in variable numbers in most effusions (Fig 2). They are large cells that may be present singly, or in clusters or rafts. They generally contain a

Figure 2. A. Mesothelial cell with a radiating corona. B. A small cluster of mesothelial cells. C. A vacuolated macrophage and a mesothelial cell. (Wright's stain, original magnification 125X)

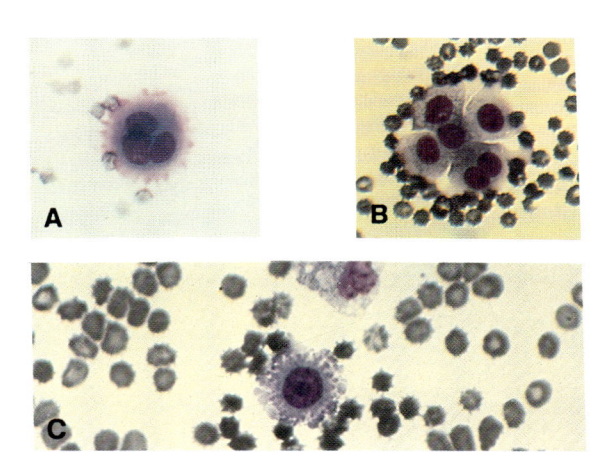

Figure 3. Lymphosarcoma. Many lymphoblasts with prominent large nucleoli, a single small lymphocyte (upper center), 3 pyknotic cells (left center, lower right, upper right), and scattered RBCs. (Wright's stain, original magnification 250X)

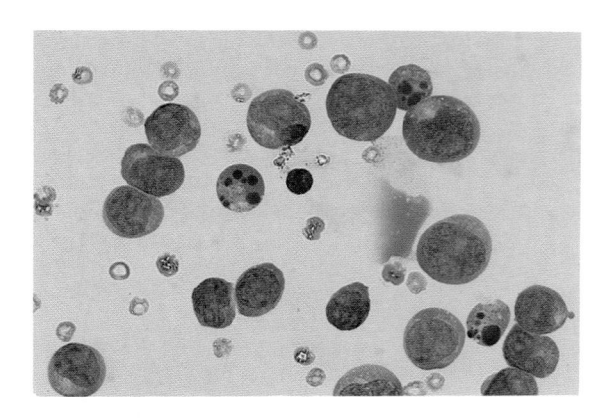

single round to oval nucleus but may be multinucleated. The nuclear chromatin has a finely reticular pattern. Nucleoli may be present in activated mesothelial cells. Activated mesothelial cells should not be confused with neoplastic cells. The cytoplasm is slightly basophilic and may contain phagocytic debris, since activated mesothelial cells may become phagocytic. A blue or red corona may be present around nucleated cells within effusions, especially mesothelial cells, as an artifact of slow drying and is of no diagnostic significance.

Peritoneal macrophages generally have a single oval to bean-shaped nucleus (Fig 2); however, multinucleation and variable nuclear shape may be present. Their nuclear chromatin is lacy and their cytoplasm is frequently vacuolated and may contain phagocytic debris.

Determining whether some cells are mesothelial cells or macrophages may be difficult. Differentiating these cells is seldom of diagnostic significance. The only time separating these 2 cell types may be helpful is in the case of a mesothelioma. However, mesotheliomas are rare and difficult to diagnose cytologically because mesothelial cells tend to hypertrophy, proliferate and exfoliate anytime fluid accumulates. With experience, mesotheliomas may be recognized cytologically. For the beginner, correct identification may be impossible.

Lymphocytes

Lymphocytes are present in small numbers in many effusions and may be the predominant cell type in chylous, pseudochylous and lymphosarcomatous effusions. With lymphosarcoma, neoplastic lymphocytes frequently, but not always, exfoliate into the fluid and are present in large numbers. Chylous and pseudochylous effusions consist primarily of small mature lymphocytes (Fig 9), while lymphosarcomatous effusions consist primarily of lymphoblasts (Fig 3). The small mature lymphocytes seen in chylous and pseudochylous effusions have a small amount of clear to blue cytoplasm, oval to bean-shaped nucleus, clumpy nuclear chromatin and no visible nucleoli, and are smaller than neutrophils. Reactive lymphocytes (Plate 1) may be seen in inflammatory effusions. These lymphocytes are larger than small lymphocytes, have a small to moderate amount of very blue cytoplasm, and may become plasmacytoid.

Care must be taken not to confuse reactive lymphocytes in inflammatory conditions with neoplastic lymphocytes. Neoplastic lymphocytes are usually lymphoblasts. They have a moderate amount of clear to blue cytoplasm, variably shaped nuclei, finely stippled nuclear chromatin, and nucleoli (often irregular in shape and size), and they are larger than neutrophils.

Eosinophils

Eosinophils (Fig 4 and Plate 2) may be present in effusions and are readily recognized by their rod-shaped (in cats) or variably sized round (in dogs) orange granules. Moderate to large numbers of eosinophils may be seen in effusions secondary to mast-cell tumors, heart-

Figure 4. Thoracic fluid from a dog with an intrathoracic mast-cell tumor. Mast cells have red-purple granules gathered to one side and a pale to nonstaining nucleus. Note the eosinophil (upper right center) with pale orange granules and nonstaining nucleus. (Wright's stain, original magnification 250X)

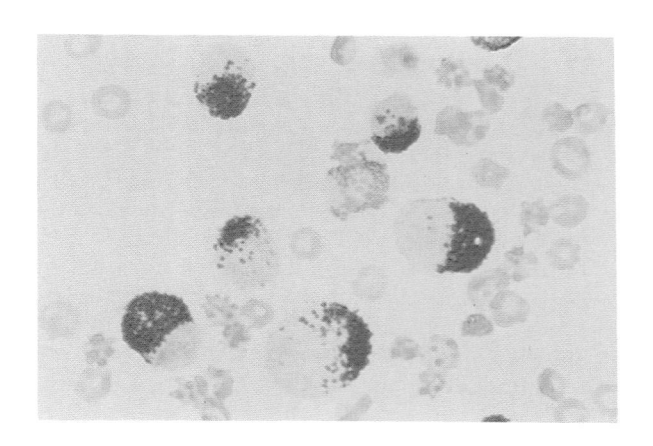

Mast Cells

Mast cells (Fig 4 and Plate 2) are readily identified by their red-purple granules. Mast-cell tumors within body cavities may be associated with effusions and frequently exfoliate large numbers of mast cells into the effusion. However, mast cells are observed in small numbers in effusions from dogs and cats with many different inflammatory disorders.

Erythrocytes

Erythrocytes may be seen cytologically within effusions secondary to overt hemorrhage or contamination with peripheral blood. It is important to differentiate bloody taps from true intracavity hemorrhage, based on clinical signs and the presence or absence of erythrophagia and platelets in the effusion, as described under hemorrhagic effusions later in this chapter.

Neoplastic Cells

Neoplastic cells may be observed in effusions with many different types of neoplasia. Various carcinomas and adenocarcinomas (epithelial-cell tumors), lymphosarcomas and mast-cell tumors (discrete-cell tumors), hemangiosarcomas (spindle-cell tumors), and mesotheliomas may exfoliate neoplastic cells into the pleural or peritoneal cavity. Identification of the neoplastic cells depends upon the viewer's ability to recognize the cell type and signs of malignancy. (See the discussion on neoplasia later in this chapter and general criteria of malignancy in Chapter 1).

Miscellaneous Findings

Glove Powder

Corn starch (glove powder) may be seen on slides made from pleural and/or peritoneal fluid (Plate 8). Typically, it is a clear-staining, large, round to hexagonal structure with a central fissure. Glove powder is an incidental finding and should not be confused with an organism or cell.[6]

Microfilariae

Microfilariae are occasionally seen within hemorrhagic effusions from dogs (Plate 8). These are generally *Dirofilaria* or *Dipetalonema* larvae that have entered the cavity with the peripheral blood.

Basket Cells

Basket cells are ruptured nucleated cells. The nuclear chromatin spreads out and stains eosinophilic. Nucleated cells may rupture due to the stresses induced in slide preparation. However, certain effusions (chylous effusions and septic exudates) cause increased cell fragility, and basket cells are frequently seen.

Classification of Effusions

In the following discussions, abdominal and thoracic fluid accumulations are classified as transudates, modified transudates or exu-

Chart 1. An algorithm to classify effusions as transudates, modified transudates or exudates, based on total protein content and total nucleated cell count.

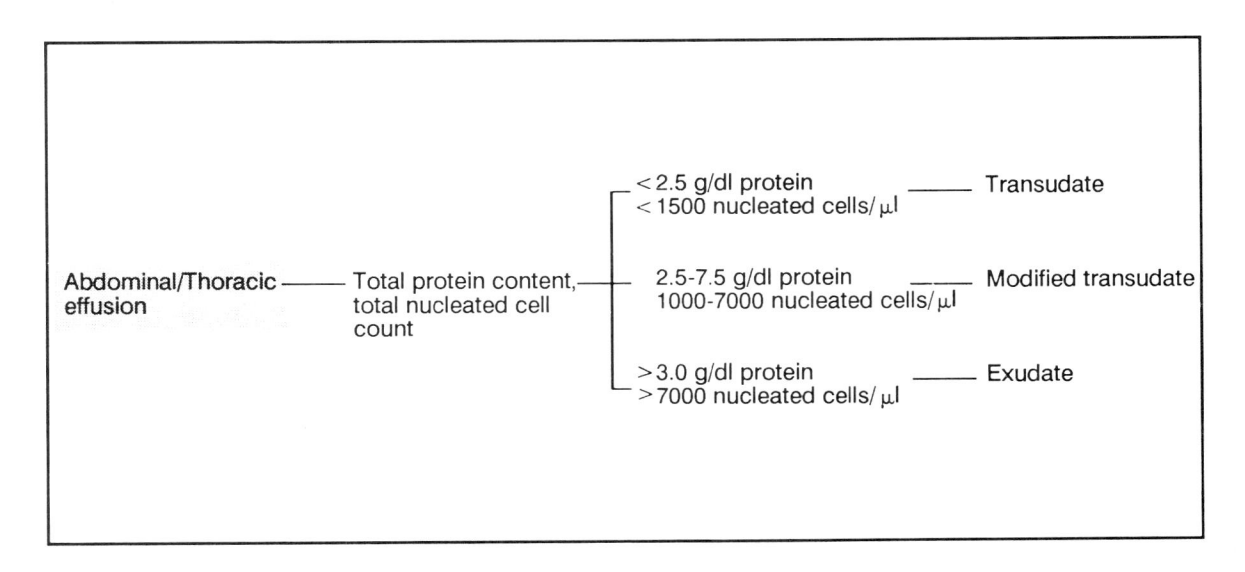

Abdominal/Thoracic effusion	Total protein content, total nucleated cell count	< 2.5 g/dl protein < 1500 nucleated cells/µl	Transudate
		2.5-7.5 g/dl protein 1000-7000 nucleated cells/µl	Modified transudate
		> 3.0 g/dl protein > 7000 nucleated cells/µl	Exudate

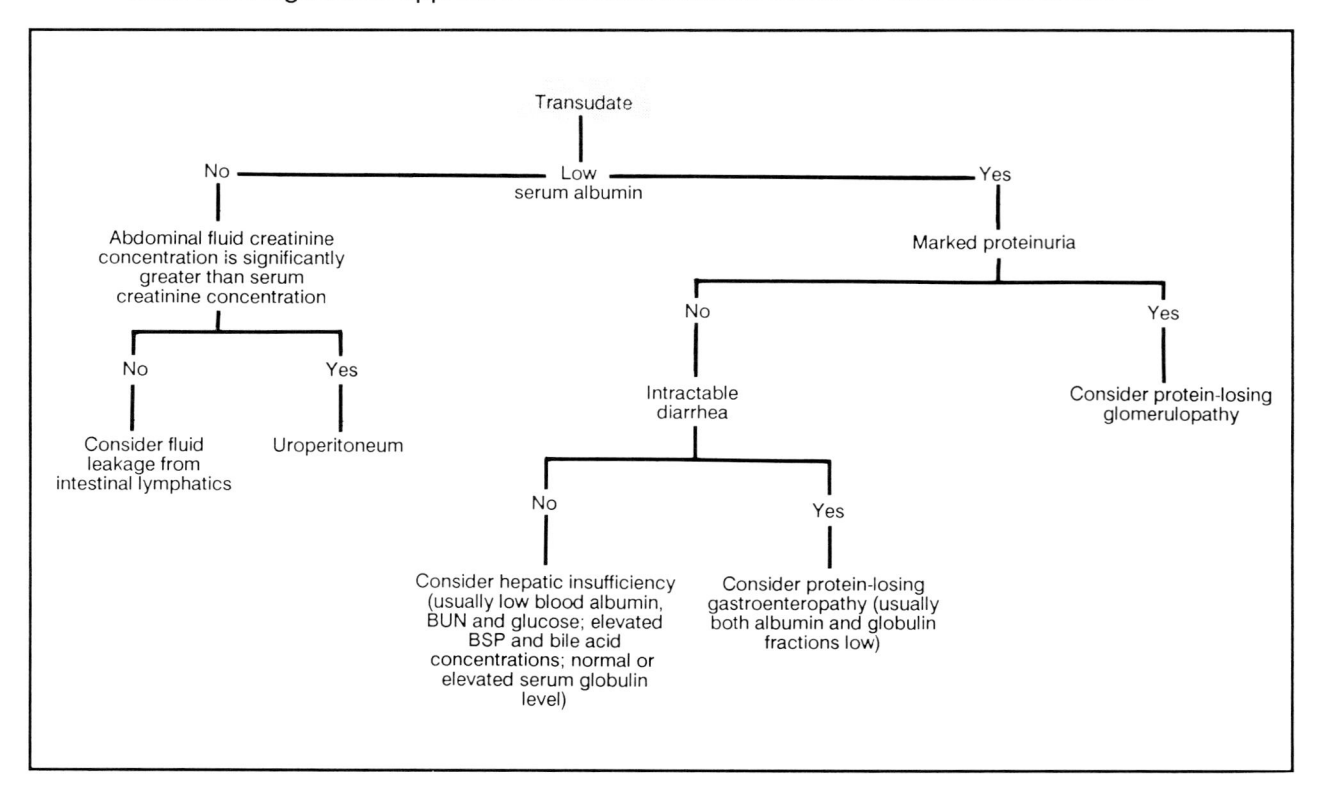

Chart 2. An algorithmic approach to the more common causes of transudative effusions.

```
                              Transudate
                                  |
         No ─────────────────── Low ─────────────────── Yes
          |                 serum albumin                |
   Abdominal fluid creatinine                    Marked proteinuria
   concentration is significantly                         |
   greater than serum                          No ─────────────── Yes
   creatinine concentration                     |                  |
          |                                Intractable       Consider protein-losing
     No ────── Yes                          diarrhea          glomerulopathy
      |         |                              |
  Consider  Uroperitoneum                No ─────── Yes
  fluid                                   |          |
  leakage from                    Consider hepatic   Consider protein-losing
  intestinal                      insufficiency      gastroenteropathy (usually
  lymphatics                      (usually low blood both albumin and globulin
                                  albumin, BUN and   fractions low)
                                  glucose; elevated
                                  BSP and bile acid
                                  concentrations; normal or
                                  elevated serum globulin
                                  level)
```

dates, based solely on their TNCC and TP concentration (Chart 1). Classifying the effusion can help determine the general mechanism of fluid accumulation. Occasionally, there is some overlap in these classifications, ie, a fluid may have a TNCC in the transudate range and a TP in the modified transudate range. If a disparity exists, TP is the more important criterion in separating transudates from modified transudates, while cellularity is more important in separating modified transudates from exudates. While evaluation of an effusion may be diagnostic for such conditions as neoplasia or infection, many effusions simply indicate a process. Historical, physical and clinical information may aid in achieving a definitive diagnosis.

Transudates

Transudates are clear, colorless effusions of low protein concentrations (<2.5 g/dl) and low TNCC (<1500 cells/μl) (Chart 2). Most transudates have protein concentrations <1.5 g/dl; however, 2.5 g/dl is used as the cutoff point because it is the lowest protein concentration at which refractometry is reliable.

Transudative effusions consist primarily of nondegenerate neutrophils and mesothelial/macrophage cell types. They generally occur due to hypoalbuminemia from such conditions as renal glomerular disease, hepatic insufficiency and protein-losing enteropathy. Hypoalbuminemia results in decreased osmotic pressure, allowing fluid to accumulate in the third space. Transudative effusions occurring due to hypoalbuminemia alone generally require serum albumin concentration to be <1.0 g/dl. However, if hypertension is also present, transudative effusions may occur with serum albumin concentrations up to 1.5 g/dl. Rarely, leakage of low-protein lymph from intestinal lymphatics, typically secondary to obstruction of intestinal lymph flow (eg, masses), may cause transudative ascites. Also, ectopic causes of fluid accumulation, such as ruptured urinary bladder and resultant uroperitoneum, can result in a low-cellularity, low-protein fluid. Therefore, classifying an effusion as a

Abdominal and Thoracic Fluid

Chart 3. An algorithmic approach to some common causes of modified transudates.

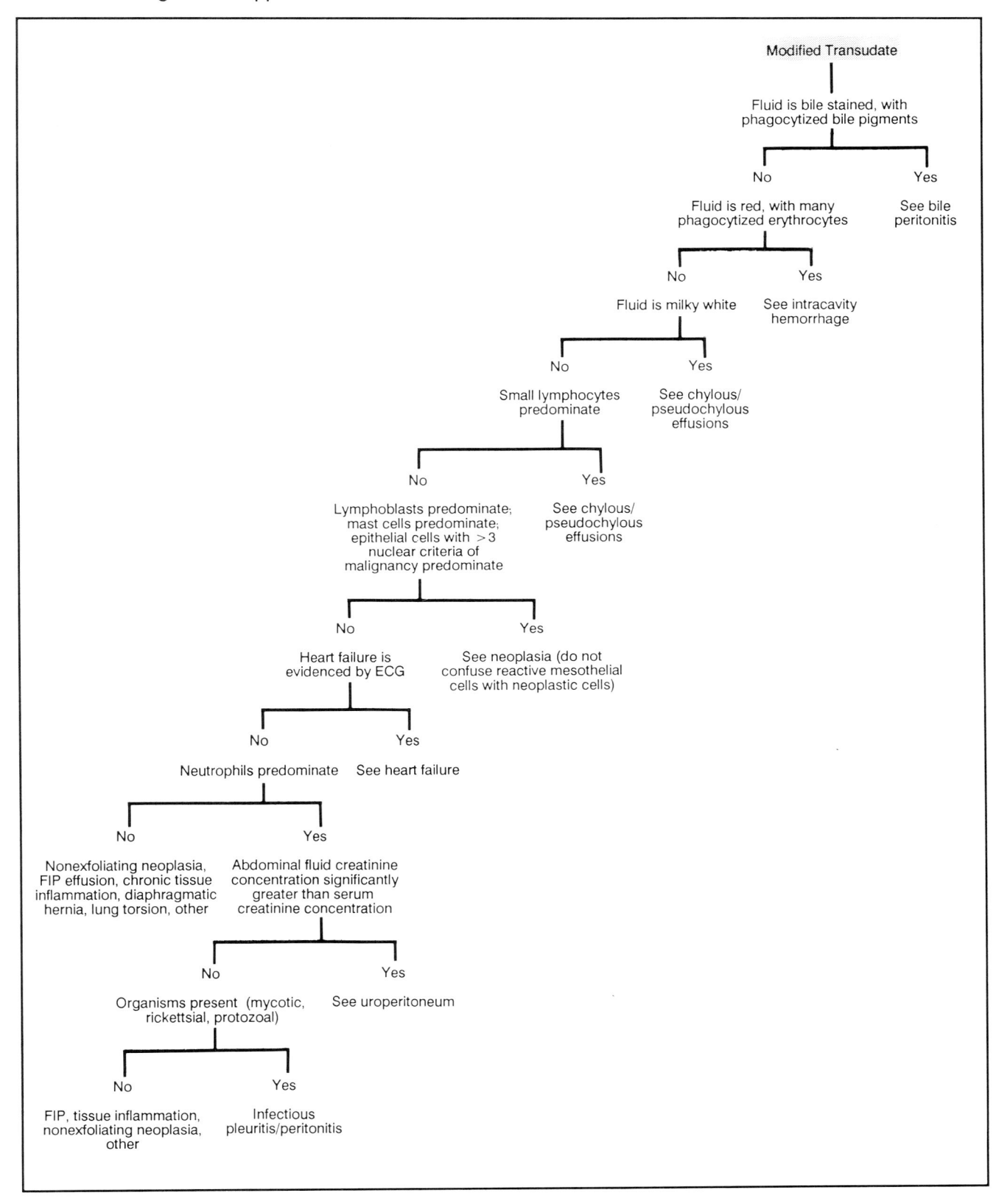

```
                                                          Modified Transudate
                                                                 |
                                                  Fluid is bile stained, with
                                                  phagocytized bile pigments
                                                       /              \
                                                     No                Yes
                                            Fluid is red, with many    See bile
                                            phagocytized erythrocytes  peritonitis
                                                /            \
                                               No             Yes
                                      Fluid is milky white   See intracavity
                                                              hemorrhage
                                          /         \
                                         No          Yes
                                Small lymphocytes   See chylous/
                                 predominate       pseudochylous
                                                     effusions
                                   /        \
                                  No         Yes
                      Lymphoblasts predominate;   See chylous/
                      mast cells predominate;    pseudochylous
                      epithelial cells with >3    effusions
                       nuclear criteria of
                       malignancy predominate
                         /           \
                        No            Yes
                  Heart failure is    See neoplasia (do not
                  evidenced by ECG    confuse reactive mesothelial
                                      cells with neoplastic cells)
                    /         \
                   No          Yes
           Neutrophils predominate   See heart failure
              /         \
             No          Yes
  Nonexfoliating neoplasia,   Abdominal fluid creatinine
  FIP effusion, chronic tissue  concentration significantly
  inflammation, diaphragmatic    greater than serum
  hernia, lung torsion, other    creatinine concentration
                                    /         \
                                   No          Yes
                        Organisms present (mycotic,   See uroperitoneum
                         rickettsial, protozoal)
                            /         \
                           No          Yes
                FIP, tissue inflammation,   Infectious
                nonexfoliating neoplasia,   pleuritis/peritonitis
                         other
```

transudate narrows the differential diagnoses (rule out hypoalbuminemia first) and eliminates consideration of exudative disease.

Modified Transudates

Most modified transudates occur as a result of fluid leakage from lymphatics carrying high-protein lymph or blood vessels. Such leakage is caused by increases in hydrostatic pressure or permeability. Both of these conditions allow high-protein ultrafiltrate fluid to pass into the cavity. Neither of these conditions results in chemotactants in the cavity; therefore, large numbers of inflammatory cells do not migrate into the fluid. Hence, high-protein, low to moderately cellular fluid develops.

The modified transudate class is the least specific classification. Effusions in this classification can develop secondary to many nonspecific disorders. Modified transudates may represent a transition stage. For example, early inflammation from a ruptured gallbladder may result in an effusion in the modified transudate range, since the accumulated fluid dilutes the cells already present. Eventually, sufficient cells accumulate to raise the fluid's cellularity to the exudate level. While modified transudates may develop from many causes, such disorders as cardiovascular disease, lung torsion, neoplasia, intracavity hemorrhage, FIP, tissue inflammation, chylous/pseudochylous effusions, urinary bladder rupture, and gallbladder or major biliary duct rupture should be considered.

Modified transudates have moderate cellularity (1000-7000 cells/μl) and protein concentration (2.5-7.5 g/dl) (Chart 3). The TNCC of the modified transudate overlaps that of the transudate. Modified transudates vary in color from amber to white to red and are frequently slightly turbid to turbid. Nondegenerate neutrophils, mesothelial/macrophage cell types, small lymphocytes or neoplastic cells may predominate, depending on the cause of the effusion.

The causes of modified transudates are many and varied. They may result from generalized disorders (*eg*, cardiovascular disease) or localized disorders (*eg*, liver disease, tumors) that cause increased capillary and/or lymphatic pressure or permeability. They are not seen with bacterial peritonitis or pleuritis unless the animal was severely leukopenic before infection. In those cases, inflammatory cells from the peripheral blood may not be present in sufficient numbers to raise the cell count of the effusion to the exudate level. While bacterial infection in these cavities may itself induce peripheral leukopenia, this is generally due to the influx of cells into the body cavity and possibly sequestration due to endotoxin. Therefore, in cases where the infection induces leukopenia, the TNCC of the effusion is typically in the exudate range.

Exudates

Since this discussion classifies fluids based solely on their TNCC and TP, the exudate classification contains some fluids not typically thought of as true exudates (*eg*, urine from ruptured urinary bladder, neoplastic effusions). However, their inclusion allows an easier, more complete diagnostic approach.

Exudates vary from amber to white to red and are turbid to cloudy fluids. Exudates have high protein concentrations (>3.0 g/dl) and a high TNCC (>7000 cells/μl) (Chart 4). The protein concentration of an exudate overlaps that of a modified transudate. Exudates occur most commonly due to chemotactants in the cavity as a consequence of an inflammatory process. Therefore, neutrophils are the predominant cell type in most inflammatory exudates. If the inflammation is due to bacterial infection, degenerate neutrophils generally predominate, unless the bacteria produce only weak or small amounts of toxin. Occasionally, an exudate develops due to abundant exfoliation of cells from a tumor or secondary to a chylous effusion, in which case neoplastic cells or small lymphocytes, respectively, may predominate.

The term "septic" denotes the presence of bacteria, while "nonseptic" denotes the absence of bacteria. In septic exudates, intracellular and/or extracellular bacteria are generally seen cytologically, while in nonseptic exudates, bacteria are not observed cytologically and culture is negative. Septic exudates typically consist primarily of degenerate neutrophils, while in nonseptic exudates the predominant cell type is variable and may be the nondegenerate neutrophil (inflammation), small lymphocyte (chylous/pseudochylous), or neoplastic cells (carcinoma or sarcoma). When degenerate neutrophils are present, a thorough search for bacteria should be performed. However, not finding organisms cytologically does not totally rule out an infectious cause. Also, since not all bacteria produce strong or

Abdominal and Thoracic Fluid

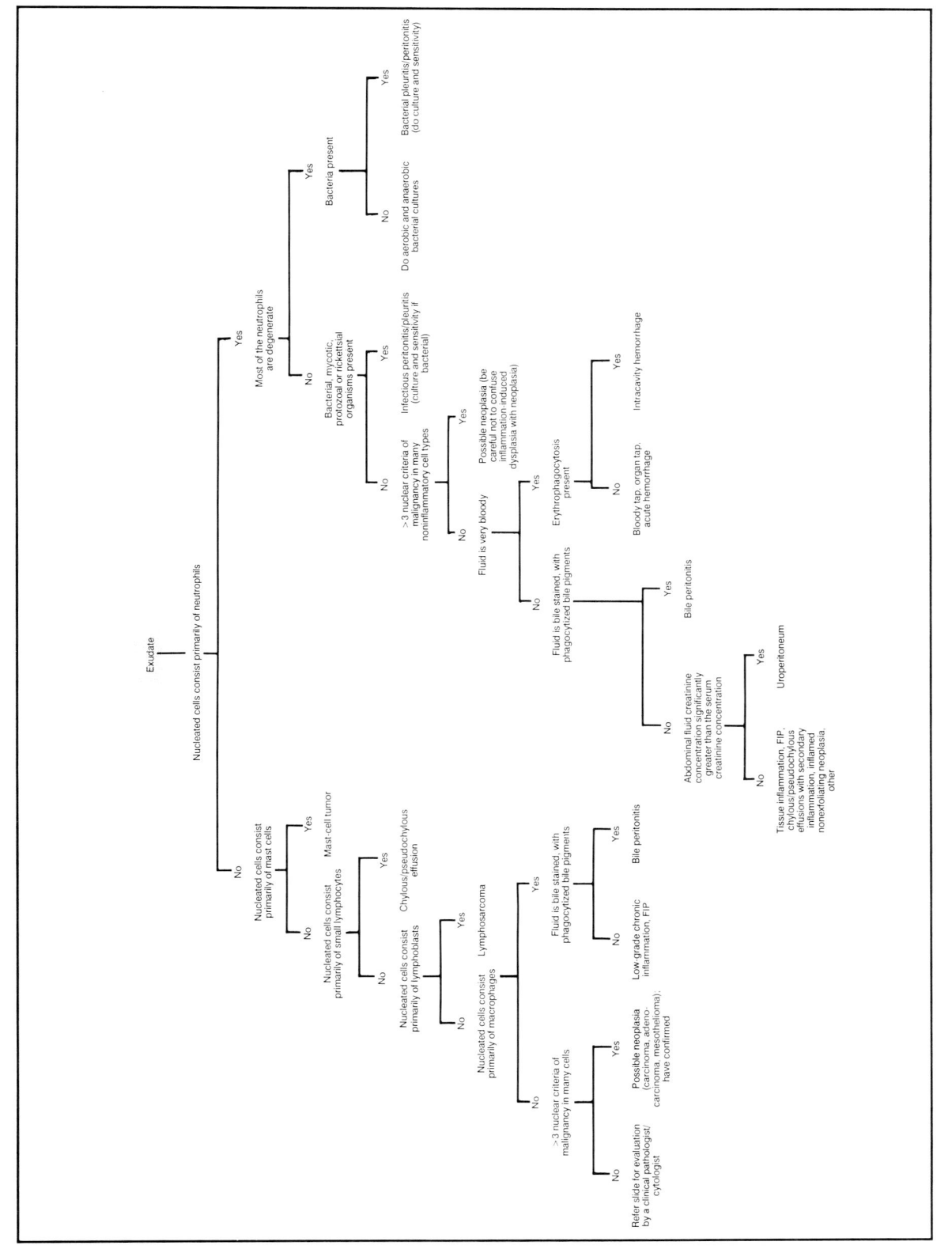

Chart 4. An algorithmic approach to the more common causes of exudative effusions.

161

Figure 5. Pleural fluid containing many degenerate neutrophils, phagocytized and nonphagocytized rods, and some extracellular spirochetes. This pleural fluid was a septic exudate. (Wright's stain, original magnification 250X)

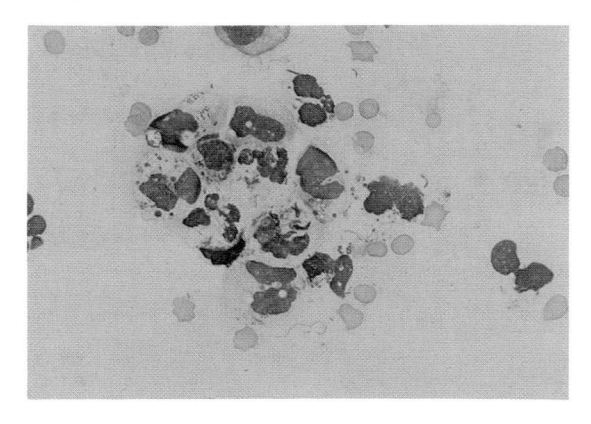

large amounts of toxin, the lack of degenerate neutrophils does not rule out the possibility of bacterial infection.

Effusions in Selected Disorders

Infectious Peritonitis/Pleuritis

Inflammation of the pleural cavity (pleuritis) and peritoneal cavity (peritonitis) are associated with chemotactants and vasoactive substances within the respective cavities. The chemotactants cause increased neutrophil and monocyte/macrophage numbers, while the vasoactive substances cause an influx of high-protein fluid. This results in an exudative effusion due to increased capillary permeability, with a massive outpouring of peripheral blood neutrophils and high-protein plasma filtrate into the cavity.[8] Neutrophils, typically degenerate neutrophils, predominate in bacterial infections; organisms are seen intracellularly and/or extracellulary (Fig 5). Spirochetes occasionally are seen in association with bacterial peritonitis and pleuritis, especially secondary to bite wounds. While bacterial infections are the most common, the authors have recognized mycotic (Plates 4 and 5), protozoal (Plate 5), and rickettsial (Plate 6) peritonitis and/or pleuritis.

Tissue Inflammation

Inflammation of an intracavity organ (eg, liver, spleen, lymph nodes, lungs, etc) or a walled-off abscess may cause an effusion. Inflammatory processes release chemotactants that cause influx of neutrophils and monocytes into the area of inflammation and vasoactive products that increase vascular permeability, causing influx of high-protein fluid. When the inflammatory process extends into the cavity or inflammatory products are released into it, the cavity becomes inflamed (pleuritis/peritonitis) and inflammatory cells tend to accumulate in large numbers. Therefore, many factors, including duration and whether or not an accompanying pleuritis or peritonitis has occurred, determine whether the effusion is in the modified transudate or exudate classification.

In effusions subsequent to tissue inflammation, nondegenerate neutrophils (Figs 1 and 6) generally predominate, but macrophages, mesothelial cells and some lymphocytes also are present. However, macrophages may become the predominant cell type in some chronic inflammatory processes. Cytologic evaluation of these effusions readily identifies the process but is typically nondiagnostic as to etiology and must be correlated with physical findings, history and other laboratory test results.

Feline Infectious Peritonitis

Clinical FIP occurs in cats of all ages, but the highest incidence is in cats <2 years of age.[9] In effusive FIP, fluid may accumulate in the abdomen and/or thorax. Evaluation of the fluid is an easy way to obtain a presumptive diagnosis of FIP. The effusion is an odorless, straw-colored to golden, tenacious fluid that may contain flecks or fibrin strands, and occasionally coagulates upon exposure to air.[9,10] Bacteriologic cultures are typically negative. Though the effusion usually has a high protein (>3.5 g/dl) concentration and a low to mod-

Figure 6. Abdominal fluid from a cat with effusive FIP. Note the nondegenerate neutrophils, RBCs and a small lymphocyte in a granular eosinophilic background. (Wright's stain, original magnification 250X)

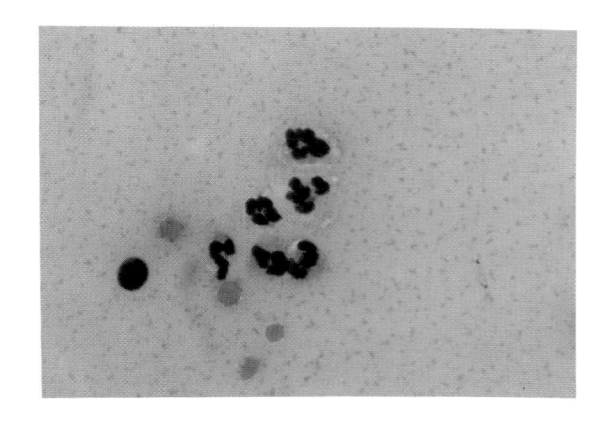

erate cell count (2000-6000/μl), cell counts of 500/μl to >25,000/μl have been reported.[9,10] Due to the high protein content, the effusion foams when shaken.

Cytologically, the typical FIP effusion has a precipitous eosinophilic background due to the high protein content and consists primarily (60-80%) of nondegenerate neutrophils (Fig 6) and lesser numbers of mesothelial/macrophage-type cells, lymphocytes and occasionally plasma cells. These effusions, consisting primarily of neutrophils but with large numbers of macrophages, are referred to as pyogranulomatous. In chronic effusions, the percentage of neutrophils may be lower as the number of mononuclear cells (mesothelial cells, macrophages, lymphocytes) increases.[10] While these findings are not diagnostic of FIP, when associated with age and clinical findings, a presumptive diagnosis of FIP can be made.

Figure 7. Abdominal fluid from a dog with bile peritonitis. A. Neutrophils and some macrophages containing pale blue-green pigment. B. Mononuclear phagocytes containing pale blue-green pigment. (Wright's stain, original magnification 125X)

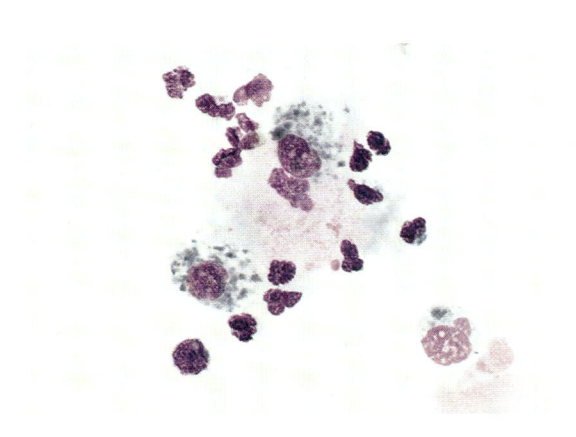

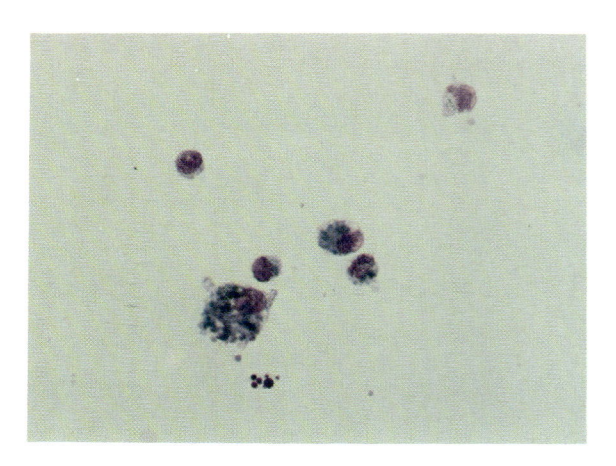

Bile Peritonitis

Release of bile into the abdominal cavity secondary to gallbladder or bile duct rupture produces peritonitis. The effusion is typically yellow-orange. Phagocytized, blue-green to yellow-green bile pigment can be seen within macrophages (Fig 7).

Uroperitoneum

Uroperitoneum may result from rupture of the kidney, ureter, urinary bladder or urethra. Measuring urea nitrogen (UN) or creatinine levels of abdominal fluid and blood collected simultaneously helps diagnose uroperitoneum. With uroperitoneum, the UN and creatinine concentration of the abdominal fluid is greater than that of the peripheral blood. Because urea equilibrates between the cavity and blood more rapidly than creatinine, measurement of creatinine level is more reliable than measurement of the UN level.

Heart Disease

Cats may develop a thoracic effusion secondary to cardiovascular disease (cardiomyopathy). These effusions are yellow to milky white and typically consist of >50% (often >80%) small mature lymphocytes (see chylous/pseudochylous effusions below). However, the proportion of neutrophils increases with repeated drainage of the effusion. The increase in neutrophil numbers is likely due to inflammation caused by thoracentesis and also possibly a proportional increase due to lymphopenia associated with lymphocyte loss.

Ascites secondary to right-sided heart failure is a common problem encountered in veterinary practice. This effusion develops secondary to increased intrahepatic pressure and leakage of high-protein hepatic lymph. Most of the nucleated cells consist of a mixture of mesothelial/macrophage-type cells, nondegenerate neutrophils and lymphocytes. There is no cytologic finding in these effusions that is pathognomonic for heart failure. Clinical, radiographic and/or electrocardiographic examinations are necessary to establish a diagnosis of heart failure. An abdominal effusion in the modified transudate range with a diagnosis of heart failure suggests the effusion is secondary to cardiovascular disease.

Chylous/Pseudochylous Effusions

Chylous effusions in dogs and cats seem to occur most frequently in the thorax, and are generally bilateral.[11] Chylous effusions may

Figure 8. Milky white pleural fluid from a cat with a chylous effusion secondary to cardiovascular disease.

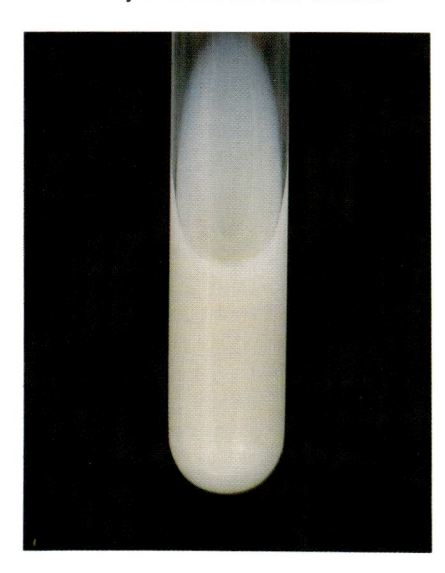

occur secondary to many causes, including heart disease, trauma, inflammation, neoplasia, diaphragmatic herniation, thoracic surgery, vomiting, chronic cough, congenital defects, heartworm infection, foreign bodies, thrombosis of the thoracic duct or terminal vein, or idiopathic causes.[11-16] Trauma and neoplasia are reportedly the most common causes of chylous effusions in dogs.[11,14] In our experience, cardiovascular disease has been the most common cause of intrathoracic chylous effusion in cats.

White milky effusions due to heart disease were originally classified as pseudochylous because no thoracic duct rupture could be demonstrated at necropsy; however, they are now thought to be due to lymphatic leakage without rupture and are classified as chylous effusions.

These effusions are odorless and vary in color from milky white (Fig 8) to yellow or pink, depending on diet and the number of RBCs in the fluid.[11-13,17]

While small lymphocytes are typically thought of as the predominant cell type (Fig 9), chylous effusions occur with neutrophils and/or macrophages predominating.[11,17] Occasionally lymphocytes are present in very small numbers.[13,16,18] With repeated thoracentesis, neutrophil numbers increase secondary to inflammation induced by thoracentesis and perhaps proportionally due to lymphopenia induced by lymphocyte loss. These nondegenerate neutrophils may become the predominant cell type and suggest inflammation, not infection. Bacterial infection in chylous effusions is uncommon due to the bacteriostatic effect of the fatty acids in chyle.[11,12,15] However, bacterial pleuritis secondary to repeated thoracentesis has been reported in dogs with chylothorax.[13]

Since many chylous effusions are not milky white nor made up predominantly of small mature lymphocytes, they are best identified by measuring triglyceride and cholesterol concentrations in both the effusion and peripheral blood.[18,19] With chylous effusions, the triglyceride concentration is higher in the effusion than in the serum, while the cholesterol concentration is higher in the serum than in the effusion.[18,19] The reverse is true for nonchylous effusions.[18,19] Also, the cholesterol concentration of the effusion divided by the triglyceride concentration of the effusion (cholesterol:triglyceride ratio) in chylous effusions is <1.0.[18]

Most milky white effusions are chylous, but occasionally they are pseudochylous. Pseudochylous effusions most commonly occur with neoplastic or inflammatory disorders, but may be associated with any chronic effusion.[12,15] While pseudochylous effusions mimic chylous effusions grossly, their white color is not due to fat but to cellular debris and protein, lecithin globulin complexes, and/or cholesterol granules.[12,15,17,19] Since the white color of pseudochylous effusions is not due to fat, identifying fat droplets cytologically on Sudan III-stained smears of the effusion confirms a diagnosis of chylous effusion.[19] However, cytologically identifiable fat may be absent from some chylous effusions; therefore, not

Figure 9. Sediment smear made from the effusion in Fig 8. Many small mature lymphocytes, vacuolated and non-vacuolated macrophages, and a neutrophil. (Wright's stain, original magnification 250X)

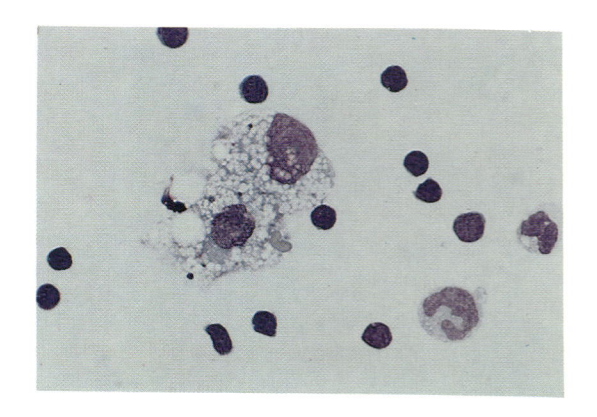

finding fat globules cytologically does not diagnose pseudochylous effusion or rule out a chylous one.[18,19] Chylous effusions often form a top "cream" layer if the fluid is left standing overnight in the refrigerator; pseudochylous effusions do not.[11] Finally, though chylous effusions reportedly clear with ether and pseudochylous effusions do not, this test has unfortunately not been reliable in our experience.[11,12]

Rarely, an effusion is white due to the large number of WBCs present. These are generally due to infectious causes, and degenerate neutrophils and bacteria are found cytologically. Also, while white, these effusions are clumpy (like curdled milk) rather than smooth (milky), as with chylous effusions.

Hemorrhagic Effusion

Hemorrhagic effusions occur with many different disorders. Hemostatic defects, trauma, heartworm infection and neoplasia are some of the more common causes. Differentiating hemorrhagic effusions from blood contamination by bloody taps and organ taps (*eg*, liver, spleen) is of diagnostic importance. Unfortunately, differentiating blood contamination from acute hemorrhage can be difficult. However, if acute hemorrhage is severe, clinical signs indicating severe blood loss should be evident.

Hemorrhage of more than one day's duration or chronic persistent hemorrhage can be differentiated from blood contamination by evaluating the smear for erythrophagocytosis and the presence or absence of platelets. When blood enters a body cavity, the platelets quickly aggregate, degranulate and disappear. Also, RBCs are phagocytized and digested by macrophages. Therefore, the *absence* of erythrophagocytosis and *presence* of platelets suggest either peracute hemorrhage or a bloody tap. The *presence* of erythrophagocytosis *and* platelets suggests either chronic persistent hemorrhage or previous hemorrhage and a bloody tap. The *presence* of erythrophagocytosis (Plate 2) and *absence* of platelets suggest chronic or previous hemorrhage.

Grossly bloody fluid occasionally is collected. In these instances, a splenic tap, puncture of a major vessel, or intracavity hemorrhage should be considered. With a major vessel or splenic tap, the PCV of the fluid generally is equal to (vessel tap) or greater than (splenic tap) the peripheral blood PCV. With severe intracavity hemorrhage, clinical signs of rapid blood loss should be evident.

Neoplasia

Effusions may occur secondary to neoplasia. If neoplastic cells are exfoliated into the effusion, a diagnosis can be made cytologically. Most effusions caused by tumors not exfoliating neoplastic cells are in the modified transudate range. However, most effusions caused by tumors that are exfoliating cells into the cavity and/or are secondarily inflamed are in the exudate category. Recognizing neoplastic cells is much more difficult if inflammation is present because cell dysplasia is readily induced by inflammation. Also, care must be taken not to confuse normal or reactive mesothelial cells with neoplastic cells.

Lymphosarcoma, mast-cell tumor, mesothelioma and various carcinomas, adenocarcinomas and sarcomas have been diagnosed by cytologic evaluation of effusions. Lymphosarcoma is diagnosed by finding large numbers of immature lymphocytes (lymphoblasts) in the effusion (Fig 3). Lymphoblasts have a moderate amount of clear to blue cytoplasm, variably shaped nuclei, finely stippled nuclear chromatin, and nucleoli (often irregular in shape and size); lymphoblasts are larger than neutrophils.

Mast-cell tumors within body cavities may cause effusions and frequently exfoliate large numbers of mast cells into the effusion (Fig 4). Mast cells are readily identified by their red-purple granules. In effusions, mast cells tend to have their granules grouped to one side. Since the granules have a high affinity for stain, the nucleus may stain poorly or not at all. Diff-Quik stain does not undergo the metachromatic reaction and, therefore, often does not stain mast-cell granules well. Eosinophils are usually present also. Neutrophils, mesothelial cells and macrophages may be present in variable numbers.

Rarely, spindle-cell tumors (sarcomas) are diagnosed cytologically in effusions. They are recognized by a characteristic spindle appearance and malignant criteria (see Chapter 1).

Mesotheliomas are uncommon tumors that are difficult to diagnose cytologically because of the variability of normal mesothelial cells. Cytologically, the neoplastic cells resemble epithelium and are present in clusters and individually. Their cytoplasm is generally clear to light blue and vacuolated, and they have

Figure 10. Thoracic effusion secondary to a carcinoma in a dog. A cluster of large carcinoma cells shows marked variation in nuclear size, large nucleoli, coarse nuclear chromatin, perinuclear vacuolation, and basophilic cytoplasm. Note the vacuolated macrophages (upper and lower left) and a mast cell (upper left center). (Wright's stain, original magnification 250X)

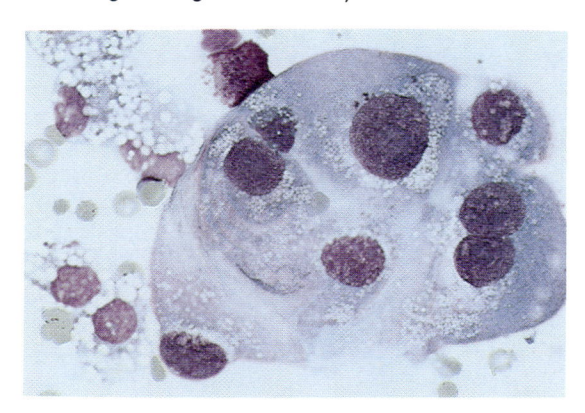

well-defined cell borders. Multinucleation, giant forms and multiple prominent angular nucleoli may be present. When mesothelioma cells are anaplastic enough to be recognized as malignant, they cannot be easily differentiated cytologically from carcinoma cells.

Carcinomas and adenocarcinomas are sometimes diagnosed by cytologic evaluation of effusions (Fig 10). These epithelial-cell tumors are identified on the basis of their nuclear criteria of malignancy. Cytoplasmic aberrations are supportive but not diagnostic. Some of the criteria of malignancy include: anisokaryosis; nuclear gigantism; coarse nuclear chromatin; large, bizarre or angular nucleoli; multiple nucleoli; nuclear molding; high nucleus:cytoplasm ratios; numerous mitotic figures; anisocytosis; basophilic cytoplasm; and abnormal cytoplasmic vacuolation. Also, cluster formation is relatively common with epithelial tumors (carcinoma). Chapter 1 contains a detailed discussion of malignant criteria.

Since many tumors do not exfoliate neoplastic cells, the absence of neoplastic cells within effusions does not rule out neoplasia. Also, differentiating neoplastic cells from reactive mesothelial cells and/or activated macrophages may be difficult. Therefore, unless the examiner is experienced in evaluating cytologic samples for neoplasia, samples interpreted as neoplastic or suspected of being neoplastic should be confirmed by a veterinary clinical pathologist or other experienced cytologist.

References

1. Sherding: Pyothorax in the cat. *Comp Cont Ed Pract Vet* 1:247-253, 1979.

2. Suter and Zinkl, in Ettinger: *Textbook of Veterinary Internal Medicine*. Saunders, Philadelphia, 1983. pp 857-861.

3. Center: Abdominal effusion in the cat. *Proc 53rd Ann Mtg AAHA*, 1986. pp 270-276.

4. Hunt: Diagnostic peritoneal paracentesis and lavage. *Comp Cont Ed Pract Vet* 2:449-453, 1980.

5. Crowe and Crane: Diagnostic abdominal paracentesis and lavage in the evaluation of abdominal injuries in dogs and cats: clinical and experimental investigation. *JAVMA* 168:700-705, 1976.

6. Cowell *et al*: Collection and evaluation of equine peritoneal and pleural effusions. *Vet Clinics No Am (Equine Pract)* 3:543-561, 1987.

7. Duncan and Prasse: *Veterinary Laboratory Medicine & Clinical Pathology*. 2nd ed. Iowa State Univ Press, Ames, 1986. pp 201-210.

8. Kock: Peritonitis. *Comp Cont Ed Pract Vet* 1:295-303, 1979.

9. Sherding: Feline infectious peritonitis. *Comp Cont Ed Pract Vet* 1:95-102, 1979.

10. Weiss and Scott: Laboratory diagnosis of feline infectious peritonitis. *Feline Pract* 10(4):16-22, 1980.

11. Quick: Chylothorax: A review. *JAAHA* 16:23-29, 1980.

12. Berg: Chylothorax in the dog and cat. *Comp Cont Ed Pract Vet* 4:986-991, 1982.

13. Fossum *et al*: Chylothorax in 34 dogs. *JAVMA* 188:1315-1318, 1986.

14. Murphie and Prescott: Chylothorax in a dog. *Mod Vet Pract* 63:484-487, 1982.

15. Walberg: Idiopathic chylothorax in a cat. *JAVMA* 182:525-526, 1983.

16. Willard and Conroy: Chylothorax associated with blastomycosis in a dog. *JAVMA* 186:72-73, 1985.

17. Lindsay: Chylothorax in the domestic cat - a review. *J Small Anim Pract* 15:241-258, 1974.

18. Fossum *et al*: Evaluation of cholesterol and triglyceride concentration in differentiating chylous and non-chylous pleural effusions in dogs and cats. *JAVMA* 188:49-51, 1986.

19. Staats *et al*: The lipoprotein profile of chylous and nonchylous pleural effusions. *Mayo Clin Proc* 55:700-704, 1980.

14

Transtracheal and Bronchial Washes

R.L. Cowell, R.D. Tyler and C.J. Baldwin

Transtracheal/bronchial (TT/B) wash is a quick, easy and inexpensive way to obtain a mucus sample from the trachea, bronchi and/or bronchioles. While complications are uncommon, subcutaneous emphysema, pneumomediastinum, hemorrhage, resultant hypoxia, needle tract infection and other complications have been reported.[1,2]

Cytologic evaluation of secretions of the tracheobronchial tree and associated structures can yield useful information (hypersensitivity reaction, inflammation, infectious agents, neoplasia) on developing or established lower respiratory tract disease. With experience, samples of tracheobronchial mucus can be readily collected without contamination from oropharyngeal organisms or cells. Avoiding oropharyngeal contamination is important because cells and commensal organisms in the oropharyngeal area may give misleading results on culture and cytologic evaluation.

A TT/B wash is indicated to obtain material for culture and/or to cytologically evaluate tracheobronchial mucus in animals with a chronic cough, unresponsive bronchopulmonary disease, or undiagnosed bronchopulmonary disease.[2,3]

Though metastatic and primary neoplasia and mycotic and protozoal infections can be demonstrated by this method, negative findings do not rule out these causes because a TT/B wash collects only material within the tracheobronchial tree. Many disorders, such as metastatic neoplasia, mycotic infections and protozoal infections, tend to localize interstitially and cannot be diagnosed by this method unless they have invaded the tracheobronchial tree. However, since this procedure is less invasive and relatively safe, and can be performed quickly, easily and without general anesthesia, it should be tried before performing a lung aspirate or biopsy.

Chart 1 presents an algorithm for evaluation of TT/B washes.

Technique

Two techniques are described below for collecting TT/B washes. The first technique is more desirable because it can be done without general anesthesia and the likelihood of oropharyngeal contamination is decreased. Bronchoscopy may be used to collect bronchial washings also, but it will not be described in detail in this chapter.

Percutaneous Technique

The skin over the cranioventral larynx is clipped and the site is prepared as for aseptic surgery. A small amount of 1-2% lidocaine is infiltrated into the subcutaneous tissue. In cats and small dogs, very light sedation may be helpful.[1] Intravenous ketamine has been recommended for sedation in cats.[2] The animal is restrained in a sitting position or in sternal recumbency, with the neck extended. Surgical gloves should be worn.

A small, triangular depression is palpated digitally just cranial to the ridge of the cricoid cartilage. This is the location of the cricothyroid ligament and of needle insertion (Fig 1). Using an 18-ga jugular catheter (Venocath: Abbott Labs or Intracath:Bard) with the needle directed slightly caudad, the skin, subcutaneous tissue and cricothyroid ligament of the larynx are penetrated. If a jugular catheter is not available, a 14-ga intravascular catheter or a 3.5-Fr polyethylene urinary catheter may be used.[2] Smaller catheters are suggested for cats and very small dogs.

Once in the tracheal lumen, the needle is positioned parallel with the trachea and the catheter is advanced through the needle and distad in the tracheal lumen to just proximal to the carina. Insertion of the needle and passage of the catheter induce coughing in most animals.[1,2] The catheter should pass easily. If

Chart 1. Flowchart for evaluation of a transtracheal/bronchial wash.

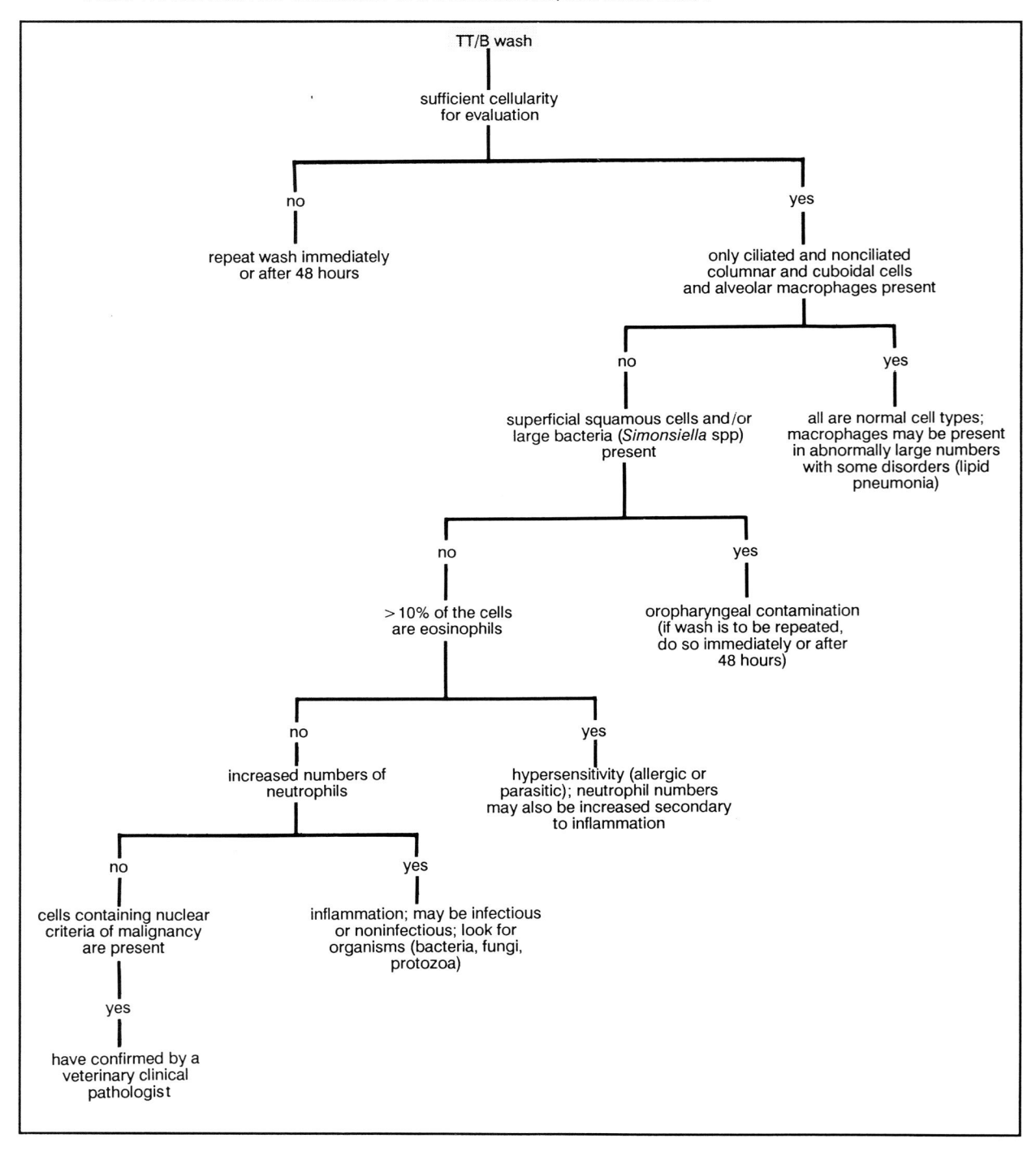

Figure 1. Diagrammatic representation of percutaneous needle placement through the cricothyroid ligament of the larynx.

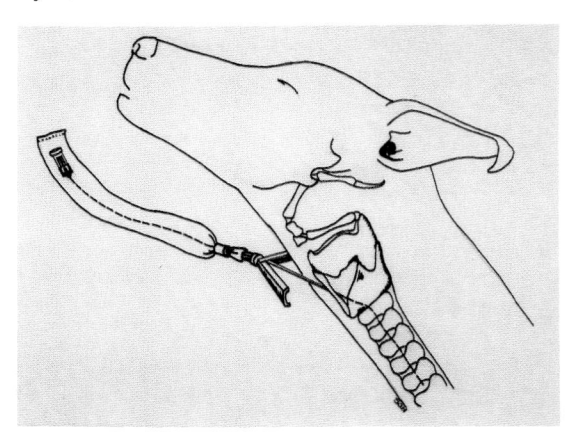

not, the catheter may have become embedded in the dorsal tracheal wall or failed to enter the trachea and is embedded in peritracheal tissue.[3] In either case, the entire catheter and needle should be withdrawn and the procedure repeated. Also, the catheter may bend, causing it to advance proximad toward the oropharynx, resulting in the oropharynx being washed instead of the bronchial tree.

Once the catheter is properly placed, the needle is withdrawn, leaving the catheter in place. With some severe pulmonary diseases, a sample can be obtained by simply aspirating after catheter positioning. However, infusion of saline into the bronchial tree before aspiration is usually necessary to obtain an adequate

Figure 2. Diagrammatic representation of catheter placement and TT/B wash collection through an endotracheal tube.

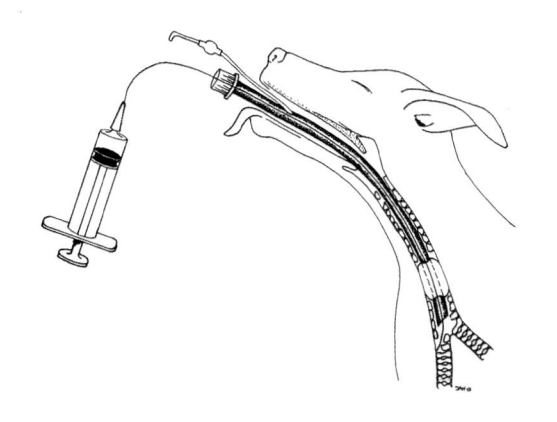

mucus sample. A 12-ml or larger syringe containing nonbacteriostatic sterile buffered saline is attached to the catheter. The saline is injected into the bronchial lumen at 1-2 ml/10 lb until the animal starts to cough or all of the fluid is injected. Typically, the animal starts coughing before all of the saline is injected; aspiration must start at this time.

Only a small portion of injected fluid will be retrieved. Injected fluid remaining in the tracheobronchial tree will be rapidly absorbed and is no cause for concern.[1] The operator aspirates for only a few seconds and then stops aspirating. Aspirating for a prolonged period results in more fluid being collected, but the chance of a contaminated wash is greatly increased because the animal will cough fluid into the oropharyngeal area and reaspirate it. Fluid reaspirated from the oropharynx contains cellular and bacterial contaminants.

After aspirating the tracheal fluid, the catheter is removed and a small portion of the fluid is placed in culture transport medium if culture is indicated. The remaining fluid should be placed in an EDTA (lavender top) tube to prevent clot formation, or slides should be prepared immediately as described for fluid samples in Chapter 1. Maintaining gentle digital pressure on the puncture site for a few minutes generally inhibits formation of subcutaneous emphysema. Applying mild pressure to the puncture site with a gauze wrap for 12-24 hours also helps prevent subcutaneous emphysema.

Endotracheal Tube Technique

Alternatively, bronchial washings may be collected through an endotracheal tube (Fig 2) as described by Moise and Blue.[4] This procedure is less desirable due to both the increased chance of oropharyngeal contamination and the need for general anesthesia. However, in certain cases (fractious or very small animals), it may be indicated.

The endotracheal tube should be sterilized. Though some tubes can tolerate steam sterilization, many require gas sterilization. Gas-sterilized endotracheal tubes can cause irritation of the tracheal mucosa if not properly aired.[4]

The animal is anesthetized and, using an endotracheal tube small enough to allow easy passage into the trachea, is intubated and the cuff is inflated. The animal need not be in a surgical plane of anesthesia. The ideal depth of anesthesia is one allowing easy intubation without inhibiting the cough reflex. To minimize oropharyngeal contamination, the endotracheal tube should be passed with minimal contact with the pharynx and arytenoid cartilages. The animal is then placed in lateral recumbency. Using sterile technique, a 14-ga catheter with stylet in place is passed part way down the endotracheal tube. The metal stylet must be removed before the catheter reaches the end of the endotracheal tube. After the metal stylet is removed the catheter is advanced until it extends 2-4 cm into the trachea. The endotracheal tube and catheter should be pre-measured to ensure that the catheter will extend beyond the endotracheal tube (Fig 2). If the catheter does not extend beyond the endotracheal tube, a good sample will not be obtained.

A 12-ml or larger syringe containing sterile buffered saline is attached to the catheter head. The saline used must not contain bacteriostatic agents. The saline is infused into the bronchi through the catheter at 1-2 ml/10 lb, and negative pressure is immediately applied to retrieve some of the saline and bronchial mucus. If the animal's cough reflex is still intact, its cough aids mucus collection by forcing bronchiolar mucus into the trachea. If the animal begins coughing, aspiration must be done quickly to minimize contamination from oropharyngeal cells and bacteria adhered to the endotracheal tube's outside surface. Also, if the endotracheal tube cuff is not sufficiently inflated, saline may be coughed proximad into the oropharyngeal region and re-aspirated into the bronchi.

If the cough reflex is not intact, retrieval of the saline/mucus mixture may be enhanced by rolling the animal over onto its other side. Since the fluid tends to flow to the dependent (down) lung, turning the animal places this lung in the superior (up) position and enhances fluid flow back to the carina. Also, gently compressing the thorax may help move the fluid toward the catheter.

After aspirating some of the infused saline, the catheter is removed from the trachea with the endotracheal tube acting as a protective shield from oropharyngeal contamination during removal. A portion of the fluid, reserved for cytologic slide preparation, should be placed in an EDTA (lavender top) tube to prevent clot formation, or slides should be prepared immediately as described for fluid samples in Chapter 1. A portion of the fluid should also be placed in culture transport medium if culture is indicated.

Bronchoscopy

Bronchial washings may also be collected through a fiberoptic bronchoscope (Olympus Corp., Lake Success, NY). Bronchoscopy has the advantage of allowing the operator to visualize the bronchi and collect biopsies, brushings or washings. The major disadvantages are the expense of the instrument and the need for general anesthesia. In the authors' experience, washings have yielded more representative and diagnostic samples of lung lesions and are preferred over brushings except when focal lesions can be visualized and brushed.

Repeating a Wash

If the TT/B wash is deemed unacceptable due to oropharyngeal contamination (or for any reason) and must be repeated, it should be repeated immediately or after a 48-hour wait. Even though a sterile saline solution is used for the wash, it induces a neutrophilic response that peaks around 24 hours after washing. If a TT/B wash is performed the next day (24 hours after the first wash), it may be difficult to tell if the inflammatory response observed is secondary to the prior wash or due to an inflammatory lung disease.[5-7]

If a contaminated wash is obtained, waiting 48 hours to collect another TT/B wash is ideal, as it allows the lungs time to clear the oropharyngeal contaminants. Sometimes, however, such a delay may not be practical. While some contaminants from the previous wash may be collected if the TT/B wash is repeated

Figure 3. Transtracheal/bronchial wash from a dog with chronic bronchial disease. A large Curschmann's spiral and scattered alveolar macrophages are present in an eosinophilic mucus background. (Wright's stain, original magnification 50X)

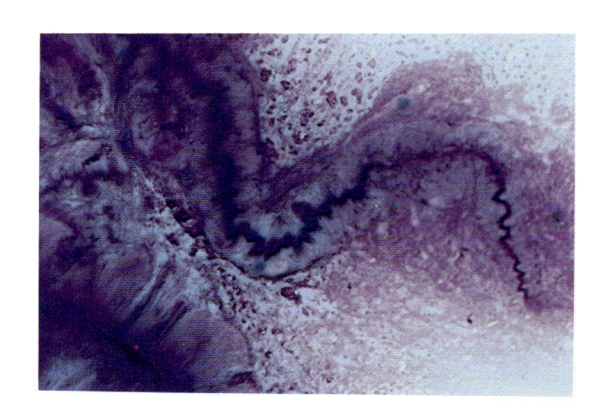

immediately, it should be minimal and may be preferable to waiting 48 hours.

Cell Counts

Cell counts on TT/B wash fluids are difficult to perform because of their mucus content and are of little diagnostic significance. Therefore, they are generally not done. Qualitative estimates (normal or increased) of cellularity on stained sediment smears and may be useful.

Slide Preparation

Diagnostic-quality smears can be made from most TT/B wash fluids by first concentrating the cells by centrifugation (see sediment procedure in Chapter 1). If the fluid is clear after centrifuging, pouring off the supernatant and resuspending the pellet, a line smear should be made as described in Chapter 1. Clear fluids may be of such low cellularity that accurate evaluation cannot be done cytologically. In this instance, the TT/B wash should be repeated. If the fluid is grossly turbid, a pull smear or squash preparation should be made as described in Chapter 1.

Cytologic Evaluation

Mucus

A small amount of mucus may be present in TT/B washes from clinically normal dogs and cats. Mucus appears as blue to pink amorphous sheets or homogeneous strands that are frequently twisted or whorled (Figs 3,6,8,11,12).[1,4] A granular appearance to the mucus is frequently associated with increased cellu-

Figure 4. Transtracheal/bronchial wash from a dog with toxoplasmosis. A ciliated columnar cell, RBC, scattered neutrophils and an extracellular *Toxoplasma gondii* organism are shown. (Wright's stain, original magnification 250X)

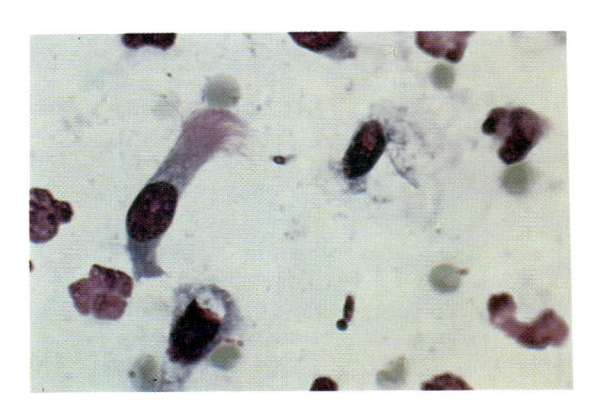

Figure 5. Transtracheal/bronchial wash from a dog. A goblet cell (arrow) and several ciliated columnar cells are shown. (Wright's stain, original magnification 250X)

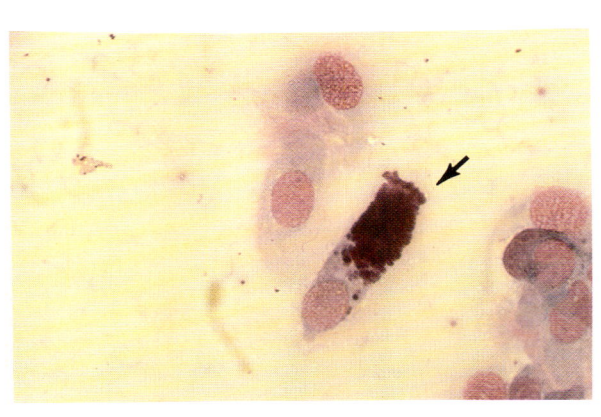

larity.[1] Inflammation from irritation, infection or upper airway damage results in increased mucus production.[5] In inflammatory conditions, mucus typically stains eosinophilic due to incorporation of inflammatory proteins and material from lysed cells into the mucus.[1]

Curschmann's spirals (Fig 3) are mucus casts of small bronchioles.[8] They appear as spirally twisted masses of mucus that may have perpendicular radiations that impart a test-tube-brush-like appearance. They may be seen in TT/B washings from patients with any disorder resulting in chronic, excessive production of mucus.

Cell Types

With TT/B washes, many different cell types may be seen, including ciliated and nonciliated columnar cells, ciliated and nonciliated cuboidal cells, alveolar macrophages, neutrophils, eosinophils, lymphocytes, mast cells, RBC, and dysplastic and neoplastic cells. Ciliated and nonciliated columnar and cuboidal cells and alveolar macrophages are the cell types seen in washings from normal dogs and cats, and also may be seen in pathologic conditions unless the area washed is filled with exudative secretions or the disease process has obliterated normal lung parenchyma.

Columnar and Cuboidal Cells: Ciliated columnar cells (Figs 4,5) are elongated or cone shaped, with cilia on the flattened end and the nucleus in the other (basal) end, frequently terminating in a tail. The nucleus is generally round to oval, with a finely granular chromatin pattern.[8] Ciliated cuboidal cells appear similar to ciliated columnar cells except cuboidal cells are as wide as they are tall. Nonciliated columnar and cuboidal cells appear identical to their ciliated counterpart, except cilia are absent.

Goblet Cells: Goblet cells (Fig 5) are mucus-producing bronchial cells. They are generally elongated (columnar) cells with a basally placed nucleus and round granules of mucin frequently distending the cytoplasm.[8] Occasionally the cytoplasm is so greatly distended that the cell appears round. The granules stain red to blue with hematologic stains. Granules from ruptured goblet cells may be seen free in the smear. Goblet cells are not commonly seen. However, any chronic pulmonary irritant may result in increased numbers of goblet cells.

Macrophages: Alveolar macrophages (Figs 6,12,13) are readily found in TT/B washings from clinically normal animals and may be the predominant cell type. Their nucleus is round to bean shaped and eccentrically positioned. A binucleate alveolar macrophage may rarely be seen in clinically normal animals. Alveolar macrophages have abundant blue-gray, granular cytoplasm. When they become activated, the cytoplasm becomes more abundant and vacuolated (foamy), and may contain phagocytized material.[9]

Neutrophils: Neutrophils in a TT/B wash look like those in peripheral blood (Figs 7,11 and Plate 1), though degenerative changes may be present. Increased numbers of neutrophils indicate inflammation. See the discussion on inflammation later in the chapter.

Figure 6. Transtracheal/bronchial wash from a dog. Many alveolar macrophages and some neutrophils in an eosinophilic mucus background are shown. (Wright's stain, original magnification 132X)

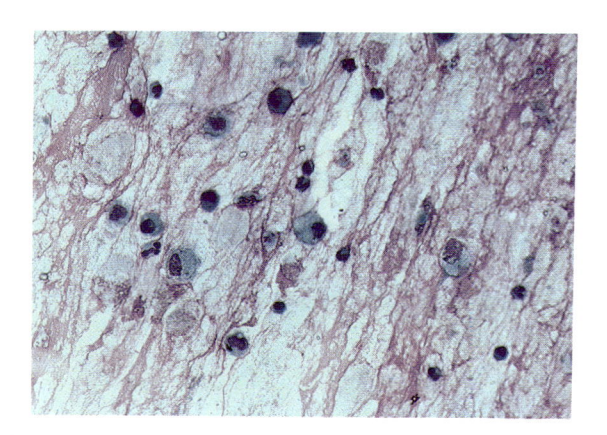

Figure 7. Transtracheal/bronchial wash from a dog. Neutrophils and superficial squamous cells are shown. Superficial squamous cells denote oropharyngeal contamination. (Wright's stain, original magnification 50X)

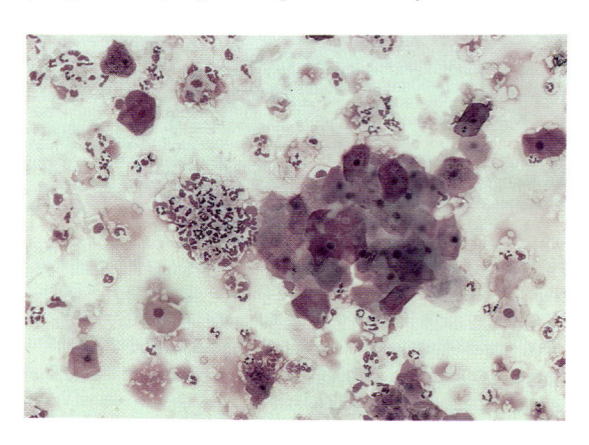

Eosinophils: Eosinophils (Fig 9 and Plate 2) are bone-marrow-derived granulocytes containing intracytoplasmic granules. These granules are lysosomes that have an affinity for the acid dye eosin (eosinophilic), which stains them red. Increased numbers of eosinophils indicate a hypersensitivity reaction, either allergic or parasitic (see hypersensitivity later in the chapter) (Fig 9).

Lymphocytes/Plasma Cells: Lymphocytes (Plate 1) may be present in small numbers in TT/B washes from normal dogs and cats. Increased numbers of lymphocytes generally denote nonspecific inflammation and are of limited diagnostic value. Mild increases in lymphocyte numbers reportedly occur with airway hyperreactivity, viral diseases of the tracheobronchial tree and chronic infections.[1,10] With immune stimulation, lymphocytes become activated. Their cytoplasm becomes more abundant and stains deep-blue because of increased protein synthesis. Also, some lymphocytes transform into plasma cells.

Mast Cells: Mast cells (Plate 2) are usually present in small numbers and are of little diagnostic significance. Mast cells are occasionally observed in TT/B washes from dogs and cats with many different inflammatory lung disorders. Mast cells are readily identified by their red-purple intracytoplasmic granules. These granules are frequently present in large numbers and may obscure the nucleus. Scattered granules from ruptured mast cells may

Figure 8. Oropharyngeal contamination in a transtracheal/bronchial wash from a dog. Mucus, alveolar macrophages and a large superficial squamous cell with bacteria adhered to its surface are present. Bacteria are also scattered throughout the slide. (Wright's stain, original magnification 250X)

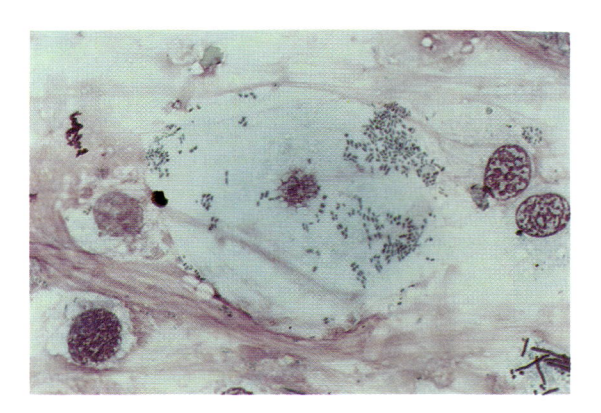

be present free on the slide and must not be confused with bacteria. A mild increase in mast cell numbers reportedly occurs with airway hyperreactivity.[10]

Superficial Squamous Cells: Superficial squamous cells are large epithelial cells with abundant, angular cytoplasm and a small round nucleus. Superficial squamous cells in a TT/B wash indicate oropharyngeal contamination (Figs 7,8). See the discussion on oropharyngeal contamination later in this chapter.

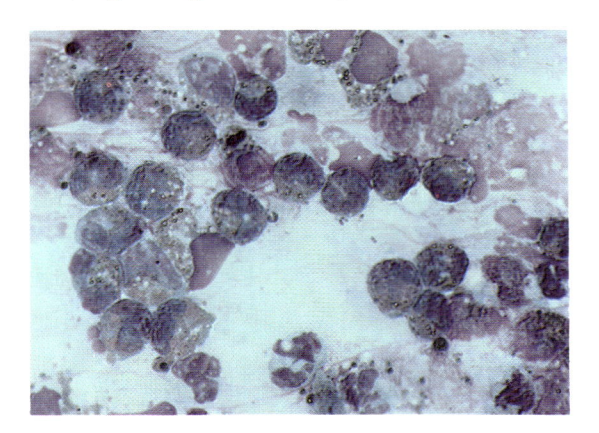

RBC: Erythrocytes may be present within macrophages or free on the slide. Erythrophagocytosis (Fig 13) indicates intrapulmonary hemorrhage. See the discussion on hemorrhage later in the chapter.

Atypical Cell Types

Atypical cells may be seen with pulmonary metaplasia, dysplasia or neoplasia (primary or metastatic). Anticancer therapy, such as irradiation and chemotherapy, may result in such severe atypia of cells of the tracheobronchial epithelium, terminal bronchial epithelium and alveolar epithelium that differentiation from neoplasia cannot be reliably made.[8] Any atypical cells observed cytologically should be evaluated for malignant criteria (Chapter 1). Transtracheal/bronchial washes collected after cancer therapy should be interpreted with caution.

Figure 10. Transtracheal/bronchial wash from a dog. A large lungworm larva is shown. (Wright's stain, original magnification 100X)

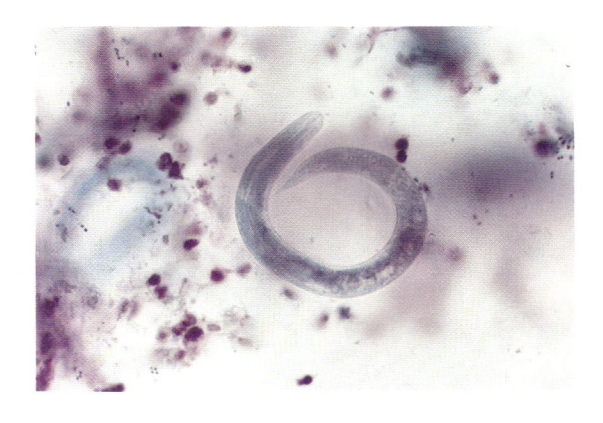

Figure 9. Transtracheal/bronchial wash from a dog. Mucus, scattered neutrophils and a large number of eosinophils are shown. Some extracellular bacterial rods, likely from oropharyngeal contamination, are also present. (Wright's stain, original magnification 330X)

Metaplasia: Metaplasia is an adaptive response of epithelial cells to chronic irritation.[8,11] Replacement of normal pulmonary epithelial cells of the trachea, bronchi and bronchioles with stratified squamous epithelium (squamous metaplasia) is an example of pulmonary metaplasia.[11] The metaplastic cells mimic maturing squamous epithelium and must not be confused with neoplastic cells.

Dysplasia: Dysplasia is, by definition, a nonneoplastic change.[11] However, severely dysplastic changes are sometimes referred to as carcinoma *in situ*.[11] Dysplastic changes include variation in cell size and shape, increased nucleus:cytoplasm ratio, darker-staining cells, and increased numbers of immature cells.[11] These changes can be difficult to differentiate from those in neoplasia and may progress to neoplasia.[11]

Neoplastic Cells: Neoplastic cells are only rarely seen on cytologic evaluation of TT/B washings. Unless the neoplasm has invaded the tracheobronchial tree and invaded bronchioles are not blocked by mucus plugs, they are not accessible for collection by TT/B wash. When neoplastic cells are observed, they are generally from adenocarcinomas. These large epithelial cells may be present as single cells or in clusters (Plates 6). Their cytoplasm is generally basophilic and vacuolated. They have a high nucleus:cytoplasm ratio, coarse nuclear chromatin, and prominent nucleoli that frequently are large and angular. Care must be taken not to confuse inflammation-induced cell dysplasia with neoplasia.

Miscellaneous Findings

Surgical glove powder (corn starch) is occasionally seen on slides from TT/B washes. This material typically appears as a large, round to hexagonal structure that stains clear to blue and has a central fissure (Fig 11). Glove powder is an incidental finding and should not be confused with an organism or cell.

Figure 11. Transtracheal/bronchial wash from a dog. Large numbers of neutrophils, an alveolar macrophage and a cluster of 4 granules of glove powder (corn starch) are present in an eosinophilic mucus background. (Wright's stain, original magnification 165X)

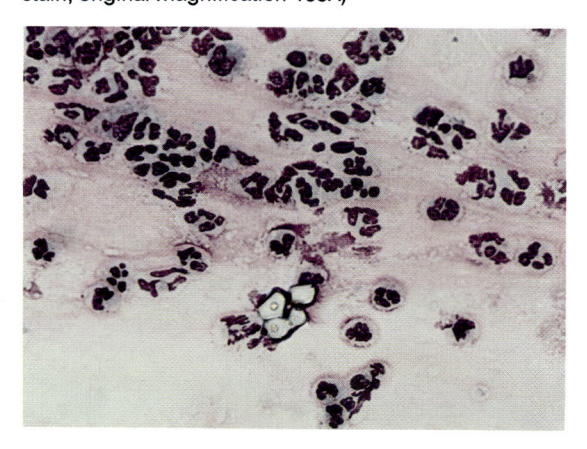

Figure 12. Transtracheal/bronchial wash from a dog with chronic lung disease. Many alveolar macrophages, 2 neutrophils and a single multinucleated giant-cell macrophage are present in an eosinophilic mucus background. (Wright's stain, original magnification 132X)

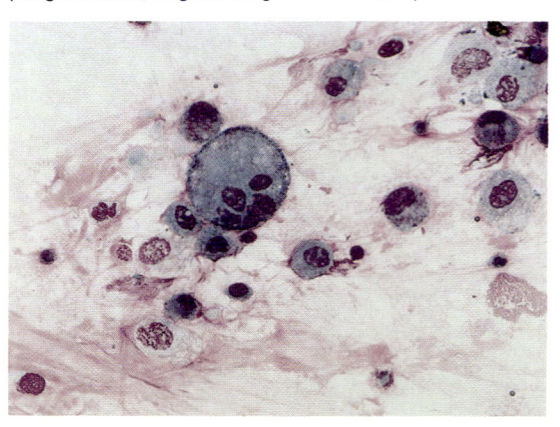

Plant pollen or plant cells may occasionally be present in TT/B washes. These should not be confused with an organism or cell.

Cytologic Interpretation

Transtracheal/bronchial washes are interpreted according to the type, quantity and proportion of cells recovered. They can generally be classified into the following categories: insufficient sample, no cells or an inadequate number of cells for evaluation; oropharyngeal contamination, superficial squamous cells and/or *Simonsiella* spp are observed (see oropharyngeal contamination below); eosinophilic infiltrate, increased numbers of eosinophils (see hypersensitivity below); neutrophilic infiltrate, increased numbers of neutrophils (see inflammation below); macrophage infiltrate, sample is very cellular and consists primarily of macrophages (see inflammation below); and atypical cells, evaluate for criteria of malignancy (see neoplasia below).

These categories, other than the first category, are not mutually exclusive. Classification of TT/B washes into one or more of the above categories allows the process(es) to be identified. Chart 1 presents an algorithm to aid in evaluation of TT/B washes. Integration of historical, physical and clinical findings may allow further refinement of the diagnosis.

Oropharyngeal Contamination

Oropharyngeal contamination is much more likely to occur when a TT/B wash is collected by passing the catheter through an endotracheal tube than by penetrating the cricothyroid ligament and bypassing the oropharyngeal area. Regardless of the procedure used, careful attention must be paid to technique to avoid oropharyngeal contamination.

Superficial squamous cells and certain large bacteria (*Simonsiella* spp) are the hallmark of oropharyngeal contamination. Superficial squamous cells (Figs 7,8) are large epithelial cells with abundant, angular cytoplasm and a small round nucleus. *Simonsiella* bacteria (Plate 3) divide lengthwise and, therefore, line up in parallel rows, giving the impression of a single large bacterium. These nonpathogenic organisms may be seen adhered to the surface of superficial squamous cells or free in the smear.

While superficial squamous cells and *Simonsiella* spp indicate oropharyngeal contamination, it must be remembered that whatever cellular constituents and bacteria are present in the oropharyngeal area may be present in a contaminated wash. Therefore, a variety of bacilli and cocci may be present in a contaminated wash (Fig 8). Bacteria without neutrophils are generally seen when the wash consists primarily of oropharyngeal contaminants. These organisms may be free or adhered to superficial squamous cells. Neutrophils may occur in a TT/B wash secondary to oropharyngeal contamination if the animal has a purulent or ulcerative oropharyngeal lesion. Therefore, oropharyngeal contamination can alter the cytologic evaluation and culture results.

Hypersensitivity

Eosinophils are important in defending against helminth infections and in modulating hypersensitivity reactions.[12] Eosinophils are present only in very small numbers (<5%) in TT/B washes from normal dogs and cats. Cytologically, eosinophils in bronchial mucus look like peripheral blood eosinophils. Eosinophil numbers >10% of inflammatory cells present in TT/B washes indicate a hypersensitivity (allergic or parasitic) response (Fig 9). Eosinophils often are the predominant cell type in these disorders. Allergic bronchitis/pneumonitis, feline asthma, lungworms, heartworms and eosinophilic granuloma or pneumonia are some of the disorders frequently causing eosinophilic lung infiltrates.

Granules may be seen free in the smear secondary to rupture of eosinophils. They stain eosinophilic and should not be confused with bacteria. Eosinophil granules may coalesce into a large crystal known as a Charcot-Leyden crystal. These elongated double pyramids can occur in any condition that causes accumulation of large numbers of eosinophils.

Circulating and, likely, tissue eosinophil numbers are decreased by glucocorticoid administration. Therefore, glucocorticoid therapy may mask the typical eosinophilic response seen cytologically with reaginic (IgE) hypersensitivity.

Transtracheal/bronchial washes should be scanned on low power (10X objective) for parasitic larvae or ova (Fig 10). Parasitic larvae (*Filaroides* spp, *Aelurostrongylus abstrusus, Crenosoma vulpis*) and ova (*Capillaria aerophila, Paragonimus* spp) are large and readily identified. Frequently an eosinophilic hypersensitivity response is noted cytologically. Inflammatory cells may predominate, especially if pneumonia is present.

Increased numbers of neutrophils and/or macrophages may be seen along with increased numbers of eosinophils if tissue irritation is sufficient to induce an inflammatory response.

Inflammation

Neutrophils are present only in very small numbers (generally <5%) in TT/B washes from normal dogs and cats.[1,9] Neutrophils in bronchial mucus look like peripheral blood neutrophils. They may show degenerative changes due to bacterial toxins or may be "smudged" (ruptured) by trauma from collection and preparation. Influx of neutrophils occurs early in an inflammatory response, making TT/B wash neutrophils a sensitive indicator of inflammation.[5] Even very mild insults, such as a sterile saline TT/B wash, result in marked influx of neutrophils. As a result, neutrophil numbers are increased in nearly all conditions that cause inflammation, both infectious and noninfectious (Fig 11). Infectious disorders include bacterial, mycotic, viral and protozoal diseases. Noninfectious disorders include tissue irritation or necrosis secondary to inhalation of toxic substances (*eg*, smoke), as well as a neoplasm that has outgrown its blood supply and developed a necrotic center.

When neutrophil numbers are increased, one should look closely for bacteria (especially intracellularly) and other microorganisms. Organisms can be found cytologically in most bacterial infections, while noninfectious inflammation or totally interstitial infections are typified by absence of microorganisms.

Increased numbers of macrophages are seen with many subacute and chronic lung disorders, such as congestive heart failure, granulomatous pneumonia and lipid pneumonia. Alveolar macrophage numbers frequently increase with chronic persistent inflammation.[5] Binucleate and multinucleate giant-cell macrophages (Fig 12) may be seen in conditions producing chronic lung disease.[8] Large, lipid-containing vacuoles may be present within macrophages in lipid pneumonia.[8] Dark or black granules (anthracotic pigment) may be present within macrophages from clinically normal animals living in large cities or other areas with polluted air. Phagocytized RBC (erythrophagia) and RBC breakdown products (hematoidin, hemosiderin) may be seen within the cytoplasm of macrophages in conditions causing pulmonary hemorrhage, such as heart failure (Fig 13 and Plate 2). Because macrophages are also important in defense against microorganisms, phagocytized microorganisms (fungi, protozoa or bacteria) may be seen.

If the causative agent can be identified, a diagnosis can be made. Otherwise, cytologic changes are interpreted as neutrophilic (purulent) or granulomatous inflammation, of which there are many causes. Bacterial tracheobronchitis, pneumonia or abscesses, necrotic tumors and inhalation of toxic substances frequently result in neutrophilic reactions. Fungi and protozoa frequently cause granuloma formation or may cause a neutrophilic response.

Bacterial Diseases: Many different bacteria can cause pulmonary infection and disease. Bacterial pneumonia is generally due to infection by a Gram-negative bacillus.[13] Cytologically, one would see bacteria phagocytized and free in TT/B washes from animals with bacterial pneumonia. Localized lung abscesses, even a small peripheral pulmonary infection, should yield organisms on TT/B wash and a neutrophilic response if bronchial communication exists.[14]

Identification of bacteria as bacilli or cocci (Plate 3) helps in choosing antibiotic therapy while awaiting culture and sensitivity results. With the hematologic stains, all bacteria (both Gram positive and Gram negative) stain blue-black. Since most pneumonias are due to infection with Gram-negative bacilli, if bacilli (especially bipolar bacilli) are seen cytologically, one should choose an antimicrobial effective against Gram-negative bacteria while awaiting culture and sensitivity results. Pathogenic cocci generally include *Staphylococcus* and *Streptococcus*; therefore, when cocci are seen cytologically, one should choose an antimicrobial effective against Gram-positive bacteria while awaiting culture and sensitivity results.

Mycotic and Protozoal Diseases: Many different fungi and protozoa can invade and colonize the lungs. Any organisms within the tracheobronchial tree can readily be collected by TT/B wash. If TT/B wash fails to yield organisms and a mycotic or protozoal infection is suspected, a lung aspirate or biopsy is indicated, since the organisms may be totally interstitial and not accessible to collection by TT/B wash.

Some of the more common fungi and protozoa that can invade pulmonary tissue are *Blastomyces dermatitidis* (Plate 4), *Cryptococcus neoformans* (Plate 4), *Coccidioides immitis* (Plate 5), *Histoplasma capsulatum* (Plate 4), *Sporothrix spp* (Plate 4), *Aspergillus* spp or other opportunistic fungi (Plate 5), *Toxoplasma gondii* (Plate 5), *Cytauxzoon felis* (Plate 5) and *Pneumocystis carinii* (Plate 5).

Viral Diseases: Many viral respiratory diseases can cause lung damage and allow secondary bacterial infection. Cytologically, one sees increased numbers of neutrophils, indicating inflammation. Lymphocyte numbers may be slightly increased, but this is a nonspecific change. If secondary bacterial infection

Figure 13. Transtracheal/bronchial wash from a dog with severe heart disease contains many free RBC. Alveolar macrophages with phagocytized RBC indicate that the RBC originate from intrapulmonary hemorrhage and not from hemorrhage secondary to collection of the TT/B wash. (Wright's stain, original magnification 250X)

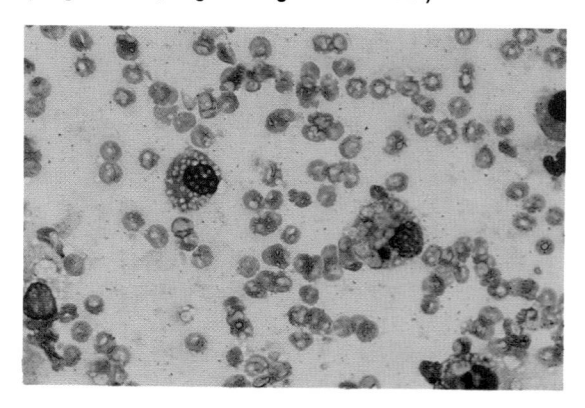

has occurred, bacteria may be seen intracellularly and free on the smear.

Hemorrhage

Erythrocytes may be seen in TT/B washes from dogs and cats with disorders causing vascular damage or RBC diapedesis into the lung. Intrapulmonary hemorrhage may be of pulmonary origin, as with trauma, infarcts (especially from heartworms), foreign bodies, lung lobe torsion, infectious diseases (bacterial, fungal, parasitic) and neoplasia. Intrapulmonary hemorrhage may also occur with disorders that are not of primary respiratory origin, such as heart failure, pulmonary embolism, hemostatic disorders and metastatic neoplasia.[15] Erythrocytes and/or RBC breakdown products (hemosiderin, hematoidin) within alveolar macrophages indicate chronic hemorrhage (Fig 13 and Plate 2). Often the hemorrhage is occult and finding hemosiderin-laden alveolar macrophages is the first indication of chronic pulmonary hemorrhage. These macrophages are frequently referred to as heart failure cells; however, they may occur with any disorder resulting in intrapulmonary hemorrhage.

Neoplasia

Neoplasia may exist as a single, solitary nodule or diffuse infiltration. Solitary lesions are rare in metastatic lung tumors but common in primary lung tumors. Most pulmonary neoplasms are metastatic nodules from malignant tumors at sites other than the lungs. Since metastatic lung tumors are generally interstitial, neoplastic cells are not collected by TT/B wash unless the tumor has invaded the bronchial tree and that portion of the bronchial tree is not clogged by secretions, or the tumor is so peripherally located its cells are uncollectable by TT/B wash. Primary lung tumors involving the bronchial tree generally exfoliate cells that are collected by routine washings. However, primary lung tumors are rare in dogs and cats.[16] Therefore, neoplastic cells are only very rarely seen on TT/B washes from dogs and cats.

Adenocarcinomas are by far the most common lung tumors, comprising 83% of all primary lung tumors in dogs and 87% in cats.[17] Lung carcinomas tend to appear in 3 sites: the hilus of the lungs; in multifocal and often peripheral locations; and involving an entire lobe or lobes.[16] Multifocal, peripheral tumors are the most common.[16] Carcinomas (Plate 6) are large-cell (epithelial) tumors. When cytologic evidence of acinus formation or production of secretory products is seen, they are classified as adenocarcinomas (Plate 6).

References

1. Creighton and Wilkins: Transtracheal aspiration biopsy: technique and cytologic evaluation. *JAAHA* 10:219-226, 1974.

2. Turnwald: Evaluation of the respiratory system in disease. *Proc 53rd Ann Mtg AAHA*, 1986. pp 52-55.

3. O'Brien: Transtracheal aspiration in dogs and cats. *MVP* 64:412-413, 1983.

4. Moise and Blue: Bronchial washings in the cat: procedure and cytologic evaluation. *Comp Cont Ed Pract Vet* 5:621-627, 1983.

5. Henderson: Use of bronchoalveolar lavage to detect lung damage. *Environ Health Perspec* 56:115-129, 1984.

6. Carre et al: Technical variations of bronchoalveolar lavage (BAL): influence of atelectasis and the lung region lavaged. *Lung* 163:117-125, 1985.

7. Damiano et al: A morphologic study of the influx of neutrophils into dog lung alveoli after lavage with sterile saline. *Am J Path* 100:349-364, 1980.

8. Johnston: Cytologic diagnosis of lung cancer: principles and problems. *Path Res Pract* 181:1-36, 1986.

9. Rebar et al: Bronchopulmonary lavage cytology in the dog: normal findings. *Vet Pathol* 17:294-304, 1980.

10. Hirshman et al: Increased metachromatic cells and lymphocytes in bronchoalveolar lavage fluid of dogs with airway hyperreactivity. *Am Rev Respir Dis* 133:482-487, 1986.

11. Slauson and Cooper: *Mechanisms of Disease*. 1st ed. Williams & Wilkins, Baltimore, 1982. pp 301-370.

12. Slauson and Cooper: *Mechanisms of Disease*. 1st ed. Williams & Wilkins, Baltimore, 1982. pp 189-192.

13. McKiernan, in Ettinger: *Textbook of Veterinary Internal Medicine*. Saunders, Philadelphia, 1983. pp 777-798.

14. Pecora: How well does transtracheal aspiration reflect pulmonary infection? *Chest* 66:220, 1974.

15. Stickles: Lower respiratory tract diseases: diagnosis and treatment. *Proc 52nd Ann Mtg AAHA*, 1985. pp 377-394.

16. Moulton et al: Classification of lung carcinomas in the dog and cat. *Vet Pathol* 18:513-528, 1981.

17. Stunzi et al: Tumors of the lung. *Bull WHO* 50:9-19, 1974.

15

The Lung Parenchyma

R.L. Cowell, R.D. Tyler and C.J. Baldwin

Percutaneous transthoracic fine-needle aspiration biopsy (FNAB) of the lung may be extremely useful in patients with generalized pulmonary disease or intrathoracic masses that can be localized radiographically.[1,2] It is a rapid, relatively safe procedure that can be used to collect material for cytologic diagnosis of neoplastic, hypersensitivity and infectious (eg, mycotic, bacterial, protozoal) lung disease, and to obtain material for culture (Table 1).[1-3] In human patients, FNAB of the lung is 96% successful in diagnosing malignant neoplams and 77% successful in obtaining material that yielded an infectious agent from immunosuppressed patients with a focal pneumonic infiltrate.[2,3]

While fine-needle aspirates can generally be obtained with little risk, less invasive procedures, such as transtracheal/bronchial wash, thoracic radiography and hematologic examination, should be performed first.[2,3] Transthoracic pulmonary aspiration is contraindicated in animals with bleeding disorders, cystic or bullous lung diseases, pulmonary hypertension, and diseases producing forceful breathing and coughing that cannot be temporarily controlled (Table 2).[1-4] The procedure is also contraindicated in intractable patients. Hemorrhage, pneumothorax and/or lung laceration are the primary complications.[1-3] In people, tumor seeding along the needle tract after fine-needle aspiration biopsy of a pulmonary mass has occurred in several instances.[5]

In generalized lung disease, the dorsal portion of the right caudal lobe is the preferred site for aspiration.[3,4] Since the lung parenchyma is thickest in the caudal lobe, parenchyma aspirates are obtained more easily from this area, and the likelihood of penetrating another vital structure is minimized.[3] Though several positions can be used, standing and sternal positions have the following advantages. The dorsal lung is in a nondependent (high) area, which results in greater negative pressure and greater distention of alveoli; therefore, fewer alveoli rupture and the biopsy site seals more rapidly. If ventilation occurs during aspiration, caudal lung motion is less; therefore, the likelihood and severity of lung laceration are reduced. Also, the chance of hemorrhage is decreased, since blood perfusion and pressure are less in nondependent lung regions.[6]

With localized lung disease, the lesion is radiographically located and proper needle placement is determined by counting the ribs and measuring from the vertebrae, sternum or costochondral junction.

Technique

Pulmonary aspirates can be obtained quickly with minimal equipment. If the lesion is localized and proper needle placement can be determined radiographically, the likelihood of obtaining a useful or diagnostic sample is high. However, in generalized lung disease, the needle may be placed in an uninvolved area and yield only normal or nondiagnostic cells on aspiration; therefore, multiple attempts are more likely to be needed.

The area to be aspirated depends on whether the lesion is localized or generalized. If generalized, the needle is inserted on the right side of the chest between the seventh and ninth ribs, two-thirds of the way dorsad between the costochondral junction and the vertebral bodies.[2,3] For localized lesions, the area

Table 1. Indications for performing a fine-needle aspiration of lung parenchyma.

Indications

- To investigate the etiology of a large, solitary pulmonary mass or consolidated area.
- To investigate the etiology of diffuse or generalized parenchymal disease.
- To detect inflammatory disease and obtain material for microbial culture.
- To detect a hypersensitivity reaction.
- To confirm metastatic neoplasia.
- To avoid the need for higher-risk procedures (thoracotomy or biopsy), especially in poor-risk patients.

Table 2. Contraindications to a fine-needle aspiration biopsy of lung parenchyma and associated complications.

Contraindication	Complication
Uncooperative patient	Lung laceration
Uncontrollable coughing or forceful breathing	Lung laceration
Any bleeding disorder	Severe bleeding
Pulmonary hypertension	Severe bleeding
Pulmonary cysts or bullous emphysema	Severe pneumothorax

of needle insertion depends on the location of the lesion, which is identified by lateral, dorsoventral and ventrodorsal radiographs.[2-4]

The hair is clipped, the area is scrubbed and draped, and an antiseptic is applied. Local anesthetic may be used if desired but is frequently not needed. Heavy sedation may be required in uncooperative patients. However, sedation should be avoided if possible because sedated patients cannot clear respiratory secretions or endobronchial hemorrhage that may result from the FNAB procedure.[2,3]

The patient is restrained in the standing, sitting, sternal or lateral recumbent position. Depending on the animal's size, a 23- to 25-ga, 5/8- to 1 1/2-inch needle, with a 10- to 20-ml syringe attached, is inserted aseptically through the chest wall at the cranial aspect of the rib, avoiding the intercostal vessels on the adjacent rib's caudal border. The nose and mouth are temporarily held closed to stop lung movement while the needle is advanced into the lung parenchyma (about 1-3 cm), and negative pressure is applied while the needle is moved back and forth (about 1 cm). Negative pressure is released and the needle is withdrawn. Some authors have advocated maintaining negative pressure while the needle is withdrawn to help avoid leaving tissue along the needle tract.[2,3]

The needle is removed from the syringe and the syringe is filled with air. The needle is reconnected to the syringe and the material in the hub of the needle is forced onto a glass slide, smeared and stained for cytologic evaluation.[1-3] Chapter 1 describes general techniques for aspirating, slide preparation and staining. An adequate sample for cytologic evaluation can generally be collected with 1-2 attempts.

The patient should be closely monitored for postaspiration complications. Thoracic radiographs, immediately and 24 hours postaspiration, have been suggested.[2,3] Pneumothorax is the most common complication, reported to occur in 20% of patients.[7] However, most involve mild asymptomatic pneumothorax, which resolves spontaneously.[2,3] Favorable patient positioning may inhibit pneumothorax progression.[6] Rotating the animal so the lung puncture site is down (dependent position) for 3 minutes markedly decreases pneumothorax formation.[6] The clinician should be prepared to insert a chest tube if severe pneumothorax develops.[2,3,5]

Scrapings and impressions of lung parenchyma taken at biopsy, lobectomy or necropsy can be useful in determining disease processes or etiology. Scrapings and impression smears are evaluated for the same changes as described for FNAB. See Chapter 1 for a general discussion on preparing scrapings and impression smears.

Cytologic Evaluation

Cell Types

With fine-needle aspirates or impression smears of pulmonary parenchyma, one may see many different cell types, such as ciliated and nonciliated columnar cells, ciliated and nonciliated cuboidal cells, goblet cells, alveolar

Figure 1. Blood, fat spaces, pulmonary epithelial cells and columnar cells in an aspirate from an atelectatic lung lobe. No signs of inflammation or neoplasia are seen. (Wright's stain, original magnification 132X)

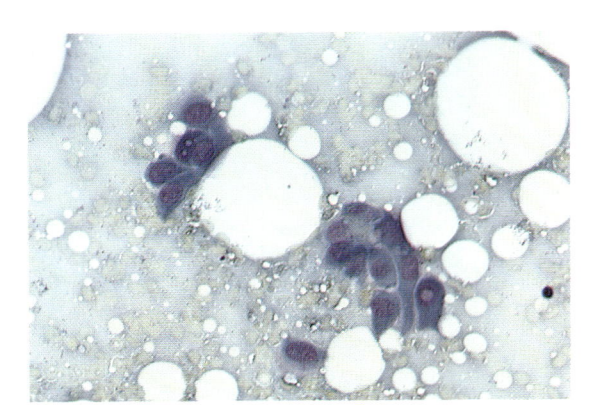

Figure 2. Dysplastic epithelial cells, eosinophils, and scattered neutrophils and macrophages in a pulmonary aspirate. The macrophages contain phagocytized RBCs and RBC breakdown products. These findings suggest hypersensitivity, inflammation and intrapulmonary hemorrhage. (Wright's stain, original magnification 132X)

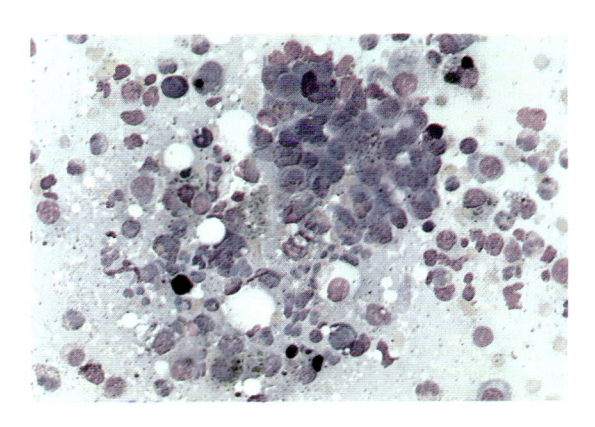

cells, alveolar macrophages, neutrophils, eosinophils, lymphocytes, mast cells, RBCs, and dysplastic and neoplastic cells. Ciliated and nonciliated columnar and cuboidal cells and alveolar macrophages are generally seen unless the disease has obliterated normal lung parenchyma. Goblet cells are only occasionally seen in pulmonary aspirates, scrapings and impression smears.

Columnar and Cuboidal Cells: Ciliated columnar cells (Chapter 14, Figs 4,5) have an elongated or cone shape, with cilia on the flattened end and the other (basal) end containing the nucleus and frequently terminating in a tail. The nucleus is generally round to oval, with a finely granular chromatin pattern.[8] Ciliated cuboidal cells appear similar to ciliated columnar cells, except cuboidal cells are as wide as they are tall. Nonciliated columnar and cuboidal cells appear identical to their ciliated counterparts, except the cilia are absent.

Goblet Cells: Goblet cells (Chapter 14, Fig 5) are mucus-producing bronchial cells. Generally, they are elongated (columnar) cells with a basally placed nucleus and round granules of mucin that frequently distend the cytoplasm.[8] Occasionally the cytoplasm is so greatly distended that the cell appears round. The granules stain red to blue with Romanowsky-type stains and may be seen free in the smear secondary to goblet cell rupture. Goblet cells are not commonly seen on pulmonary aspirate cytology preparations.

Alveolar Cells: Alveolar cells (Fig 1) are cuboidal to round epithelial cells that line alveoli. They have centrally to basally located round to oval nuclei. The nuclear chromatin is midly coarse and the cytoplasm is light blue. Occasionally the cells appear elongated, especially in FNAB, due to mechanical distortion during slide preparation. Some alveolar cells are present in most pulmonary cytology smears.

Macrophages: Alveolar macrophages (Chapter 14, Figs 6,12,13) are readily found in pulmonary aspirates and impression smears from clinically normal animals, and may be the predominant cell type. The nucleus is round to bean-shaped and eccentrically positioned. Occasionally a binucleate alveolar macrophage is seen in smears from clinically normal animals. Alveolar macrophages have abundant blue-gray, granular cytoplasm. When they become activated, the cytoplasm becomes more abundant and vacuolated (foamy), and may contain phagocytized material.[9]

Neutrophils: Neutrophils in pulmonary aspirates or impression smears look like peripheral blood neutrophils (Plate 1 and Chapter 14, Fig 11), though degenerative changes may be present. Some neutrophils are generally present due to blood contamination during aspiration or making of impression smears. The number of neutrophils present secondary to blood contamination depends on the degree of contamination and the number of neutrophils present in the peripheral blood. Generally, there is 1 WBC/500-1000 RBCs. Increased numbers of neutrophils indicate inflammation. (See the discussion on inflammation later in the chapter.)

Eosinophils: Eosinophils (Plate 2 and Chapter 14, Fig 9) are bone marrow-derived granulocytes containing intracytoplasmic lysosome granules. These granules have an affinity for the acid dye eosin, which stains them red or eosinophilic. Increased numbers of eosinophils indicate an allergic or parasitic hypersensitivity reaction. (See the discussion on hypersensitivity later in the chapter).

Lymphocytes/Plasma Cells: Lymphocytes (Plate 1) may be present in small numbers in pulmonary aspirates, scrapings and impression smears from normal dogs and cats. With immune stimulation, lymphocytes become activated. Their cytoplasm becomes more abundant and stains deep blue due to increased protein synthesis. Also, some lymphocytes develop into plasma cells. Slightly increased numbers of small or reactive lymphocytes generally denote nonspecific inflammation and are of limited diagnostic value. Cellular aspirates consisting primarily of small lymphocytes may occur when a reactive pulmonary lymph node or thymona is aspirated. Large numbers of lymphoblasts (>50% of the cell population) indicate lymphosarcoma (Plate 7).

Mast Cells: Mast cells (Plate 2) are occasionally observed in pulmonary aspirates, scrapings and impression smears from dogs and cats with many different inflammatory lung disorders. In small numbers, they are of little diagnostic significance. However, mast cells are usually found in very large numbers with pulmonary mast-cell neoplasia (Plate 7). Mast cells are readily identified by their red-purple intracytoplasmic granules. These granules are frequently present in large numbers and may obscure the nucleus. Scattered granules from ruptured mast cells may be present free on the slide and must not be confused with bacteria.

Erythrocytes: Erythrocytes are always present in pulmonary aspirates, scrapings and impression smears. Blood contamination during collection must be differentiated from true intrapulmonary hemorrhage. The presence of pulmonary macrophages with phagocytized RBCs or RBC breakdown products, such as hematoidin, biliverdin or hemosiderin, (Plate 2 and Chapter 14, Fig 13) denotes intrapulmonary hemorrhage.

Neoplasia: Pulmonary neoplasia may be primary or metastatic. Carcinomas and adenocarcinomas (Plate 6) seem to be the most common form of pulmonary neoplasia. Cells retrieved on pulmonary aspirates, scrapings or impression smears are evaluated for the criteria of malignancy described in Chapter 1. Evaluating cells for neoplastic criteria is easier if inflammation is absent because inflammation readily induces metaplastic and dysplastic changes, which must be differentiated from neoplastic changes. Also, one must be careful not to confuse cells obtained by accidental aspiration of nonpulmonary tissue, such as accidental aspiration of the liver, with neoplastic cells. Cytologic evaluation of atypical cell types is further described later in the chapter.

Miscellaneous Findings: Corn starch (glove powder) is frequently seen on slides from pulmonary aspirates, scrapings and impression smears. Typically, these are clear-staining, large, round to hexagonal particles with a central fissure (Chapter 14, Fig 11). Glove powder is an incidental finding and should not be confused with an organism or cell.

Cytologic Interpretation

Pulmonary aspirates, scrapings and impression smears are interpreted according to the type, quantity and proportion of cells recovered. They can generally be classified into the following categories:

Insufficient sample: No cells are seen other than those from blood contamination.

Only normal cell types: Blood and alveolar cells and macrophages (possible columnar cells, etc) are the only cells present.

Eosinophilic infiltrate: The proportion of eosinophils in the aspirate is greater than the number of eosinophils expected due to blood contamination (see hypersensitivity below).

Neutrophilic infiltrate: The number of neutrophils in the aspirate is significantly greater than would occur from blood contamination alone, and the neutrophil is the predominant cell type (see inflammation below).

Granulomatous inflammation: Inflammatory giant cells or epithelioid macrophages are present (see inflammation below).

Macrophage infiltrate: The sample is very cellular and consists primarily of macrophages (see atelectasis under normal cell types and inflammation below).

Hyperplasia/dysplasia/neoplasia (benign or malignant): Atypical cells are seen but insufficient criteria of malignancy are present for establishing a diagnosis of malignant neoplasia (see atypical cell types below).

Malignant neoplasia: Cells with sufficient criteria of malignancy to diagnose malignant neoplasia are present (see neoplasia under atypical cell types below).

Ectopic aspirate: Cells typical of an organ other than the lung are present (see abdominal organ aspiration under atypical cell types below).

These categories, other than the first category, are not mutually exclusive. Classification of pulmonary aspirates and impressions into 1 or more of the above categories allows the process(es) to be identified. Chart 1 presents an algorithm to aid evaluation of pulmonary aspirates, scrapings or impression smears. Integration of the historical, physical and clinical findings may allow further refinement of the diagnosis.

Only Normal Cell Types Present

If the area of involvement is missed, only blood and normal cell types (alveolar cells, macrophages, and cuboidal and columnar cells) may be seen. In this instance, reaspiration is warranted. If an area of involvement cannot be aspirated, a lung biopsy is indicated.

Large numbers of pulmonary macrophages and alveolar cells are frequently present when an area of atelectasis is aspirated (Fig 1). Due to the high cellularity of the aspirate and lack of inflammatory response, one may be suspicious of neoplasia. However, on careful evaluation of cell morphology, sufficient criteria of malignancy (Chapter 1) are not present to warrant a diagnosis of neoplasia.

Figure 3. A fine-needle aspiration biopsy of a radiographically identified pulmonary mass. A. Many neutrophils and some inflammation-induced dysplastic epithelial cells are present. Bacteria were evident elsewhere in the smear, indicating an infectious etiology. (Original magnification 40X)

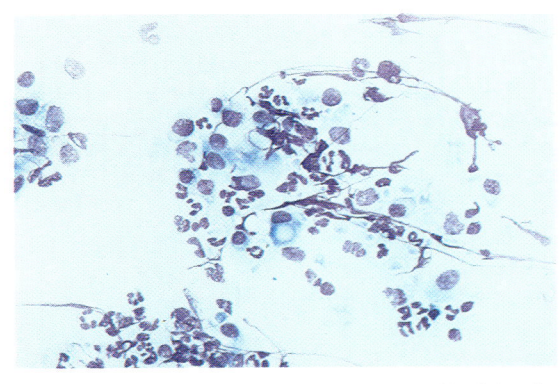

B. Higher magnification shows dysplastic epithelial cells. (Wright's stain, original magnification 250X)

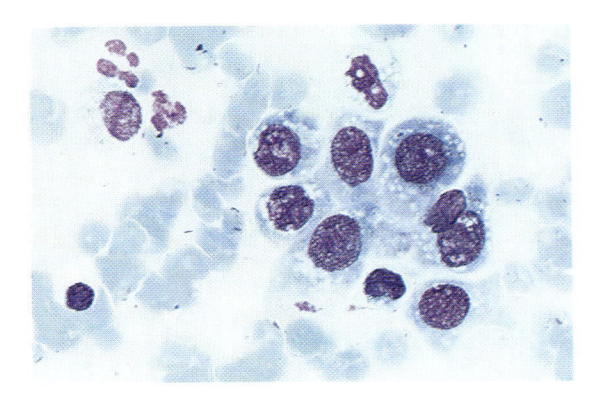

Hypersensitivity

The eosinophil is important in defending against helminth infections and in modulating hypersensitivity reactions.[9] Eosinophils are present only in very small numbers (<5%) in pulmonary aspirates and impression smears from normal dogs and cats. Increased numbers of eosinophils (>10% of the inflammatory cells) in pulmonary aspirates, scrapings or impression smears indicate an allergic or parasitic response (Fig 2 and Chapter 14, Fig 9). Rarely, increased numbers of eosinophils may be associated with certain tumors or some hyphating fungal infections. These diseases can be diagnosed by identifying the mycotic agent or neoplastic cells present.

Increased numbers of neutrophils and/or macrophages may be seen along with increased numbers of eosinophils if tissue irritation is sufficient to induce an inflammatory response. Circulating and likely tissue eosinophil numbers are decreased by glucocorticoid administration. Therefore, glucocorticoid therapy can mask the typical eosinophilic response seen cytologically with reaginic (IgE) hypersensitivity.

Inflammation

Increased numbers of inflammatory cells, neutrophils or macrophages, denote inflammation (Plate 3). Eosinophilic inflammation is described above under hypersensitivity. While alveolar macrophages are normal inhabitants of the lung, even in the absence of an inflammatory response, neutrophils are present in large numbers only when inflammation is present (Chapter 14, Fig 11). Neutrophils may show degenerative changes due to bacterial toxins or may be smudged (ruptured) secondary to trauma from collection and preparation. Neutrophil numbers are considered increased when their concentration exceeds that expected by the degree of blood contamination. Typically, 1 WBC/500-1000 RBCs is the expected WBC concentration due to blood contamination. However, this WBC number may increase with peripheral leukocytosis.

Inflammation may be present due to infectious or noninfectious processes. Infectious disorders include bacterial, mycotic, viral and protozoal diseases. Some examples of noninfectious disorders include tissue necrosis secondary to inhalation of a toxic substance, and neoplasia that has outgrown its blood supply and developed a necrotic center. Identification of neoplastic cells or the infectious agent allows diagnosis.

Pulmonary aspirates containing large numbers of neutrophils and small to moderate numbers of macrophages suggest acute or chronic-active inflammation. If the causative agent can be identified, a diagnosis can be made. Otherwise, the cytologic changes are interpreted as neutrophilic (purulent) inflammation, of which there are many causes. Bacterial pneumonia or abscesses, necrotic tumors and inhalation of toxic substances frequently result in a neutrophilic reaction. Mycotic and protozoal agents frequently result in granuloma formation but may be associated with a neutrophilic response.

Very cellular samples consisting almost totally of pulmonary macrophages and alveolar cells are common when areas of atelectasis are aspirated or imprinted. Such diseases as lipid pneumonia and granulomatous pneumonia can result in cellular aspirates or imprints consisting primarily of macrophages. Large, lipid-containing vacuoles may be present within macrophages in lipid pneumonia.[8] Phagocytized RBCs and/or RBC breakdown products within macrophages may be seen with intrapulmonary hemorrhage (Fig 2 and Plate 2). Nonphagocytized RBCs are always present due to blood contamination. Macrophages are important in defending against microorganisms; phagocytized microorganisms, especially mycotic or protozoal organisms, may be seen.

Granulomatous reactions are characterized by the presence of neutrophils, many macrophages and occasionally binucleated and multinucleated inflammatory giant cells. Though many disorders can cause granulomatous inflammation, in dogs and cats, foreign bodies and mycotic and protozoal agents are most common.

Bacterial Diseases: Many different bacteria can cause pulmonary infection and disease. Bacterial pneumonia is generally due to infection by a Gram-negative rod.[1] Phagocytized and nonphagocytized bacteria may be found in aspirates, scrapings and impression smears of lung parenchyma from animals with bacterial pneumonia or a lung abscess. Identifying the bacteria as rods or cocci (Plate 3) helps in choosing initial antibacterial therapy while awaiting culture and sensitivity results. With hematologic stains, bacteria (both Gram-positive and Gram-negative) stain blue-black.

Since most pneumonias are due to infection with Gram-negative rods, if bacterial rods (especially bipolar rods) are seen cytologically, a drug effective against Gram-negative bacteria should be used while awaiting culture and sensitivity results. Filamentous rods (Plate 3) suggestive of either *Actinomyces* spp, *Nocardia* spp or rarely *Fusobacterium* spp are occasionally seen. *Mycobacterium* spp may infect dogs or cats and are more difficult to identify cytologically because they do not stain with routine hematologic stains. However, on careful examination, the negative images of the bacterium can be seen (Plate 4). The pathologic bacterial cocci are generally *Staphylococcus* spp and *Streptococcus* spp; therefore, when bacterial cocci are seen cytologically, a drug effective against Gram-positive bacteria should be used while awaiting culture and sensitivity results.

Mycotic and Protozoal Diseases: Many different mycotic and protozoal organisms can colonize the lungs. A lung aspirate or biopsy and scraping or impression smear is indicated when generalized lung disease or a localized mass cannot be confirmed by less invasive means. Some of the more common mycotic and protozoal organisms that can invade pulmonary tissues are *Blastomyces dermatitidis* (Plate 4), *Cryptococcus neoformans* (Plate 4), *Coccidioides immitis* (Plate 5), *Histoplasma capsulatum* (Plate 4), *Sporothrix spp (Plate 4)*, *Aspergillus* spp or other opportunistic fungi (Plate 5), *Toxoplasma gondii* (Plate 5), *Cytauxzoon felis* (Plate 5) and *Pneumocystis carinii* (Plate 5).

Figure 4. This aspirate from a dog with a pulmonary adenocarcinoma shows a group of large epithelial cells with variation in cell and nuclear size, coarse nuclear chromatin, large nucleoli, basophilic cytoplasm and cytoplasmic vacuolation. (Wright's stain, original magnification 250X)

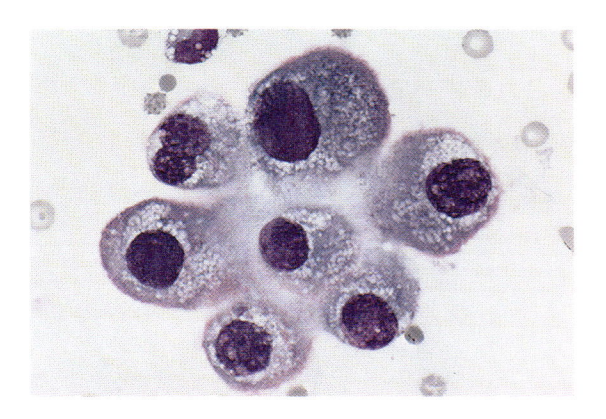

Viral Diseases: Many viral respiratory diseases can cause lung damage and allow secondary bacterial infection. Cytologically, viral diseases frequently cause nonspecific neutrophilic (purulent) inflammation. With secondary bacterial infection, large numbers of neutrophils and bacterial organisms are present.

Feline infectious peritonitis (FIP) is a coronavirus infection that causes multifocal, discrete areas of necrosis and inflammation in numerous organs. Scrapings, impressions and aspirates consist of necrotic debris, many neutrophils and macrophages, and scattered lymphocytes and plasma cells.[10] While there is no cytologic finding that is diagnostic of FIP, demonstration of necrosis and inflammation supports a presumptive diagnosis of FIP.

Atypical Cell Types

Atypical cells may be seen with pulmonary metaplasia, dysplasia, neoplasia (primary or metastatic), anticancer therapy or accidental aspiration of abdominal or nonpulmonary thoracic organs. Any atypical cells should be evaluated for malignant criteria (Chapter 1).

Metaplasia: Metaplasia is an adaptive response of epithelial cells to chronic irritation.[8,11] Replacement of normal pulmonary epithelial cells of the trachea, bronchi and bronchioles with stratified squamous epithelium (squamous metaplasia) is an example of pulmonary metaplasia.[11] These metaplastic cells mimic maturing squamous epithelium and must not be confused with neoplasia.

Dysplasia: By definition, dysplasia is a non-neoplastic change.[11] It occurs due to external alteration of cell proliferation, differentiation and maturation. Such conditions as inflammation and tissue irritation can cause dysplasia. However, severely dysplastic changes are sometimes referred to as carcinoma *in situ*.[11] Dysplastic changes (Fig 3) indicate asynchrony in cell and tissue development. They include variation in cell size and shape, increased nucleus:cytoplasm ratio, darker-staining cells, and increased numbers of immature cells.[11] These changes can be difficult to differentiate from neoplasia and may progress to neoplasia.[11]

Neoplasia: The macroscopic appearance of pulmonary neoplasia ranges from solitary nodules, to multiple nodules, to diffuse infiltrations. Most pulmonary neoplasias are metastatic nodules from malignant tumors in sites other than the lungs. Solitary lesions are rare in metastatic lung tumors but common in primary lung tumors. However, primary lung tumors are rare in dogs and cats.[12] When evaluating cells for criteria of malignancy, care must be taken not to confuse inflammation-induced dysplasia (described above) or abnormal organ aspiration (described below) with neoplasia.

While many different neoplasms may invade the lungs, carcinomas and adenocarcinomas are most common. Lung carcinomas tend to appear in 3 sites: the hilus of the lungs; multifocal and often peripherally; and involving an entire lobe or lobes.[12] Multifocal, peripheral sites tend to be the most common.[12] Adenocarcinomas are by far the most common primary lung tumor, comprising 83% of all primary lung tumors in dogs and 87% in cats.[13] Carcinomas and adenocarcinomas are large-cell (epithelial) tumors that show the criteria of malignancy listed in Chapter 1. When cytologic evidence of acinus formation or production of secretory products is seen,

Chart 1. An algorithmic approach to evaluation of pulmonary aspirates, scrapings or impression smears.

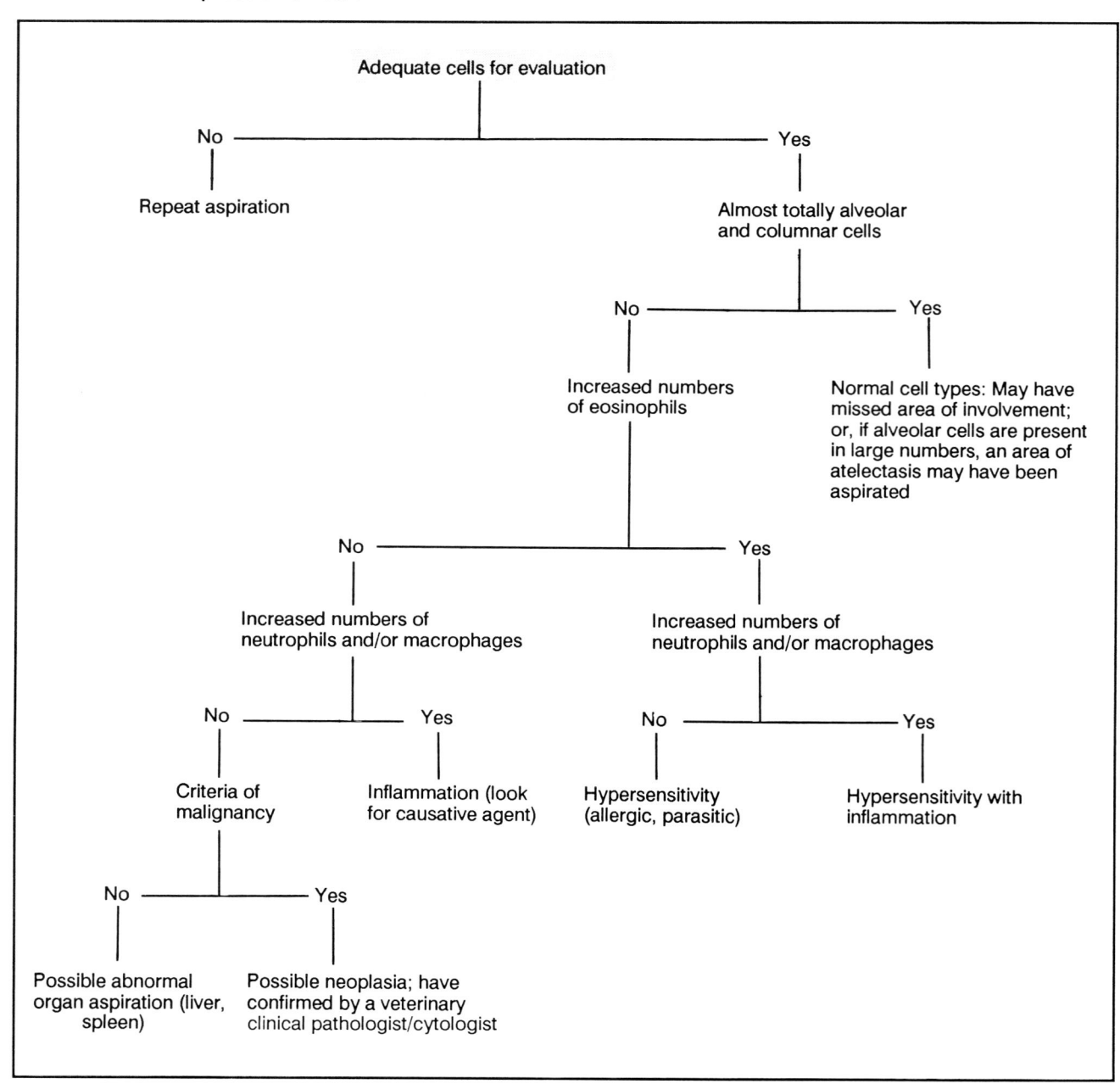

```
                         Adequate cells for evaluation
                         /                            \
                       No                              Yes
                        |                                |
                 Repeat aspiration            Almost totally alveolar
                                                and columnar cells
                                               /                  \
                                             No                    Yes
                                              |                     |
                                   Increased numbers       Normal cell types: May have
                                    of eosinophils          missed area of involvement;
                                    /          \            or, if alveolar cells are present
                                  No            Yes         in large numbers, an area of
                                   |             |          atelectasis may have been
                                                            aspirated

                    Increased numbers of          Increased numbers of
                  neutrophils and/or macrophages  neutrophils and/or macrophages
                      /            \                  /            \
                    No              Yes             No              Yes
                     |               |               |               |
                Criteria of     Inflammation (look  Hypersensitivity  Hypersensitivity with
                malignancy      for causative agent) (allergic,        inflammation
                /      \                             parasitic)
              No        Yes

    Possible abnormal    Possible neoplasia; have
    organ aspiration     confirmed by a veterinary
    (liver, spleen)      clinical pathologist/cytologist
```

they are classified as adenocarcinomas (Fig 4 and Plate 6).

Other tumors, such as lymphosarcoma and mast-cell tumors, are readily recognized cytologically by large numbers of lymphoblasts (Plate 7) and mast cells (Plate 7), respectively. Connective tissue tumors, such as hemangiosarcoma, also occur in the lungs and appear cytologically identical to their counterparts described in Chapter 2.

Anticancer Therapy: Irradiation and chemotherapy may result in such severe atypia of cells of the tracheobronchial epithelium, terminal bronchial epithelium and alveolar epithelium that differentiation from neoplasia cannot be reliably made.[8] Pulmonary aspirates obtained after cancer therapy should be interpreted with caution.

Lymph Nodes: Enlarged pulmonary lymph nodes may appear radiographically as intrathoracic masses. Cytologic interpretation of aspirates of pulmonary lymph nodes is the same as interpretation of peripheral lymph nodes as described in Chapter 8.

Thymus: A thymoma may appear radiographically as an intrathoracic mass. Cytologically, one finds many small lymphocytes and variable numbers of thymic epithelial cells. Thymic epithelial cells are medium to large, and may vary in shape from round to oval to stellate. They have a round to oval nucleus, with mildly coarse nuclear chromatin. Invasive and noninvasive thymonas cannot be differentiated by cytologic examination alone.

Fat: Mediastinal lipomas may appear radiographically as intrathoracic masses. Aspirated intrathoracic fat (lipoma or otherwise) grossly appears as a greasy, nondrying material. Cytologically, it appears identical to subcutaneous lipomas (described in Chapter 2), with fat spaces and some lipocytes constituting the majority of the smear (Plate 8).

Abdominal Organ Aspiration: Though the distal dorsal portion of the lung is the thickest, the needle can be forced too deeply and abdominal organs aspirated. The liver is the abdominal organ most frequently aspirated accidentally. Hepatocytes are large (epithelioid) cells with a single, round nucleus and single to multiple, small, round nucleoli. The cytoplasm is blue-gray and often granular. Bile may be present. Cytoplasmic vacuoles may be present in fatty deposition or corticosteroid hepatopathy. Care must be taken not to confuse accidentally aspirated hepatocytes with neoplastic cells. Hepatic aspirates are fully described in Chapter 16.

References

1. McKiernan, in Ettinger: *Textbook of Veterinary Internal Medicine.* Saunders, Philadelphia, 1983. pp 777-798.

2. Roudebush, in Kirk: *Current Veterinary Therapy VIII.* Saunders, Philadelphia, 1983. pp 228-230.

3. Roudebush *et al*: Percutaneous fine-needle aspiration biopsy of the lung in disseminated pulmonary disease. *JAAHA* 17:109-116, 1981.

4. Kirk and Bistner: *Handbook of Veterinary Procedures and Emergency Treatment.* 3rd ed. Saunders, Philadelphia, 1981. pp 518-519.

5. Anderson and Arentzen: Carcinoma of the lung. *Surg Clin No Am* 60:794-813, 1980.

6. Zidulka *et al*: Position may stop pneumothorax progression in dogs. *Am Rev Respir Dis* 126:51-53, 1982.

7. Shure *et al*: Transbronchial needle aspiration in the diagnosis of pneumonia in a canine model. *Am Rev Respir Dis* 13:290-291, 1985.

8. Johnston: Cytologic diagnosis of lung cancer: principles and problems. *Path Res Pract* 181:1-36, 1986.

9. Slauson and Cooper: *Mechanisms of Disease.* 1st ed. Williams & Wilkins, Baltimore, 1982. pp 189-192.

10. Pedersen, in Greene: *Clinical Microbiology and Infectious Diseases of the Dog and Cat.* Saunders, Philadelphia, 1984. pp 514-526.

11. Slauson and Cooper: *Mechanisms of Disease.* 1st ed. Williams & Wilkins, Baltimore, 1982. pp 301-370.

12. Moulton *et al*: Classification of lung carcinomas in the dog and cat. *Vet Pathol* 18:513-528, 1981.

13. Stunzi *et al*: Tumors of the lung. *Bull WHO* 50:9-19, 1974.

16

The Liver

D.J. Meyer and T.W. French

Recent articles indicate that guided fine-needle aspiration is an accurate, safe and relatively inexpensive method for diagnosis of hepatic neoplasia.[1-4] A clinical study evaluating the diagnostic utility of cytologic examination in nonneoplastic disease showed it was often possible to differentiate normal from abnormal, but definitive diagnosis was uncommon.[5] Cytologic examination of human hepatic tissue was found to be an acceptable procedure for detection and quantification of fatty change, a finding we may be able to extrapolate to veterinary medicine.[3,5] Histologic examination of liver tissue remains a valuable aid in differential diagnosis of liver disease; however, cytologic examination of aspirates is a practical initial choice in approaching selected liver disorders.

Indications

Hepatomegaly is the principal indication for aspiration and cytologic examination of the liver. Generalized organomegaly suggests a diffuse process, infiltrative or vacuolar, from which a representative cytologic specimen may be obtained without visual guidance. An asymmetric mass may be aspirated by using radiographic landmarks. Focal lesions, identified by ultrasonography, laparoscopy or laparotomy, are best sampled by visual guidance. Slides for immediate cytologic interpretation can be made by imprinting liver biopsy specimens before formalin fixation.

Technique

A 1 1/2-inch, 22-ga needle attached to a 12-ml syringe is satisfactory for aspiration of the liver. When available, we prefer to use a 2 1/2-inch spinal needle with a stylet. The stylet prevents obstruction of the needle by tissue as it is advanced through the body wall. The stylet is removed after the abdominal cavity is entered, but suction is not applied until the liver is penetrated. About 5-6 ml of negative pressure is applied as the needle is advanced through the liver parenchyma. The suction is gently released before removing the needle from the abdominal cavity. Frequently, little or no material is observed in the hub of the syringe. Negative pressure should be released promptly if much blood appears in the syringe. Continued aspiration in this situation often dilutes the specimen with blood, which may clot rapidly and thereby hinder smear-making.

The needle is carefully removed from the syringe, 1 ml of air is drawn into the syringe, and the needle is replaced on the syringe. While holding the tip of the needle over a clean glass slide, a small amount of air is gently forced through the needle to expel a small drop of material onto the slide. Blood-tinged fluid, which may or may not contain small bits of tissue, is usually observed.

Smears can be made from the fluid in the same manner used to make blood films. "Squash" preparations can be made from any small tissue fragments present.[6] Occasionally, when a spinal needle is used, small cores of tissue (1-1.5 cm long) are obtained. Touch imprints can be made from the tissue core and the remaining tissue placed in neutral buffered formalin for subsequent histologic processing if desired. Unstained cytologic preparations should be protected from formalin vapors because such exposure alters the tinctorial characteristics of the commonly used Romanowsky stains. Slide preparation and staining techniques are further discussed in Chapter 1.

Nonguided aspiration of the liver usually is performed from the left side. The left hepatic lobe is largest and the gallbladder is located to the right of midline. The patient generally is restrained in right lateral recumbency, though the standing position works well in large dogs. An enlarged liver often can be delineated by digital palpation, as the caudal border extends beyond the last rib. Percussion can be used to estimate the location of the liver under the rib cage. Intercostal percussion over the thorax produces a resonant sound. As the percussion proceeds caudad, a dull sound is heard when the liver is encountered. An aspirate can usually be obtained using the next intercostal space.

Precautions

As with any biopsy procedure, fine-needle aspiration requires consideration of hemostasis. The aspiration technique, however, causes only minimal cutting of tissue. Consequently, significant hemorrhage is unlikely. The platelet count, however, should be evaluated before aspiration, since platelet function is very important in occluding defects in vessel walls. On a blood film, a platelet count of >10 platelets per oil-immersion (100X objective) field is adequate. We also find it prudent to question the client regarding recent use of aspirin and aspirin-containing compounds because of their effect on platelet function. If bleeding tendencies are perceived during routine venipuncture, coagulation studies should be done.

Figure 1. Oval hepatocytes with round, central to eccentric nuclei and abundant basophilic cytoplasm. A binucleate hepatocyte is located to the right. (Wright's-Giemsa, 1000X)

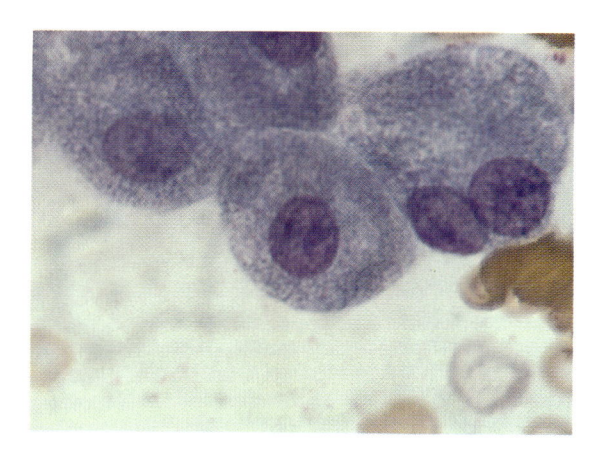

Figure 2. An intranuclear crystalline structure distorts the nucleus of a hepatocyte. (Wright's-Giemsa, 1000X)

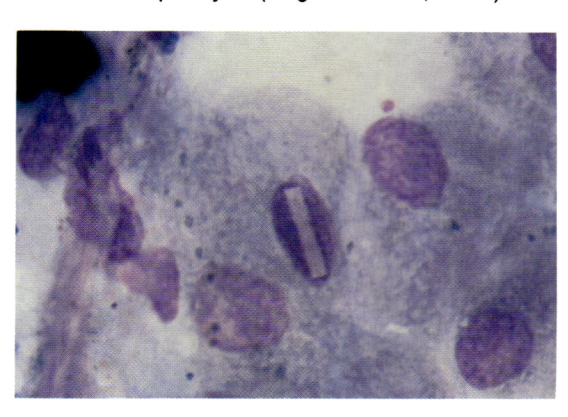

Cytologic Examination

Microscopic evaluation of cytologic preparations usually is performed on Romanowsky-stained specimens. The following descriptions are based on Wright's-Giemsa-stained cells. The commonly used Diff-Quik stain (American Scientific Products) is another Romanowsky stain with similar tinctorial properties. Cellular detail, however, is better with the Wright's-Giemsa stain, so it is recommended for cytologic examination with suspected neoplasia.

Normal Findings

Recognition of the normal hepatocyte serves as the basis for examination of the liver aspirate. These large, oval to polygonal cells constitute the majority on slides prepared from normal livers. Hepatocytes are readily aspirated, and may be seen as individual cells or in variably sized clusters. The round, often centrally located nucleus contains stippled to ropey chromatin and usually a single, light blue nucleolus. Occasional binucleate forms may be seen normally. The abundant cytoplasm is lightly basophilic, though cytoplasmic granules may impart an eosinophilic hue (Fig 1). Intranuclear cytoplasmic inclusions and intranuclear crystalline structures may be observed in aspirates from apparently normal canine livers (Figs 2,3).[7] The significance of these latter findings is unknown.

Figure 3. The uppermost hepatocyte contains an intranuclear vacuole, which should not be mistaken for a viral inclusion body. (Wright's-Giemsa, 1000X).

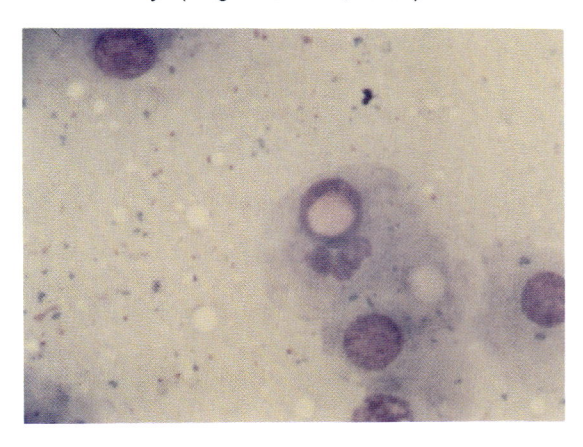

Epithelial cells originating from the intrahepatic biliary tract also may be encountered. These are relatively small cells with round nuclei and scant cytoplasm that usually exfoliate in sheets or clusters (Fig 4). As with normal hepatocytes, normal epithelial cells are notable for their uniform appearance.

The normal canine liver contains mast cells scattered throughout the parenchyma. Observation of a few mature, well-granulated mast cells in an otherwise normal cytologic preparation of liver should not cause alarm (Plate 2).

Bile Pigment

Retention of bile pigment is a common cytologic finding in many hepatobiliary disorders and precedes development of clinically recognizable jaundice. The dark pigment is observed as fine granules or clumps within the cytoplasm of the hepatocyte (Fig 5). Extracellular accumulations of bile may be seen as "casts" of the intrahepatic biliary system, which courses between hepatocytes (Fig 6). Accumulations of hemosiderin/iron within the liver may appear as yellow to golden pigment within hepatocytes or macrophages. We have seen this pigment in aspirates from patients with immune-mediated hemolysis and concurrent extramedullary hematopoiesis. One author has seen iron-filled macrophages in aspirates from livers with various inflammatory diseases. Prussian blue stain differentiates hemosiderin from other yellow pigments.

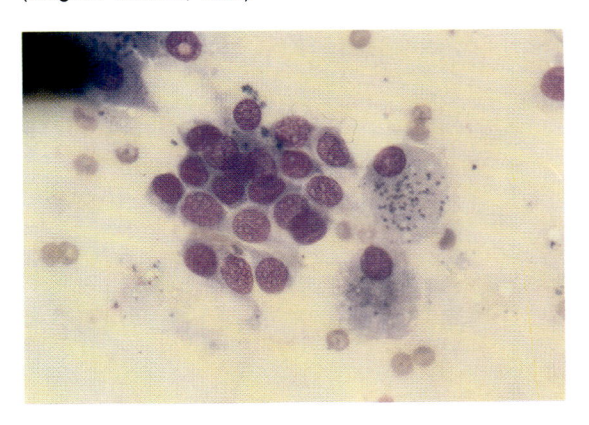

Figure 5. Clumps of dark pigment (presumably bile) are in the cytoplasm of these hepatocytes from an icteric dog. (Wright's-Giemsa, 400X)

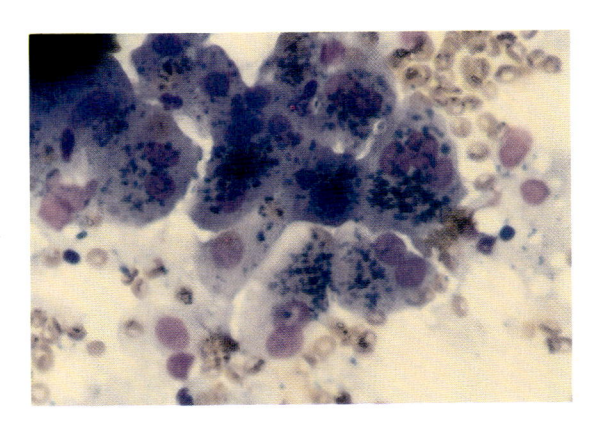

Figure 4. A sheet of epithelial cells from the biliary system, contrasted with 2 hepatocytes located to the right. (Wright's-Giemsa, 400X)

Neoplasia

Lymphosarcoma: Lymphosarcoma (lymphoma) is the most common neoplastic cause of generalized hepatomegaly in dogs and cats. Such infiltration often impairs intrahepatic bile flow, resulting in jaundice. Cytologic examination of aspirates generally is diagnostic because the clearly ectopic, readily aspirated cells tend to be diffusely distributed throughout the liver. Neoplastic lymphocytes comprise a monotonous population of discrete, round cells with a moderate amount of deeply basophilic cytoplasm (Fig 7). Their nuclei are generally round and contain diffuse chromatin: one or more prominent nucleoli may or may not be observed.

Liver aspirates containing normal-appearing, small to medium-sized lymphocytes, however, may pose more of a diagnostic dilem-

Figure 6. Dark bile forms canalicular "casts" among the hepatocytes in this liver aspirate from an icteric cat with suppurative cholangitis. Note the numerous neutrophils surrounding the clump of hepatocytes. (Wright's-Giemsa, 400X)

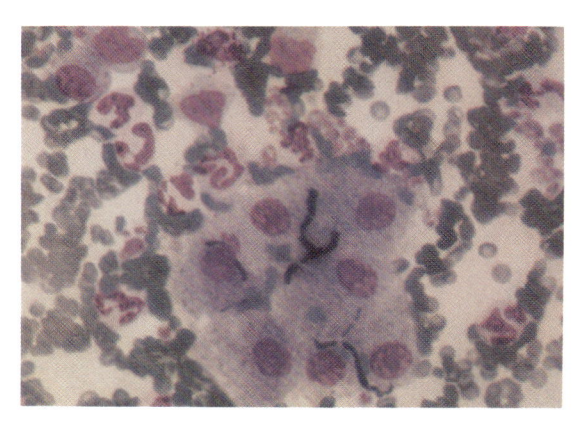

ma. Certain chronic inflammatory liver diseases may have a predominance of lymphocytes constituting the infiltrate. This situation is most common in cats, in which chronic lymphocytic cholangitis may be associated with dramatic infiltration causing hepatomegaly (Fig 8).[9,10] Examination of blood, bone marrow and histologic sections of liver may be needed to distinguish this entity from a well-differentiated lymphoid neoplasm.

Acute Myelogenous Leukemia: Neoplastic blast cells of acute myelogenous leukemia (AML) also can infiltrate the liver, and may be indistinguishable from lymphoblasts on routinely stained cytologic preparations (Fig 9).

Figure 7. Numerous immature lymphocytes are located to the left of a clump of hepatocytes in this liver aspirate from a dog with hepatic lymphosarcoma. (Wright's-Giemsa, 400X)

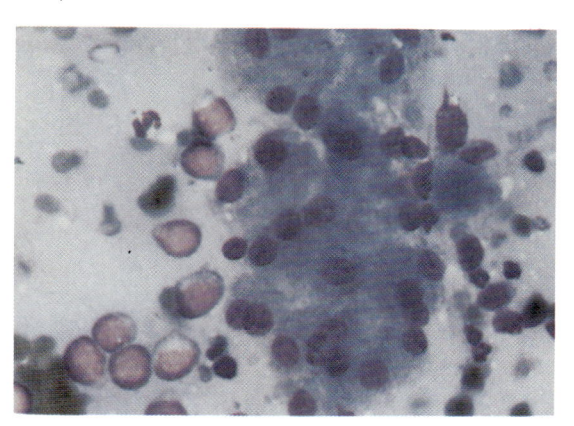

In dogs, the incidence of AML is relatively low as compared to that of lymphosarcoma. In cats, however, greater consideration should be given to this diagnosis. Cytochemical staining may help differentiate these cells from lymphoblasts. Pertinent hemogram findings, such as nonregenerative macrocytic anemia, leukopenia and thrombocytopenia, are commonly observed even when circulating blasts are not present in great numbers. Bone marrow examination usually is diagnostic in that morphologic evidence of concurrent abnormalities in all marrow cell lines (*eg,* dysplastic erythroblasts and megakaryocytes) often can be demonstrated.[8]

Mast-Cell Neoplasia: Hepatomegaly is present in 70% of dogs with systemic mastocytosis.[11] As previously mentioned, mast

Figure 8. This liver aspirate from an icteric cat contains many small lymphocytes scattered around a clump of hepatocytes. The histologic diagnosis was lymphocytic cholangitis, and the infiltrate had replaced an estimated 70% of the parenchymal cells in the surgical specimen examined. (Wright's-Giemsa, 400X)

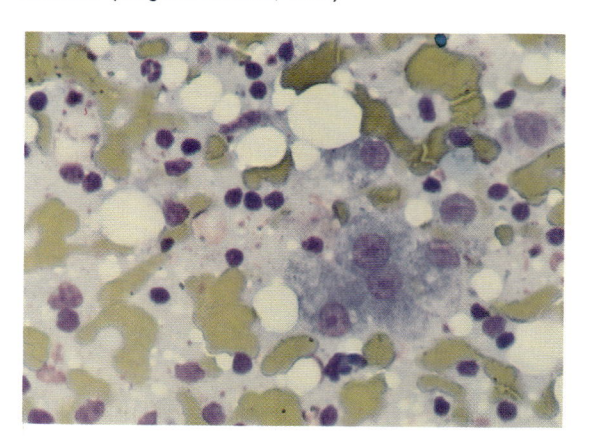

cells may be seen in small numbers in aspirates of normal livers. Finding more numerous mast cells, however, especially when immature or atypical in appearance, supports the diagnosis of mast-cell neoplasia as the cause of hepatomegaly. (Neoplastic mast cells are depicted in Plate 7). Examination of bone marrow and peripheral blood buffy coat smears is indicated to help stage the disease.[11]

Hepatocellular Carcinoma: Neoplastic proliferation of hepatocytes can result in hepatomegaly that usually is asymmetric and involves the left hepatic lobe.[12,13] This diagnosis is likely when cytologically malignant cells resembling hepatocytes are aspirated from a large hepatic mass. Cytologic indications of malignancy include marked variation in cell

Figure 9. Numerous blast cells surround a hepatocyte in this aspirate from an anemic, FeLV-positive cat. Peripheral blood contained many nucleated RBC and small numbers of blast cells. A bone marrow aspirate contained dysplastic erythroid precursors and megakaryocytes, and a high proportion of blast cells like those in the liver. This pattern was diagnostic of acute myelogenous leukemia. (Wright's-Giemsa, 400X)

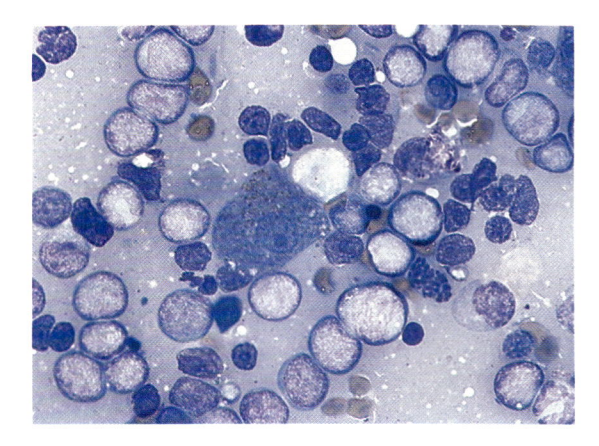

and nuclear size, prominent nucleoli of varying size, and variable nucleus:cytoplasm ratios (Fig 10). This diagnosis should be reserved for specimens with dramatically anaplastic features, since mild variability in hepatocytes may be observed in benign conditions, such as regenerating hepatic tissue (Fig 11) and nodular hyperplasia.

Bile Duct Carcinoma: Like hepatocellular carcinoma, canine bile duct carcinoma (cholangiocellular carcinoma) commonly causes asymmetric hepatomegaly involving the left

Figure 10. Large hepatocytes containing variably sized nuclei with prominent, bizarre nucleoli predominate in this liver aspirate from a cat with hepatocellular carcinoma. (Wright's-Giemsa, 400X)

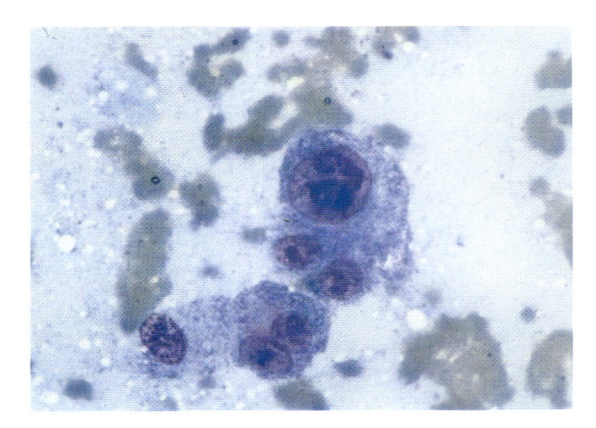

hepatic lobe.[14] However, more recent study found that the right side of the liver was more commonly involved.[30] The reason for this discrepancy is not known. Likewise, the serum aspartate aminotransferase and alanine aminotransferase ratio (AST:ALT) is usually <1, whereas it is usually >1 in cases with carcinoid and sarcoma.[12] These neoplastic cells often exfoliate in dense clusters, which may obscure cellular detail. These cells are usually smaller than hepatocytes, vary in overall and nuclear size, and have only a thin rim of cytoplasm (Fig 12). This appearance is in contrast to that of normal bile duct epithelium (Fig 4).

Other Primary Hepatic Neoplasms: Leiomyosarcoma, fibrosarcoma and osteogenic sarcoma are uncommon hepatic tumors in

Figure 11. Numerous binucleate hepatocytes with mild anisocytosis and anisokaryosis are seen in this touch imprint from a liver biopsy taken from an icteric dog. Histopathologic examination indicated hepatocellular regeneration, probably secondary to an unidentified toxic insult. (Wright's-Giemsa, 400X)

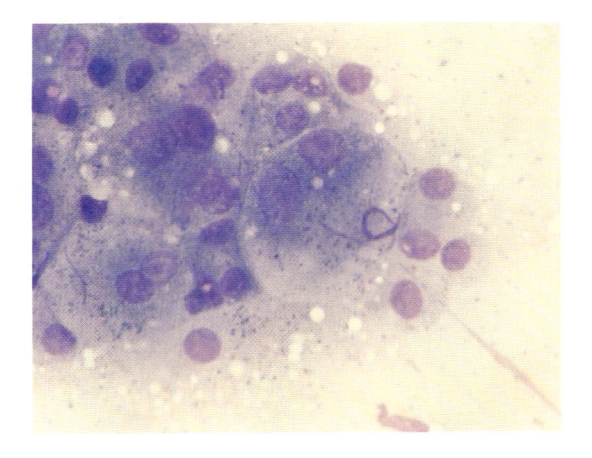

dogs and generally are difficult to diagnose cytologically due to their tendency to yield poorly cellular aspirates.[12-15] Dogs appear to have a relatively high incidence of carcinoid neoplasms.[16] Our experience in cytologic recognition of this neoplasm in other tissues is limited but indicates that, while it does exfoliate well, the cell type is difficult to specifically identify. Consequently, histologic examination should be used to confirm these tumor types.

Metastatic Neoplasia: Hepatomegaly is not a frequent consequence of metastatic cancer.[17] Focal metastatic lesions are best recognized and aspirated with aid of ultrasound, laparoscopy or laparotomy.[18] While various ultrasonographic patterns have been described for hepatic neoplasia, none is specific for cell type, nor do they differentiate between benign and malignant lesions.[19] Cytologic examination may not always provide definitive diagnosis of cell types but, in our experience, it usually can differentiate between benign and malignant conditions. Histologic evaluation of the tumor often is needed for definitive diagnosis as to cell type. Splenic, pancreatic and intestinal neoplasms are the most common malignancies to metastasize to the liver.

Nonneoplastic Disorders

Glucocorticoid-Induced Hepatopathy: Administration of glucocorticoids to dogs frequently causes increased serum liver enzyme activities and, occasionally, hepatomegaly secondary to accumulation of glycogen.[20-23] We have also observed hepatomegaly in association with hyperadrenocorticism. Clinically, it is important to note that these patients are not icteric and, biochemically, the serum bilirubin concentration is normal. Cytologically, glycogen-related hepatomegaly should be suspected when most hepatocytes contain a "feathery" cytoplasmic change. Fixation of the cytologic specimen during the staining process removes glycogen, leaving variably sized cytoplasmic vacuoles laced with wisps of blue cytoplasm (Fig 13). While cats apparently are more resistant to this morphologic change, prednisolone and megestrol acetate occasionally induce a similar vacuolar change.[24]

Feline Hepatic Lipidosis: Diffuse deposition of lipid within the liver is a common cause of icterus and hepatomegaly in cats.[25] The

Figure 12. Dense clusters of large, neoplastic epithelial cells predominate in this liver aspirate from an icteric cat. For comparison, note the 2 hepatocytes located to the left of center. Bile duct carcinoma was confirmed histologically. (Wright's-Giemsa, 400X)

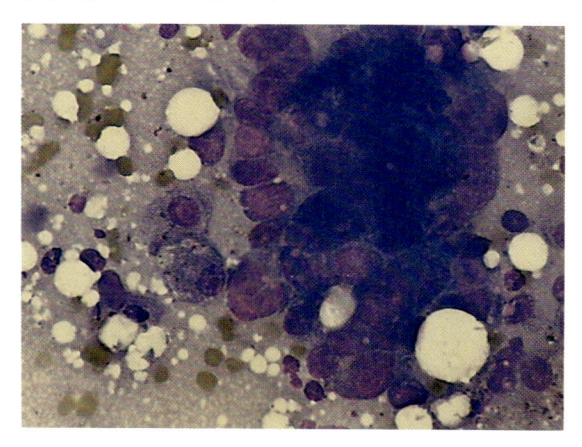

Figure 13. Vacuolated hepatocytes predominate in this aspirate from a dog with hepatomegaly. The indistinct vacuolar cytoplasmic change suggested glycogen. Corticosteroid-induced hepatopathy was confirmed histologically. (Wright's-Giemsa, 1000X)

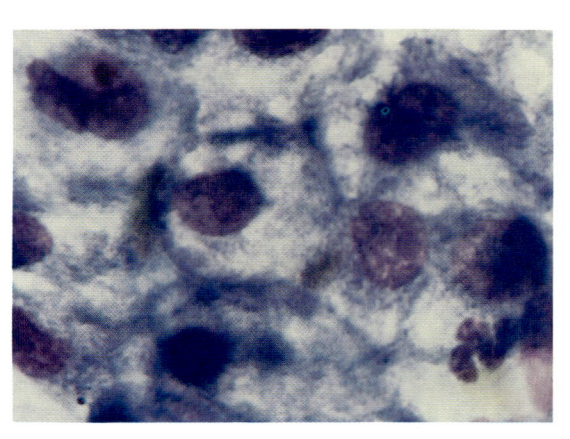

etiopathogenesis remains unknown, but probably involves multiple factors. Cytologically, hepatic lipidosis is recognized by a large cytoplasmic vacuole displacing the hepatocyte nucleus to the periphery (Fig 14). Fixation during the staining process removes the lipid, leaving a crisp, clear cytoplasmic space in contrast to the indistinct vacuolar change associated with glycogen (Fig 13). Numerous small, well-delineated vacuoles also may be observed in this syndrome (Fig 14). Histologically, we have seen both patterns in the same biopsy specimen. Finding numerous lipid-laden hepatocytes in aspirates from an icteric patient with hepatomegaly and high serum alkaline phosphatase activity supports the diagnosis.[3,25] Cats with sphingomyelin lipidosis and alpha-mannosidosis also have severe vacuolar changes in their liver.[26,27] While these conditions appear to be rare, hepatic lipidosis in a young cat should prompt consideration of such inborn errors of metabolism.

Inadvertent aspiration of intraabdominal fat also yields tissue with a fatty appearance. Such adipose tissue usually contains more stroma and lacks the crisp, uniform oval vacuoles typical of hepatic lipidosis. Sheets of mesothelial cells also may be seen, further indicating lack of hepatic penetration (Plate 8).

Feline Cholangitis/Cholangiohepatitis: Inflammation of the intrahepatic biliary tree may be described as suppurative if the predominant inflammatory cell is the neutrophil (Fig 6), and lymphocytic (nonsuppurative) if lymphocytes predominate (Fig 8). Lympho-

The Liver

Figure 14. Liver aspirates from icteric cats with hepatomegaly and histologic diagnoses of hepatic lipidosis (top to bottom) A. Most of these hepatocytes contain large, clear cytoplasmic vacuoles, indicating macrovesicular fatty change (400X). B. Discrete cytoplasmic vacuoles may displace the nucleus to the periphery of the hepatocyte (1000X). C. Multiple small, discrete vacuoles in the cytoplasm of these hepatocytes indicate microvesicular fatty change. (Wright's-Giemsa, 400X)

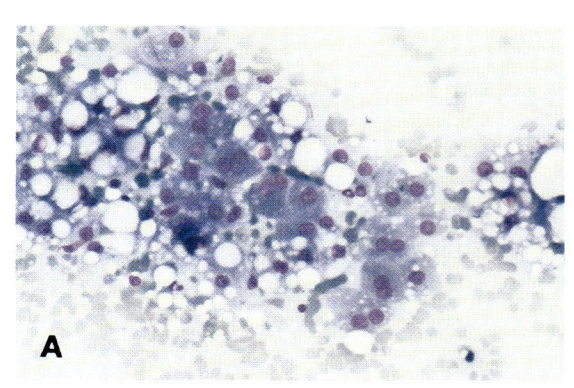

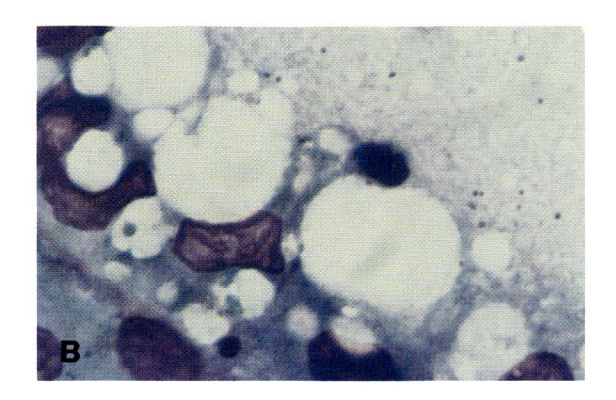

Figure 15. Pink, amorphous extracellular material is observed among the hepatocytes in this aspirate from a dog with hepatomegaly and osteomyelitis of several months' duration. Hepatic amyloidosis was confirmed histologically. (Wright's-Giemsa, 1000X)

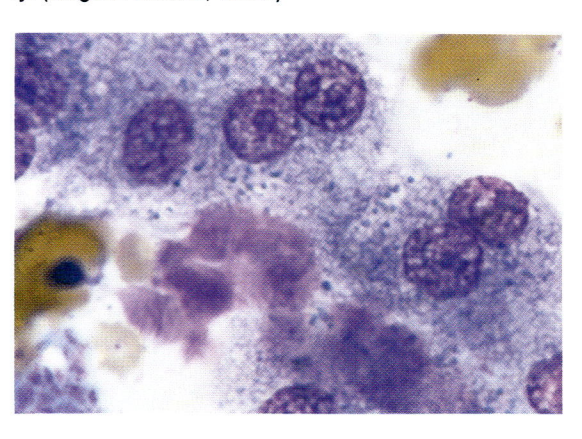

recurrent, may be an early clinical sign. The cause of the periportal lymphocytic infiltrate is not known. Variation in clinical characteristics of the disease suggests more than one factor may be involved.[10,25] The difficulty in cytologic distinction from well-differentiated lymphosarcoma is discussed above.

Amyloidosis: Deposition of amyloid in the liver can result in generalized hepatomegaly. Hepatic amyloidosis, in our experience, is most commonly a sequel to a chronic inflammatory process elsewhere in the body. The presence of amyloid is suggested by amorphous, pink-staining material swirled among relatively

Figure 16. Touch imprint of a dark liver nodule identified during an exploratory laparotomy. Hepatocytes appear normal except for an increased number of binucleate forms (left) and occasional mitotic figures (right). The cytologic pattern suggested nodular hyperplasia, and subsequent histologic examination confirmed the diagnosis. (Wright's-Giemsa, 400X)

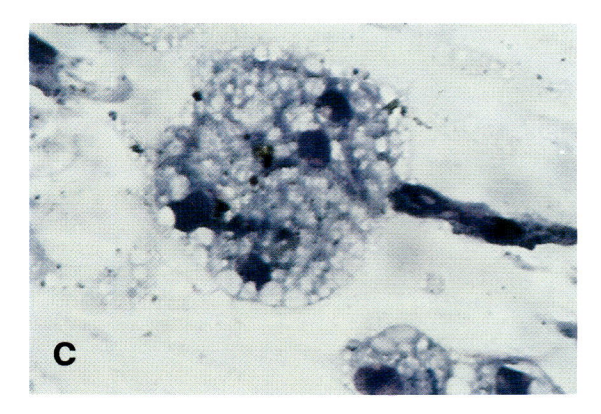

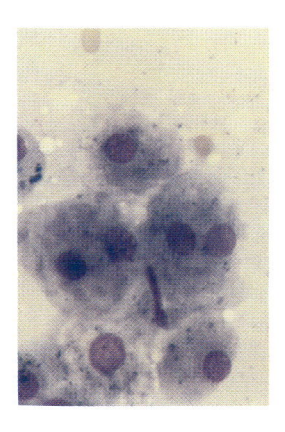

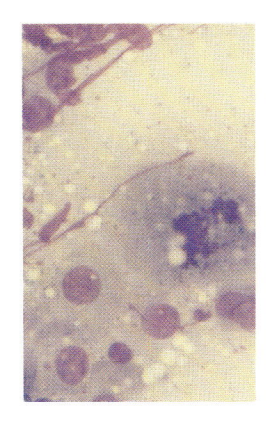

cytic cholangitis/cholangiohepatitis is a common cause of icterus and hepatomegaly in cats. Since the portal area is the primary site of the inflammatory infiltrate, icterus, sometimes

195

Figure 17. Neutrophils, eosinophils and lymphocytes are prominent in this liver aspirate from an icteric cat. Histologic examination revealed cholangitis with a mixture of these same cell types, and parasite ova compatible with those of the liver fluke, *Platynosomum fastosum*. (Wright's-Giemsa, 1000X)

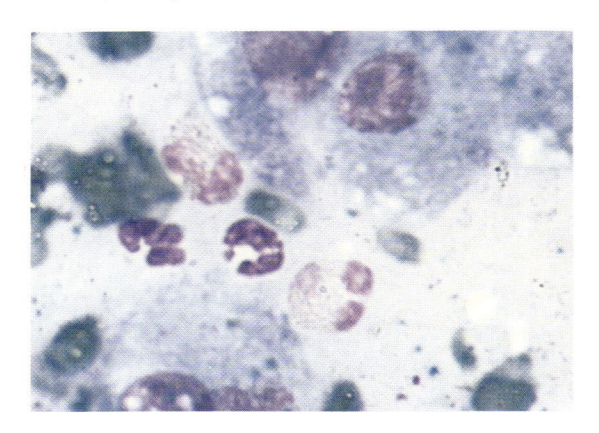

normal-appearing hepatocytes (Fig 15). Histologically, Congo red staining produces birefringence of the material when viewed with polarized light. We have not attempted this procedure with cytologic specimens.

Nodular Hyperplasia/Adenoma: Benign, focal proliferation of hepatocytes, resulting in a nodular hepatic surface, is a common finding in aged dogs. In one study, all dogs over the age of 15 years had nodular hyperplasia, which grossly may resemble metastatic disease.[28] Cytologically, adenoma and nodular hyperplasia are indistinguishable. Hepatocytes appear relatively normal except for mild variation in size and increased numbers of binucleate cells (Fig 16).[29] The mild variation in size should not cause confusion with hepatocellular carcinoma, which has a more anaplastic cytologic appearance and usually appears as a large, solitary mass involving a single hepatic lobe.

Inflammatory Liver Disease: Cytologic diagnosis of inflammatory liver disease by aspiration biopsy in people has been reported to be less than satisfactory.[5] In our experience, this is the case in veterinary medicine as well. In such conditions as chronic active hepatitis, for example, relatively few inflammatory cells are diffusely scattered throughout the paren-

Figure 19. A large, mature megakaryocyte is located adjacent to a cluster of hepatocytes in this liver aspirate from a dog with regenerative anemia. Erythroid and granulocytic precursors were seen in other fields. (Wright's-Giemsa, 400X)

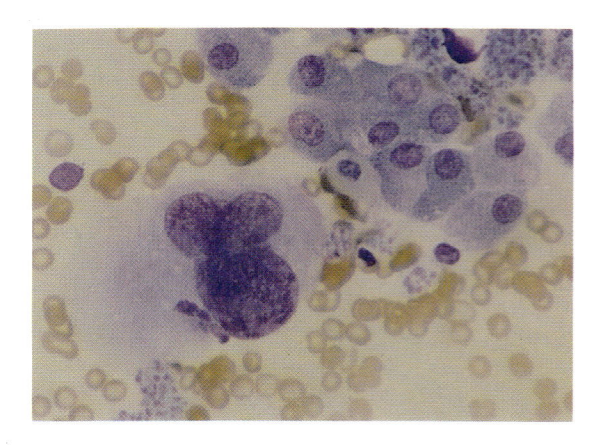

Figure 18. Liver aspirate from an unvaccinated dog with clinical and biochemical evidence of acute hepatitis. Large, pink intranuclear inclusions are present in 2 hepatocytes. Small, round, slightly blue nucleoli are visible in the other hepatocytes. Normal nucleoli should not be confused with the large, eosinophilic intranuclear inclusions. (Wright's-Giemsa, 1000X) (Courtesy of Dr. R.L. Cowell, Oklahoma State University).

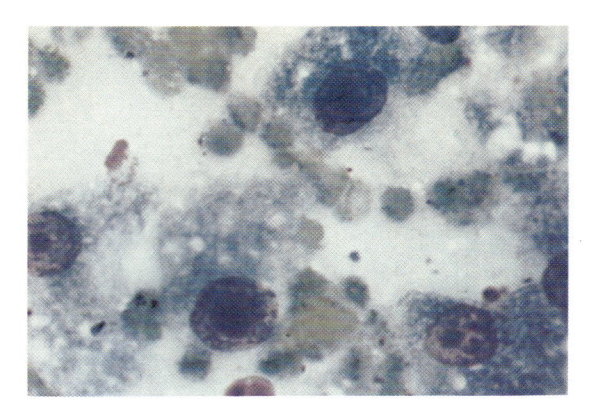

chyma, and therefore are not reliably detected. In this disease, histologic examination is essential to characterize the time course and prognosis based on cell type, amount of fibrosis and number of remaining viable hepatocytes.

In some other inflammatory conditions, however, characterization of the cellular response, and perhaps definitive diagnosis, can be achieved. We have seen a cytologic pattern of eosinophilic inflammation in aspirates from livers of cats infected with liver flukes, common in southern Florida and Hawaii (Fig 17). Intranuclear inclusions associated with infectious canine hepatitis have been seen on occasion (Fig 18). Certain other infectious causes of inflammation of the liver may also be identifiable in cytologic preparations. Histoplasmosis, cytauxzoonosis and toxoplasmosis, for example, may at times be diagnosed in this manner (Plates 4 and 5).

Extramedullary Hematopoiesis: The presence of normal hematopoietic cells in the liver is a common, nonspecific finding in animals with accelerated erythropoiesis in response to anemia. Cellular elements of the granulocytic, erythroid and megakaryocytic lines may be observed (Fig 19). These cells have a normal appearance, with the more mature stages being most numerous. Similar nonneoplastic proliferation of hematopoietic cells has been observed in livers of animals with abnormal bone marrows, such as in cats with myelodysplastic syndromes.[8] Mild extramedullary hematopoiesis and occasionally small numbers of circulating nucleated RBC may also be observed in nonanemic dogs with chronic inflammatory liver disease. The pathogenesis of these last findings is not known.

References

1. Perman et al: *Cytology of the Dog and Cat.* AAHA, Denver, CO, 1979. pp 152-155.

2. Rebar: *Handbook of Veterinary Cytology.* Ralston Purina, St. Louis, 1978. pp 22, 50.

3. Meyer and Center: Approach to the diagnosis of liver disorders in dogs and cats. *Comp Cont Ed Pract Vet* 8:880-888, 1986.

4. Whitlatch et al: Fine needle aspiration biopsy of the liver—a study of 102 consecutive cases. *Acta Cytologica* 28:719-725, 1984.

5. Johnston: Needle biopsy of the liver for the diagnosis of nonneoplastic liver diseases. *Acta Cytologica* 29:385-390, 1985.

6. Meyer: The management of cytology specimens. *Comp Cont Ed Pract Vet* 9: 10-17, 1987.

7. Smith et al, in Jones: *Veterinary Pathology.* 4th ed. Lea & Febiger, Philadelphia, 1972. pp 1235-1236.

8. Blue et al: Non-lymphoid hematopoietic neoplasia in cats: a retrospective study of 60 cases. *Cornell Vet* 78:21-42, 1988.

9. Prasse et al: Chronic lymphocytic cholangitis in three cats. *Vet Pathol* 19:99-108, 1982.

10. Lucke and Davies: Progressive lymphocytic cholangitis in the cat. *J Small Anim Pract* 25:249-260, 1984.

11. O'Keefe et al: Systemic mastocytosis in 16 dogs. *J Vet Int Med* 1:75-80, 1987.

12. Patnaik et al: Canine hepatic neoplasms: a clinicopathologic study. *Vet Pathol* 17:553-564, 1980.

13. Patnaik et al: Canine hepatocellular carcinoma. *Vet Pathol* 18:427-438, 1981.

14. Patnaik et al: Canine bile duct carcinoma. *Vet Pathol* 18:439-444, 1981.

15. Griffiths et al: Fine needle aspiration cytology and histologic correlation in canine tumors. *Vet Clin Pathol* 13:13-17, 1984.

16. Patnaik et al: Canine hepatic carcinoids. *Vet Pathol* 18:445-453, 1981.

17. Strombeck: Clinicopathologic features of primary and metastatic neoplastic disease of the liver in dogs. *JAVMA* 173:267-269, 1978.

18. Hager et al: Ultrasound-guided biopsy of the canine liver, kidney, and prostate. *Vet Radiol* 26:82-88, 1985.

19. Feeney et al: Two-dimensional, gray-scale ultrasonography for the assessment of hepatic and splenic neoplasia in the dog and cat. *JAVMA* 184:68-81, 1984.

20. Rogers and Reubner: A retrospective study of probable glucocorticoid-induced hepatopathy in the dog. *JAVMA* 170:603-606, 1977.

21. Fittschen and Bellamy: Prednisone-induced morphologic and chemical changes in the liver of dogs. *Vet Pathol* 21:399-406, 1984.

22. Badylak and van Vleet: Sequential morphologic and clinicopathologic alterations in dogs with experimentally-induced glucocorticoid hepatopathy. *Am J Vet Res* 42:1310-1318, 1981.

23. DeNovo and Prasse: Comparison of serum biochemical and hepatic functional alterations in dogs treated with corticosteroids and hepatic duct ligation. *Am J Vet Res* 44:1703-1709, 1983.

24. Middleton et al: Suppression of cortisol responses to exogenous adrenocorticotropic hormone, and the occurrence of side effects attributable to glucocorticoid excess in cats during therapy with megestrol acetate and prednisolone. *Can J Vet Res* 51:60-65, 1987.

25. Center: Feline liver disorders and their management. *Comp Cont Ed Pract Vet* 8:889-903, 1986.

26. Baker et al: Sphingomyelin lipidosis in a cat. *Vet Pathol* 24:386-391, 1987.

27. Jezyk et al: Alpha-mannosidosis in a Persian cat. *JAVMA* 189:1483-1485, 1986.

28. Bergman: Nodular hyperplasia in the liver of the dog: an association with changes in the Ito cell population. *Vet Pathol* 22:427-438, 1985.

29. Fabry et al: Nodular hyperplasia of the liver in the beagle dog. *Vet Pathol* 19:109-119, 1982.

30. Evans: The radiographic appearance of primary liver neoplasia in dogs. *Vet Radiol* 28:192-196, 1987.

17

The Splenic Parenchyma

P.S. MacWilliams

The spleen is part of the hemolymphatic system and consists of a cellular parenchyma of red and white pulp supported by a stroma of reticular fibers. It is surrounded by a connective tissue capsule containing variable amounts of smooth muscle. As a component of the hemolymphatic system, the spleen serves several purposes. In addition to an important role in the immune response, functions of the spleen include: storage of platelets and mature RBC; maturation of reticulocytes; phagocytosis and destruction of RBC, platelets, WBC and foreign particles; and extramedullary hematopoiesis.[1] The nature of these functions causes the gross and microscopic appearance of the spleen to be affected by a variety of systemic inflammatory diseases and hematologic disorders. As with other organs, the spleen is subject to disturbances of cell growth (hyperplasia, atrophy), circulatory abnormalities (hematoma, congestion, thrombosis, infarction), inflammation and neoplasia (primary and metastatic).[2] Several of these processes, either alone or in combination, may result in splenic enlargement.

Splenomegaly is a common clinical abnormality in small animal practice and is usually detected by palpation. Minor degrees of splenomegaly can be revealed by radiography or ultrasonography. Depending on the cause, splenomegaly may be accompanied by hematologic abnormalities, such as hemolytic anemia, thrombocytopenia, leukemia or hemolymphatic neoplasia.[3] Causes of splenomegaly in dogs and cats are listed in Table 1.[2-4]

Once splenomegaly is detected, the specific cause should be determined, since splenic enlargement is usually a secondary manifestation of some other clinical problem. A complete physical examination and history are essential. Careful palpation and radiographic studies should reveal the severity of splenomegaly and whether the enlargement is diffuse and symmetric or localized to one area of the spleen (asymmetric). A CBC and careful examination of RBC, WBC and platelet morphology on a peripheral blood film are indicated.

Depending on presentation, a variety of diagnostic procedures may be useful. Immune-mediated causes of splenomegaly may be detected by tests for RBC antiglobulins (Coombs' test), antinuclear antibodies or rheumatoid factor. Serologic tests may suggest fungal or protozoal infections. Blood films should be carefully searched for atypical WBC and RBC parasites, such as *Hemobartonella*, *Cytauxzoon* or *Babesia*. Cytologic examination of bone marrow or lymph node is very useful in diagnosis of hemolymphatic neoplasia and sometimes reveals infectious agents responsible for splenomegaly. Collection and cytologic evaluation of abdominal fluid are always indicated when splenomegaly is accompanied by peritoneal effusion. Serum chemistry assays and additional radiographic procedures may also contribute information to the diagnostic process.

Collection of Splenic Specimens

Specimens for cytologic assessment of the spleen are derived from 3 sources: fine-needle aspirates, impression smears of surgical biopsies, and impression smears collected at necropsy.

Fine-Needle Aspiration

Aspiration of splenic samples through the abdominal wall of the live animal should be carefully considered. An enlarged spleen is usually turgid, friable and engorged with blood. Profuse intraabdominal hemorrhage and tumor metastasis within the abdominal cavity are 2 significant complications of this procedure.[3,5] For these reasons, aspiration of the spleen is contraindicated when hemangiosarcoma is suspected. In live dogs and cats, aspiration of the spleen is indicated when the cause of splenomegaly cannot be determined by other means. In general, splenic aspiration should only be attempted in dogs and cats with symmetric splenomegaly. The technique is especially useful in detecting splenic enlargement due to hemolymphatic neoplasia and has some value in splenomegaly due to infectious, immunologic or hemolytic disease (Table 1).

Aspiration of the spleen can usually be done without general anesthesia. The size and location of the spleen within the abdominal cavity determine the actual site for aspiration. The surgical site on the abdomen is determined by where the spleen can be most easily apposed to the abdominal wall. The site is clipped and washed, and surgical disinfectant is applied. Infiltration of the area with local anesthetic may be helpful. Use of a 22- to 23-ga needle with an attached 6- or 12-ml syringe is recommended. Needle length is determined by the size of the animal, but usually a 1- or 1 1/2-inch needle is adequate.

The spleen is pressed gently against the abdominal wall at the prepared site. The needle with attached syringe is inserted through the skin and muscle layer into the spleen. Withdrawing the syringe plunger produces negative pressure while the needle is moved within the spleen along several axes. Maintaining suction while redirecting the needle in the parenchyma collects cells and tissue fragments from several areas. Negative pressure on the plunger should be released when a small amount of bloody fluid appears in the syringe tip. Excessive hemorrhage and dilution of the sample with blood should be avoided. It is very important to release the syringe plunger before the needle is withdrawn from the spleen. Immediately after withdrawing the needle from the animal, small drops of the aspirate are applied to glass slides. The consistency of the aspirated specimen determines the method of smear preparation.[6] Most splenic aspirates have the consistency of blood, and slides are prepared in the same manner as

Table 1. Causes and characteristics of splenomegaly in dogs and cats.

Cause	Type of Enlargement	Severity of Enlargement

Hyperplasia
    infection
    immunologic disease
	symmetric	mild to moderate

Extramedullary Hematopoiesis	symmetric	mild to moderate

Hemolymphatic Neoplasia
    lymphoproliferative neoplasms
    myeloproliferative disorders
	symmetric	moderate to severe

Splenic Neoplasia
    hemangioma/hemangiosarcoma
    fibrosarcoma
    leiomyosarcoma
    metastatic neoplasms
	asymmetric or nodular	mild to severe

Circulatory Disturbances
    hematoma
    portal hypertension
    torsion
	asymmetric
	symmetric
	symmetric
		mild to moderate
		mild to moderate
		severe

blood films. Specimens that are thick or contain tissue fragments are prepared by the squash technique, gently compressing the material between 2 slides. The cells are spread by pulling the slides across each other. Chapter 1 contains a detailed description of slide preparation techniques.

Impression smears of splenic tissue from surgical biopsies or necropsy specimens have several uses. In some situations, an immediate diagnosis may be obtained. For example, a homogeneous population of large lymphoblasts (Fig 4 and Plate 7) or a pure population of mast cells (Plate 7) confirms a diagnosis of lymphoma and mastocytoma, respectively. In other cases, cytologic findings may eliminate neoplasia from the differential diagnoses and allow immediate pursuit of other causes of splenomegaly.

Figure 1. Impression smear of normal feline splenic tissue. A. The cell population is a mixture of small and large lymphocytes. The large cells in the center are lymphoblasts. The smaller cells with a small amount of light-blue cytoplasm and smooth nuclear chromatin are small lymphocytes. (Wright's stain, 480X) B. Higher magnification reveals several small lymphocytes and one lymphoblast (upper left). (Wright's stain, 1200X)

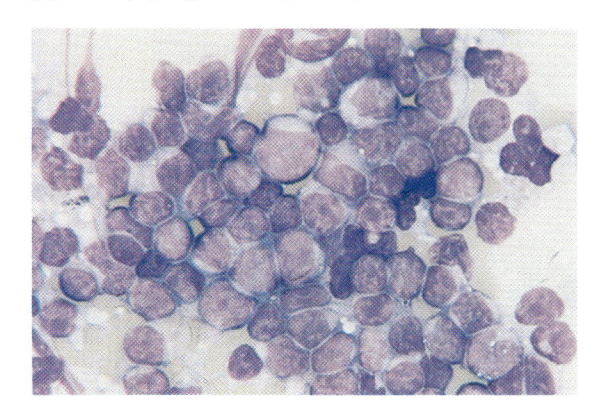

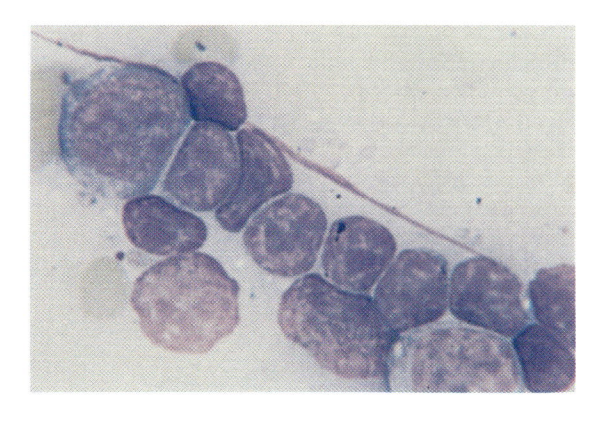

Impression Smears

Impression smears of splenic tissue are a valuable adjunct to histopathologic examination by revealing cellular details not visible in tissue sections. Though tissue architecture is lost in collection, recognition of individual cell types, fungi, protozoa, RBC parasites and neoplastic cell lines is sometimes easier on Wright's-stained slides and can complement histologic assessment. Impression smears and aspirates of spleen are especially valuable in differentiating various cell types (erythroid, granulocytic, lymphoid) of hemolymphatic neoplasms.

The most important aspect of making impression smears of splenic tissue is blotting the tissue on a paper towel to remove excess blood and tissue fluid before making tissue imprints on glass slides. A fresh-cut surface of the spleen is exposed by trimming the tissue with a scalpel blade. Cells are exfoliated by gently touching the blotted tissue surface to a glass slide.[6,7] Further details are described in Chapter 1.

Wright's stain or a similar Romanowsky stain (eg, Diff-Quik:American Scientific Products) is the preferred stain for splenic cytology because most veterinarians are familiar with its staining characteristics and it provides excellent definition of cytoplasmic features. Staining times with Wright's or Diff-Quik may need to be increased for slides that are more densely cellular than blood films. Chapter 1 contains specific information on staining techniques.

Microscopic Examination

Systematic examination of a well-stained slide that is representative of splenic parenchyma provides valuable information to identify the cause of splenomegaly. Low-power objectives (4X and 10X) are used to assess cellularity and stain quality, locate cell clusters, and select slides and microscopic fields for further examination under higher magnification. The 40X and 100X objectives are used to assess general composition of the cell population and study nuclear and cytoplasmic details of individual cells. At these magnifications, it is helpful to find a small lymphocyte or segmented neutrophil for size and color comparisons (Figs 1,2,6).

Interpretation of cytologic findings and differentiation of the various causes of splenomegaly require knowledge of the history, clinical signs and laboratory results. Table 1 lists 5 general causes of splenic enlargement. One should bear in mind that more than one mechanism may be operative in a given animal. For example, a dog with immune-mediated hemolytic anemia may have splenomegaly due to reactive hyperplasia and extramedullary hematopoiesis. Fine-needle aspirates of a symmetrically enlarged spleen are useful in identifying hyperplasia, extramedullary hematopoiesis, hemolymphatic neoplasia and infectious agents, such as *Histoplasma, Cytauxzoon* and *Babesia*. For impression smears of biopsy or necropsy specimens, cytologic assessment is most useful for identifying protozoa and fungi, and for differentiating hyperplasia, extramedullary hematopoiesis, hemolymphatic neoplasia and splenic neoplasia. Cytologic findings attributable to circulatory disturbances causing splenomegaly are equivocal.

Chart 1 presents an algorithm for classification of splenic cytologic findings.

Normal Cytologic Features

Cytologic features of normal splenic aspirates and impression smears must be understood before abnormalities can be detected. Impression smears of normal splenic tissue have microscopic features similar to those of normal lymph nodes. Slides are usually very cellular due to a mixed population of small lymphocytes and lymphoblasts.[3,7] Small lymphocytes predominate in most fields. However, because the spleen contains numerous lymphoid follicles with germinal centers, lymphoblasts may predominate in some microscopic fields using the 100X objective. Small lymphocytes are smaller than segmented neutrophils and have a round or slightly indented nucleus, dark condensed chromatin, and a thin rim of pale-blue cytoplasm (Fig 1). Lymphoblasts are identified by their large size, large irregular or indented nucleus, light-staining vesicular chromatin, multiple nucleoli and lightly basophilic cytoplasm. In addition to the lymphocyte population, a few macrophages and plasma cells may be observed, along with lesser numbers of neutrophils, mast cells and platelet clumps. Some macrophages may contain cytoplasmic hemosiderin. The numbers of RBC in the background vary with the degree of splenic congestion and how well the cut surface was blotted.

The microscopic appearance of fine-needle aspirates of splenic tissue is affected by the amount of hemodilution in the specimen. Ex-

Figure 2. Impression smear of hyperplastic splenic tissue from a dog. A. Lymphoblasts and a few small lymphocytes surround 2 macrophages with eccentric oval nuclei and a large amount of vacuolated cytoplasm containing cellular debris and dark pigment. A mast cell is adjacent to the macrophage in the bottom portion of the field. (Wright's stain, 480X) B. Higher magnification reveals lymphoblasts with multiple nucleoli, surrounded by small lymphocytes and one neutrophil. Compare the sizes of the neutrophil, small lymphocyte and lymphoblast. A plasma cell is located in the upper left hand corner. (Wright's stain, 1200X)

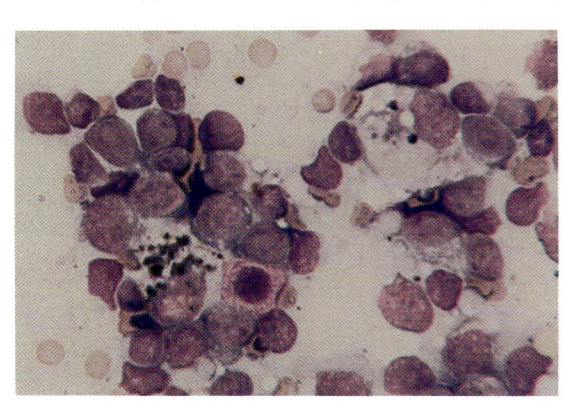

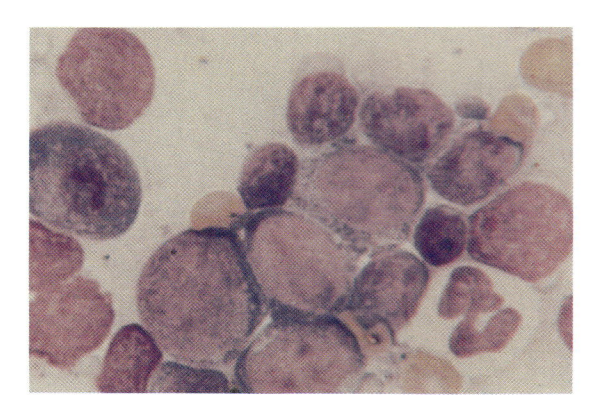

perience with fine-needle aspirates of normal spleen is limited. Depending on the amount of blood contamination, the background contains varying numbers of RBC, WBC and platelets. As in impression smears, the lymphoid population is mixed, with small lymphocytes predominating. Lesser numbers of lymphoblasts are present, along with a few macrophages and plasma cells. Neutrophils, mast cells, endothelial cells and fibrocytes are noted occasionally.[3]

Hyperplasia

Though considered a single category of splenomegaly, splenic hyperplasia results from a variety of inflammatory diseases, both septic and nonseptic. Mild to moderate degrees of splenomegaly are found in immune-mediated disorders and in systemic infectious diseases caused by bacteria, rickettsiae, protozoa and fungi. Cytologic findings in hyperplastic splenomegaly depend on the causative agent, mechanism of disease, and host immune response. In general, splenic hyperplasia is characterized by increased numbers of macrophages, plasma cells and lymphoblasts at the expense of small lymphocytes (Fig 2).[3] However, reduction in numbers of small lymphocytes is relative, and these cells remain the predominant cell type. A slight increase in neutrophil numbers is expected. With chronic infections, the increase in macrophage and plasma cell numbers is often pronounced. When macrophages are prominent, it is important to examine their cytoplasm for cellular debris, pigment, phagocytized RBC, bacteria and such organisms as *Histoplasma* (Plate 4) and *Leishmania* (Plate 5). The RBC in the background or within macrophages should be examined for *Hemobartonella, Babesia, Cytauxzoon* (Plate 5) and Heinz bodies.[8] Leukocytes should be scrutinized for morulae of *Ehrlichia*.

Extramedullary Hematopoiesis

Extramedullary hematopoiesis is the development of sites of hematopoiesis outside of bone marrow. This phenomenon is observed frequently in dogs and cats with chronic hemolytic anemias and in those with severe bone marrow disorders compromising production of blood cells. The spleen is a frequent site of involvement, and splenomegaly is not unusual in animals with extramedullary hematopoiesis, either alone or in combination with reactive hyperplasia or neoplasia. In most situations, the predominant hematopoietic cell line is erythroid, with lesser numbers of megakaryocytes and granulocyte precursors.

Hematologic disorders frequently associated with extramedullary hematopoiesis include chronic hemolytic anemias, myeloproliferative disorders, lymphoproliferative neoplasia and myelodysplastic syndromes.[2] In hemolytic anemias due to immunologic disease or infectious agents, the cytologic appearance is characterized by erythroid precursors (metarubricytes, rubricytes, prorubricytes and a few rubriblasts) with a background of small and large lymphocytes (Fig 3). Macrophages containing hemosiderin and phagocytized RBC are present. Metarubricytes are numerous and recognized easily, but the more immature cells can be confused with lymphoid cells. Features of immature RBC that differentiate them from lymphoid cells include a nearly round nucleus with irregularly clumped chromatin imparting a wheel-spoke or checkerboard appearance (Fig 3). The cytoplasm is dark blue to blue-gray, depending on the stage of maturity, and may contain a juxtanuclear clear zone. When these cells are found in conjunction with myeloproliferative disease or lymphoid neoplasia in the spleen, erythroid precursors are mixed with the neoplastic cells.

Figure 3. Feline splenic tissue with extramedullary hematopoiesis. A. Most of the cells are erythroid precursors at various stages of development, with a few neutrophils and several lymphocytes (lower left). The large round cells in the center are rubriblasts and prorubricytes. (Wright's stain, 480X) B. Comparison between lymphoid cells (lower left) and erythroid precursors. Immature erythroid cells at the rubriblast and prorubricyte stage have a round nucleus, dark basophilic cytoplasm, coarse granular or loosely clumped chromatin and, when present, a single nucleolus. The metarubricyte at the top of the field has an immature nucleus in well-differentiated cytoplasm (nuclear-cytoplasmic asynchrony). (Wright's stain, 1200X)

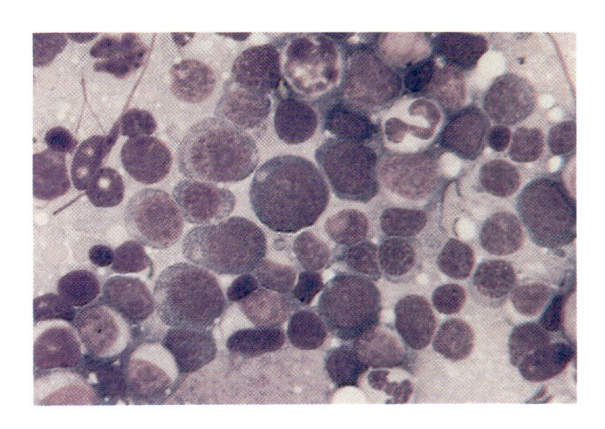

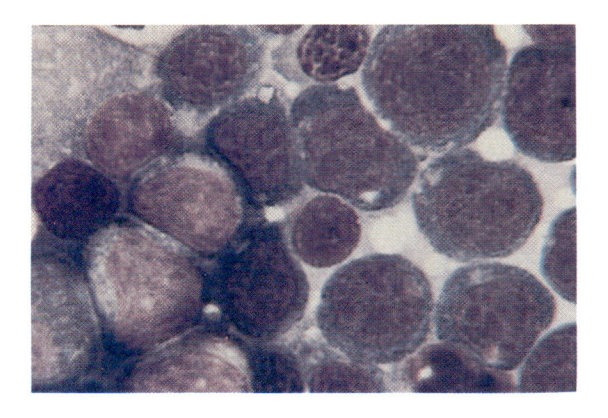

Asynchronous development of nucleus and cytoplasm is often present, especially in cats (Fig 3).

Hemolymphatic Neoplasia

The normal spleen contains a mixed population of cells with a variety of sizes, shapes and colors. When the spleen is enlarged due to lymphoproliferative neoplasia or a myeloproliferative disorder, the hallmark of the cytology specimen is a very cellular slide containing a homogeneous population of neoplastic cells.[9] Replacement of parenchyma with these cells is nearly complete, leaving only a few normal lymphoid cells and macrophages. The microscopic appearance of neoplastic cells depends on their cell type. Neoplasms identified frequently in the spleen include those derived from lymphocytes, erythroid precursors, granulocytes and undifferentiated cells. Hematologic assessment, including blood and bone marrow and a battery of special stains, is sometimes necessary for definitive diagnosis.

In most dogs and cats with lymphoma and acute lymphocytic leukemia, normal cells are replaced by a homogeneous population of large, hyperchromatic lymphoblasts with abundant dark-blue cytoplasm and large round or indented nuclei containing multiple nucleoli (Fig 4 and Plate 7).

Splenic impression smears from cats with erythremic myelosis have numerous large round cells with round eccentric nuclei, fine granular chromatin, a single nucleolus and dark-blue cytoplasm containing a few fine red granules. In some cells, the cytoplasm contains a small localized clear zone (Fig 5). A few rubricytes and metarubricytes are present, with frequent examples of asynchronous maturation of the nucleus and cytoplasm.

Neoplastic cells can be derived from granulocytes, monocytes, plasma cells, mast cells or primitive, undifferentiated cells. Splenic cytology is characterized by a monotonous population of the involved cell type displacing normal cells (Figs 6, 7 and Plate 7).

Splenic Neoplasia

Hemangiosarcoma can be recognized on impression smears. The specimen must be blotted well to remove excess blood, since these neoplasms have a rich blood supply. Slides

Figure 4. Impression smear of splenic tissue from a dog with lymphoma reveals a homogeneous population of lymphoblasts. Nucleoli are multiple and prominent. (Wright's stain, 480X)

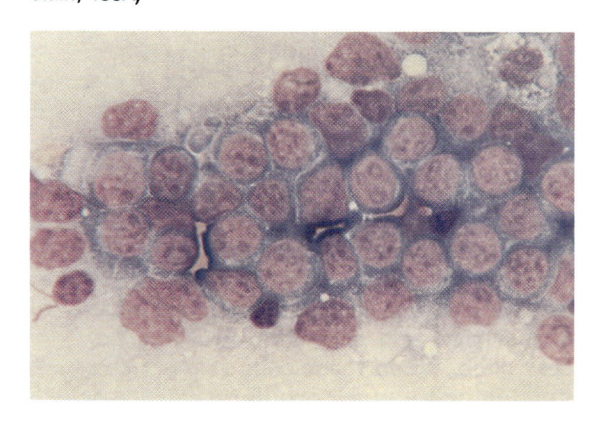

Figure 5. Impression smear of splenic tissue from a cat with erythremic myelosis. A. The normal cell population is displaced by numerous large hyperchromatic round cells. There is no differentiation toward more mature forms in the erythroid series. (Wright's stain, 480X) B. The primitive cells in this myeloproliferative disorder are similar to rubriblasts. Morphologic features include a round nucleus, with coarse granular chromatin, a large single nucleolus and dark-blue cytoplasm with a prominent clear zone. (Wright's stain, 1200X)

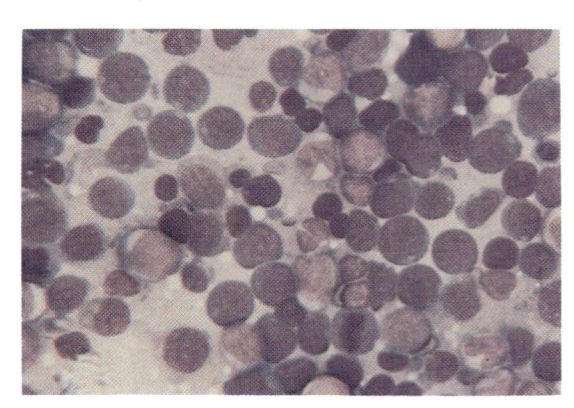

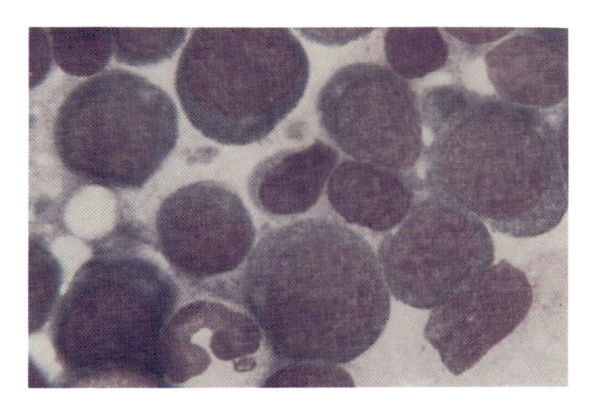

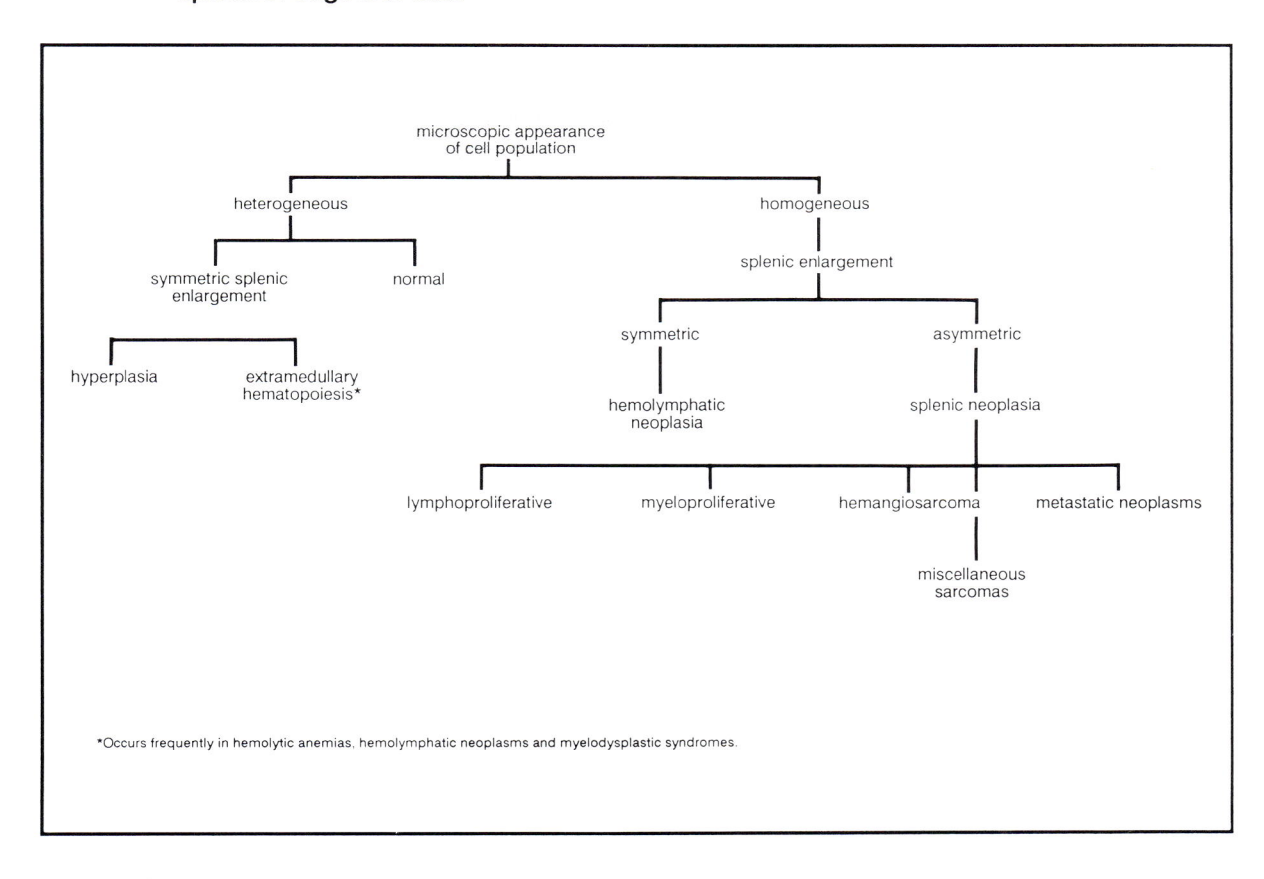

Figure 6. Impression smear of splenic tissue from a dog with multiple myeloma. The spleen is diffusely infiltrated by neoplastic plasma cells. With the exception of a small lymphocyte in the center, all of the cells are plasma cells. (Wright's stain, 480X)

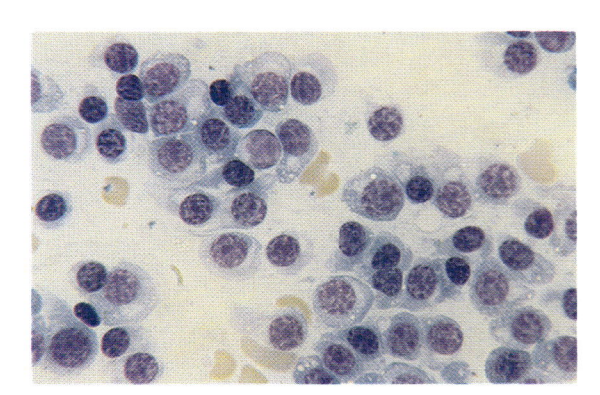

Figure 7. Impression smear of splenic tissue from a cat with an undifferentiated hemolymphatic neoplasm. A neutrophil and several small lymphocytes in the center are surrounded by primitive cells with indistinct cell margins, round nuclei, vesicular chromatin and a single prominent nucleolus. (Wright's stain, 480X)

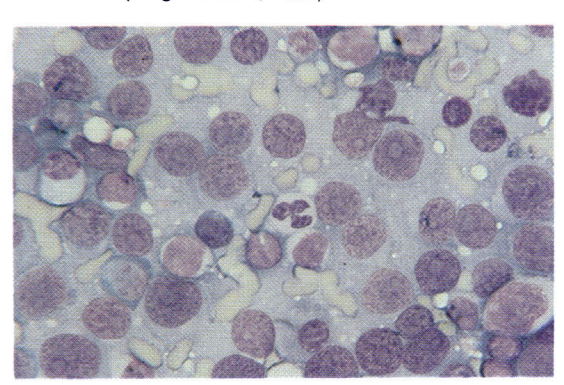

Chart 1. Cytologic classification of fine-needle aspirates and impression smears from the spleen of dogs and cats.

```
                    microscopic appearance
                       of cell population
                    ┌──────────┴──────────┐
               heterogeneous          homogeneous
               ┌─────┴─────┐               │
        symmetric splenic  normal    splenic enlargement
           enlargement                ┌────┴────┐
        ┌──────┴──────┐           symmetric  asymmetric
   hyperplasia   extramedullary       │          │
                 hematopoiesis*   hemolymphatic splenic
                                   neoplasia   neoplasia
        ┌─────────────┬──────────────┬─────────────┐
  lymphoproliferative myeloproliferative hemangiosarcoma metastatic neoplasms
                                          │
                                    miscellaneous
                                      sarcomas
```

*Occurs frequently in hemolytic anemias, hemolymphatic neoplasms and myelodysplastic syndromes.

Figure 8. Impression smear of splenic tissue from a dog with hemangiosarcoma. The cells are very pleomorphic, with indistinct cell margins and variable amounts of blue cytoplasm. Variation in nuclear size and shape is marked. Nucleoli are prominent and vary in size, shape and number. (Wright's stain, 480X)

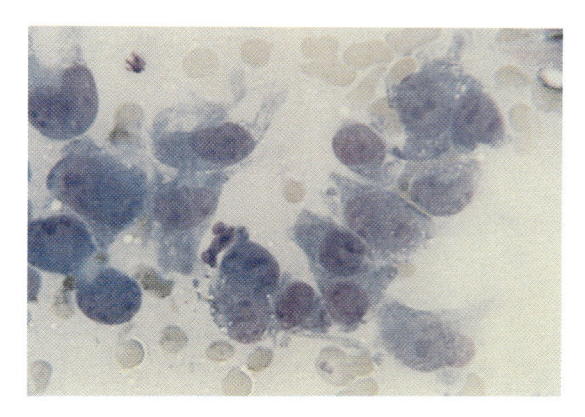

made from scrapings of fresh-cut surfaces of tissue are frequently superior. The microscopic appearance of a hemangiosarcoma is typical of a mesenchymal neoplasm. Cells exfoliate individually or as aggregates associated with vascular structures. Tumor cells are very pleomorphic and hyperchromatic, with marked anisokaryosis. Some cells are fusiform, with indistinct borders, while others are irregularly shaped, with angular margins. Giant forms are not unusual. Nuclei are round to oval, with a variable chromatin pattern and multiple large pleomorphic nucleoli. The cytoplasm is light blue and clear (Fig 8).

Fibrosarcomas and leiomyosarcomas occur less frequently than hemangiosarcomas, and have the cytologic appearance of spindle-cell tumors. The diagnostic criteria discussed in Chapter 1 can be used to identify these tumors. Fibrosarcomas are further discussed in Chapter 2.

References

1. Banks: *Histology and Comparative Organology: A Text-Atlas.* Krieger, Huntington, 1980. pp 131-143.

2. Valli, in Jubb *et al*: *Pathology of Domestic Animals,* Vol 3. 3rd ed. Academic Press, Orlando, 1985. pp 94-114, 194-200.

3. Feldman and Zinkl, in Ettinger: *Textbook of Veterinary Internal Medicine.* 2nd ed. Saunders, Philadelphia, 1983. pp 2067-2076.

4. Lipowitz *et al*, in Slatter: *Textbook of Small Animal Surgery.* Saunders, Philadelphia, 1985. pp 1204-1218.

5. Osborne *et al*: Needle biopsy of the spleen. *Vet Clin No Am* 4:311-316, 1974.

6. Meyer: The management of cytology specimens. *Comp Cont Ed Pract Vet* 9:10-17, 1987.

7. Rebar: *Handbook of Veterinary Cytology.* Ralston Purina, St. Louis, 1979.

8. MacWilliams: Erythrocytic rickettsiae and protozoa of the dog and cat. *Vet Clin No Am* 17:1443-1461, 1987.

9. O'Keefe and Couto: Fine-needle aspiration of the spleen as an aid in the diagnosis of splenomegaly. *J Vet Int Med* 1:102-109, 1987.

18

The Renal Parenchyma

J.H. Meinkoth, R.L. Cowell and R.D. Tyler

Fine-needle aspiration biopsy (FNAB) can be very useful in diagnosis of renal neoplasia, mycosis and hydronephrosis in dogs and cats. Fine-needle aspiration biopsy of the kidney is easier in cats than in dogs because cat kidneys are more easily palpated and immobilized against the body wall. Impression smears from renal biopsy or necropsy specimens allow rapid evaluation of renal disease.

During the last 2 decades, FNAB has been used with increasing frequency in human medicine to determine the nature of renal masses.[1-3] An accurate diagnosis can be made in most cases by augmenting ultrasonography or radiography with cytologic examination. This often eliminates the need for more invasive and costly biopsy procedures.[1]

The primary indication for renal FNAB is abnormally sized or shaped kidneys. While cytologic specimens collected by FNAB lack the cellular architecture necessary to characterize many lesions as completely as by full tissue biopsy, it is much safer and often yields sufficient diagnostic information to aid clinical management. The information from FNAB helps determine the nature of the pathologic process (*ie*, inflammatory, neoplastic, cystic), rather than a specific diagnosis.[1,2]

Both fluid and solid lesions may be encountered. Fluid lesions can often be identified as hydronephrosis, benign cysts or cystic neoplasia. With a solid lesion, neoplasia or inflammation may be detected.

The most common occurrences limiting cytologic evaluation are samples that do not contain sufficient numbers of cells, samples that are not from the lesion and samples whose cells are ruptured during slide preparation.[2] Radiographs to determine the location and extent of the lesion, and multiple (4-5) aspirations improve the chances of obtaining a diagnostic sample. When available, real-time ultrasound can be used to guide needle placement during sample collection.

In human medicine, FNAB has been reported to be practically free of major complications.[1] However, FNAB is contraindicated in animals with bleeding disorders, distended bowel loops and dispositions that prevent adequate restraint during sample collection. Hematuria, fever and pain are the most common side effects in people.[1] Perirenal hemorrhage, pneumothorax, seeding the needle tract with neoplastic cells, and infection have also been reported.[1,2] In a review of over 6000 human renal aspirations, no deaths or life-threatening complications were reported.[1,4]

Technique

A blind, percutaneous technique can be used if the kidney can be manually immobilized against the wall of the abdomen.[1] This is usually possible with cats and sometimes with dogs. Sedation or anesthesia is used only to the extent needed for adequate restraint of the patient to prevent unexpected movement during the procedure. If anesthesia is needed, agents excreted in the urine in active form (*eg*, ketamine) should be avoided in patients with renal failure. Inhalation anesthetics and narcotics have been suggested for use in these patients.

The skin over the site at which the kidney is to be positioned is clipped and prepared as for surgery. The patient is restrained in lateral recumbency and the kidney is manually immobilized against the body wall. A 22- or 23-ga needle, attached to a 10- to 20-ml syringe, is inserted through the body wall into the kidney. If the lesion is focal, the needle is directed into it. If the kidney is diffusely enlarged, the needle is directed through the cortex. Care should be taken to avoid the renal hilus, which contains the renal artery and vein. As mentioned earlier, ultrasound or radiographs may help direct the needle to the proper site for aspiration.

Negative pressure is applied with the syringe while the needle is moved back and forth (about 1 cm) several times.[1] If blood is aspirated, the procedure should be stopped. Negative pressure is released before the needle is withdrawn from the kidney to prevent aspiration of the sample into the syringe and aspiration of unwanted material.[1] The needle is removed from the syringe and the syringe is filled with air. The needle is then replaced on the syringe and the material in the hub of the needle is sprayed onto a glass slide, smeared and stained. (See Chapter 1 for a complete discussion of slide preparation.) If fluid is obtained and a sufficient volume of sample is collected, direct smears and a smear of the sediment following centrifugation with a low-speed urine centrifuge should be made.

Impression smears can be made when abnormal kidneys are removed surgically or discovered on necropsy. See Chapter 1 for further discussion of slide preparation techniques.

Cytologic Evaluation

Evaluating aspirates or impression smears of renal parenchyma can be very useful in determining what process(es) are occurring. For efficient and thorough evaluation, a logical and methodical approach should be used. Chart 1 presents an algorithm to aid evaluation of renal cytologic preparations.

Normal Cells

Renal tubular epithelial cells are the predominant cell type seen in renal FNAB. They are rather large polygonal to round cells that occur singly and in clusters (Fig 1).[1] They have a round, centrally placed nucleus and abundant light-blue cytoplasm. In cats, they are frequently vacuolated due to the presence of lipid droplets in the cytoplasm (Fig 1). This may also occur in dogs with diabetes mellitus or long-term exposure to corticosteroids. Cells of the distal convoluted tubules and ascending limb of Henle may contain dark intracytoplasmic granules.[1] Differentiation of the various epithelial cell types is not important. The cells and their nuclei should be relatively uniform in size and shape; however, the different types of epithelial cells differ slightly in size.[1] Nucleoli, if present, should be small and round.

Cells from the loop of Henle often remain together in the shape of recognizable tubules (Fig 2). Glomeruli, which are less frequently seen, are multilobulated, multilayered structures containing capillaries.[1]

Other Cells Present

Neutrophils (Plate 1) are present to some degree in all aspirates due to peripheral blood contamination (1 WBC/500-1000 RBCs). In inflammatory conditions, neutrophils are typically present in numbers greatly exceeding those seen with peripheral blood contamination (Plate 3). Morphologically, they are similar to peripheral blood neutrophils; however, degenerative changes may be seen, especially with infections due to Gram-negative bacteria. Phagocytized bacteria can be seen in septic conditions.

Macrophages (Plate 2) are large mononuclear cells with abundant blue-gray cytoplasm. The cytoplasm is often vacuolated and may contain phagocytized debris. The nucleus is round to bean-shaped, occasionally trilobed and eccentrically located within the cell. Macrophages often phagocytize large microorganisms (fungi, protozoa) and effete cells. Irregularly shaped nuclei and vacuolated cytoplasm

Figure 1. Fine-needle aspiration biopsy of a normal cat's kidney. A. Bare nucleus (lower left) and a renal tubular epithelial cell. B. Fat-filled renal tubular epithelial cell. Fatty renal tubular epithelial cells are typically larger than their nonfatty counterparts due to cytoplasmic distention from accumulated fat. (Wright's stain, original magnification 250X)

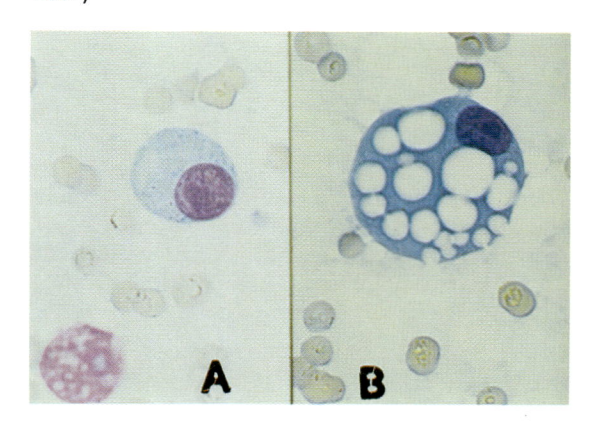

help distinguish these cells from renal epithelial cells.

Lymphoid cells can be seen in inflammatory and neoplastic processes. Small, mature lymphocytes are about 10 μ in diameter and slightly smaller than a neutrophil (Plate 1). They have a round, slightly indented, deep purple nucleus, with smudged nuclear chromatin. There is usually only a thin rim of light-blue cytoplasm that does not encircle the entire nucleus. Nucleoli are not discernible.

In contrast, lymphoblasts are larger than neutrophils (Plate 7). Their nuclear chromatin is less dense and lighter in color; multiple nucleoli are frequently present. The cytoplasm is more abundant, sometimes completely encircling the nucleus, and is a deeper blue. Compared to renal tubular epithelial cells, lymphoblasts have deeper-blue cytoplasm, a higher nucleus:cytoplasm ratio and prominent nucleoli.

Plasma cells are B-lymphocytes that have been stimulated to produce antibodies (Plate 1). Their nucleus is eccentrically placed and their cytoplasm is moderately abundant and deep blue. A clear area representing the Golgi apparatus abuts the nucleus in the center of the cell. The deep-blue cytoplasm, eccentric nucleus and perinuclear clear areas help distinguish plasma cells from renal tubular epithelial cells.

Cytologic Characteristics of Fluid Lesions

Fluid aspirated from renal lesions is evaluated on gross appearance, selected biochemical tests and cytologic appearance.

Cysts

Renal cysts are one of the more common space-occupying lesions of the human kidney.[1,2] They have also been reported in domestic animals. Renal cysts can be single or multiple, congenital or acquired.[1] Renal cysts usually do not cause symptomatic disease. However, they can enlarge and induce local tissue hypoxia, causing overproduction of erythropoietin and resultant polycythemia, or sufficient parenchyma may be lost due to pressure atrophy that renal failure eventually develops. Benign cysts contain clear, straw-colored fluid. The fluid is of low cellularity but may contain a few cuboidal epithelial lining cells.[1] These cells occur singly and generally have foamy cytoplasm. The nucleus:cytoplasm ratio is low and nucleoli are absent or small.[2] A few neutrophils and macrophages may also be present.

A small percentage of renal-cell carcinomas are cystic in nature, and benign cysts must be differentiated from these. If hemorrhage has occurred into a cyst, neoplasia should be suspected.[1] Intracystic hemorrhage is documented by finding macrophages containing phagocytized RBCs or RBC breakdown products (Plate 2). This can be used to help differentiate existing hemorrhage from peripheral blood contamination during the aspiration procedure. Exfoliated cells should be evaluated for malignant changes (Chapter 1);[1] however, not all cystic neoplasms exfoliate recognizably malignant cells into the fluid. Lipid and cholesterol content has been used in human medicine to help differentiate between benign cysts and malignant neoplasia.[6] Benign cysts have less lipid and cholesterol than cystic neoplasms; however, this has not been studied in animals.

Hydronephrosis

Hydronephrosis is the dilation of the renal pelvis and the associated parenchymal atrophy and cystic enlargement of the kidney that result from obstruction of urine outflow. The obstruction can be complete or partial, can arise suddenly or be progressive, and can be at any level of the urinary tract.

Hydronephrotic lesions generally yield a variable amount of clear fluid. Cytologically, the smears contain few cells. There may be a few inflammatory cells and epithelial lining cells. Large numbers of inflammatory cells are seen with secondary infections. Hydronephrosis may be distinguished from renal cysts by radiography.

Reported causes of hydronephrosis include ectopic ureters, calculi, neoplasia, prostatic hyperplasia, pregnancy and inadvertent surgical ligation of the ureter.

Abscesses

Renal abscesses are uncommon in dogs and cats but may occur secondary to a septic process, such as pyelonephritis. The aspirated material grossly resembles any other purulent exudate.[1] Cytologically, the smears are very cellular and typically consist of >85% neutrophils, with varying numbers of macrophages. A search should be made for infectious agents, and material should be submitted for culture and sensitivity tests. Identification of bacterial rods or cocci (Plate 3) helps in choosing initial antibacterial therapy while awaiting culture and sensitivity results. With the hematologic stains, bacteria (both Gram-positive and Gram-negative) stain blue-black. If bacterial rods (especially bipolar rods) are seen cytologically, a drug effective against Gram-negative bacteria should be used while awaiting culture and sensitivity results. The pathologic cocci are generally *Staphylococcus* spp and *Streptococcus* spp; therefore, when cocci are seen cytologically, a drug effective against Gram-positive bacteria should be used while awaiting culture and sensitivity results.

Cytologic Characteristics of Aspirates of Solid Lesions

Solid lesions are evaluated cytologically to determine whether the lesion is inflammatory or neoplastic. Finding malignant cells is diagnostic of neoplasia. Finding only inflammatory cells does not totally rule out neoplasia, since tumors can incite an inflammatory response, and overtly malignant cells may be missed in the collection procedure. Also, inflammation can cause dysplastic changes in cells, making the evaluation of malignancy difficult. Finding an infectious agent along with inflammatory cells increases the likelihood that the lesion is strictly inflammatory.

Inflammation

Increased numbers of neutrophils, macrophages, eosinophils and/or lymphocytes denote inflammation. Because the kidney is highly vascular, most renal aspirates contain some inflammatory cells secondary to peripheral blood contamination (about 1 WBC/500-1000 RBCs). Cytologic preparations from inflammatory lesions contain neutrophil numbers that are markedly increased in comparison to RBC numbers. Inflammation can be due to infectious agents or noninfectious causes, such as toxins, trauma or neoplasia.

A marked predominance of neutrophils (usually >90%) with only a few macrophages (usually <5%) is typical of the inflammation produced by pyogenic bacteria, but can be produced by any of the causes listed above.

Many species of pyogenic bacteria have been cultured from dogs with acute pyelonephritis. They usually ascend from the lower urogenital tract but occasionally may be hematogenous in origin. Phagocytized and/or nonphagocytized bacteria may be found in bacterial pyelonephritis.

Smears of inflammatory lesions containing increased numbers of macrophages (>15%), and especially those containing multinucleated giant inflammatory cells, warrant a search for fungal spores, fungal hyphae and protozoa. Spores of *Blastomyces dermatitidis* (Plate 4), *Cryptococcus neoformans* (Plate 4), *Coccidioides immitis* (Plate 5), *Histoplasma capsulatum* (Plate 4) and the alga *Prototheca zopfii* (Plate 5) have all been found in kidneys of animals with disseminated disease, though they are more consistently found in other tissues.

Aspergillus spp, *Candida* spp and other opportunistic fungi can infect immunocompromised animals. Fungal hyphae (Fig 2 and Plate 5) may be found in imprints or aspirates. Culture is necessary to further identify the fungus.

Figure 2. Impression smear taken at necropsy from a dog's kidney. *Top:* Highly cellular smear showing recognizable tubules and fungal hyphae (Wright's stain, original magnification, 33X). *Bottom:* Higher magnification of same area (Original magnification 200X).

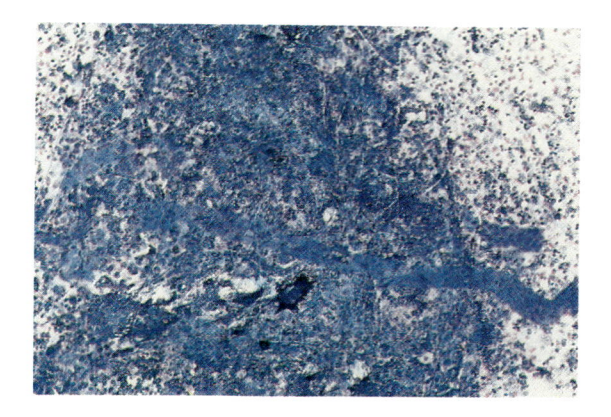

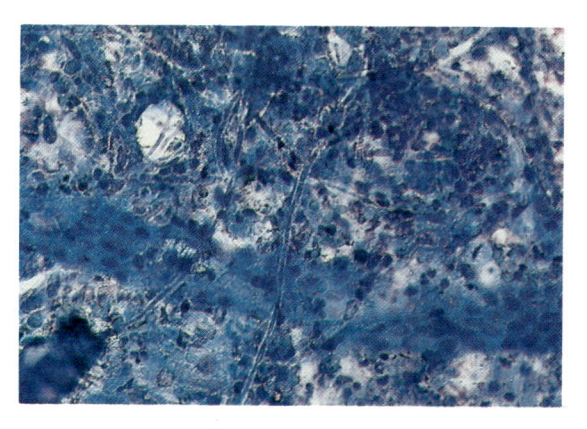

The Renal Parenchyma

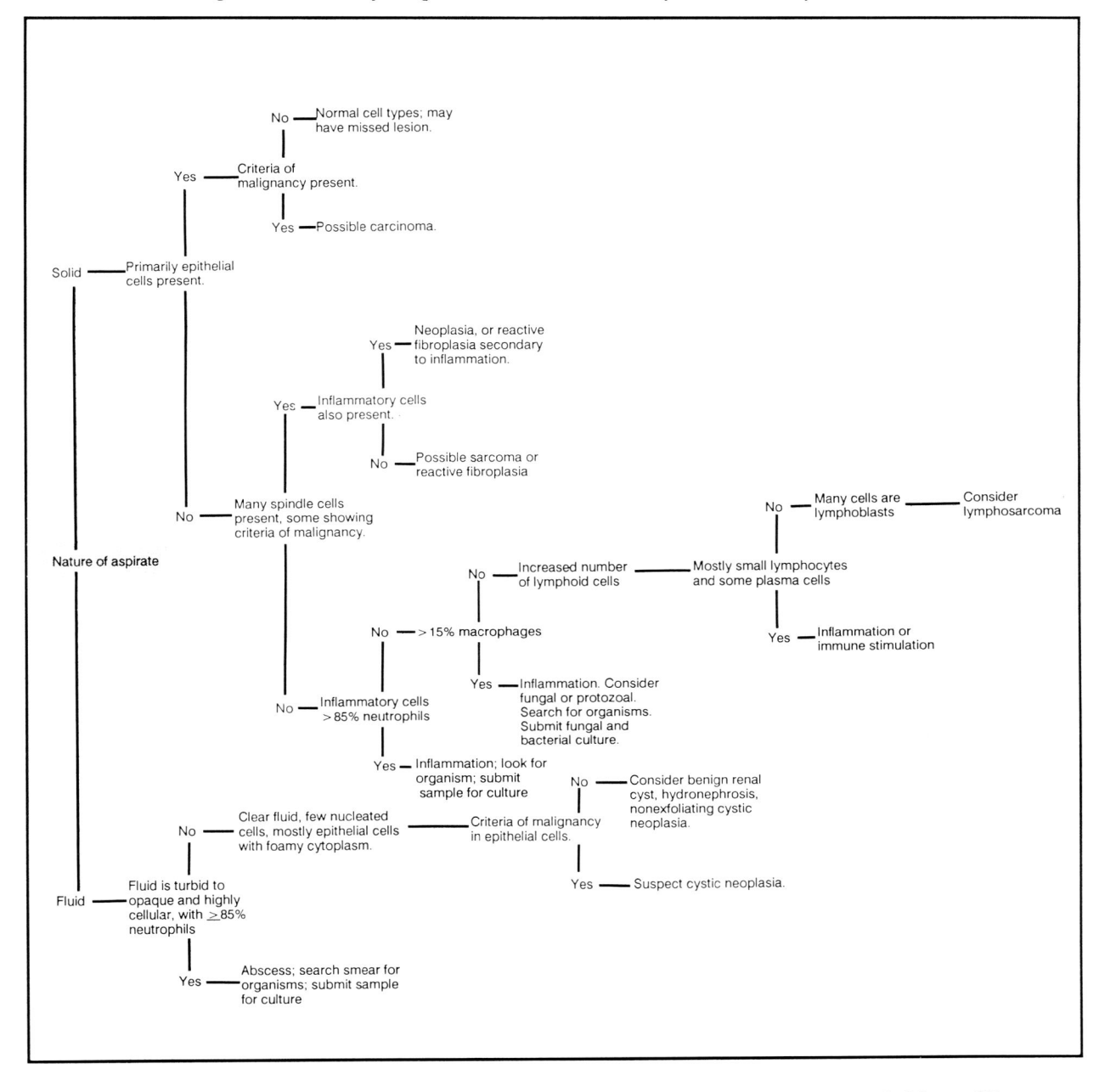

Chart 1. An algorithm to aid cytologic evaluation of renal aspirates and impression smears.

```
                                         No ── Normal cell types; may
                                                have missed lesion.
                                          │
                              Yes ── Criteria of
                           │          malignancy present.
                           │              │
                           │          Yes ── Possible carcinoma.
              Primarily epithelial
   Solid ──── cells present.
     │
     │                                    Neoplasia, or reactive
     │                              Yes ── fibroplasia secondary
     │                                 │    to inflammation.
     │                                 │
     │                            Yes ── Inflammatory cells
     │                             │      also present.
     │                             │      │
     │                             │      No ── Possible sarcoma or
     │                             │              reactive fibroplasia
     │              Many spindle cells
     │         No ── present, some showing                                              No ── Many cells are ──── Consider
     │              criteria of malignancy.                                              │     lymphoblasts         lymphosarcoma
Nature of aspirate                                                                       │
     │                                    No ── Increased number ──── Mostly small lymphocytes
     │                                     │     of lymphoid cells     and some plasma cells
     │                                     │                                             │
     │                            No ── >15% macrophages                                 │
     │                             │                                                 Yes ── Inflammation or
     │                             │     Yes ── Inflammation. Consider                     immune stimulation
     │                             │             fungal or protozoal.
     │              Inflammatory cells        Search for organisms.
     │         No ── >85% neutrophils         Submit fungal and
     │              │                         bacterial culture.
     │              │
     │              Yes ── Inflammation; look for
     │                      organism; submit           No ── Consider benign renal
     │                      sample for culture.        │     cyst, hydronephrosis,
     │              Clear fluid, few nucleated         │     nonexfoliating cystic
     │         No ── cells, mostly epithelial cells    │     neoplasia.
     │              with foamy cytoplasm.   Criteria of malignancy
     │              │                       in epithelial cells.
     │              │                              │
     │              │                              Yes ── Suspect cystic neoplasia.
     │         Fluid is turbid to
   Fluid ──── opaque and highly
              cellular, with ≥85%
              neutrophils
              │
              │     Abscess; search smear for
              Yes ── organisms; submit sample
                     for culture
```

Chronic inflammation and immune stimulation can result in increased numbers of lymphocytes and plasma cells in the kidney. In these instances, aspirates may yield many lymphoid cells. These aspirates must be differentiated from aspirates of renal lymphosarcoma. The lymphoid cells in aspirates from areas of chronic inflammation are mostly small, mature lymphocytes, with variable numbers of plasma cells and some lymphoblasts. Lymphosarcoma aspirates typically yield a large number of lymphoblasts (Plate 7), with scattered or no renal epithelial cells. Plasma cells are rare.

Neoplasia

Primary neoplasia of the kidney represents 0.6-1.7% of tumors in dogs.[7,8] Benign renal tumors are rare in dogs and cats.[9] In dogs, renal-cell carcinomas, other carcinomas and nephroblastomas are the most common primary tumors of the kidney.[8,9] In cats, alimentary lymphosarcoma often involves the kidneys;[8] however, renal-cell carcinoma is the most common primary tumor.[8] Sarcomas (other than lymphosarcoma) are rare in kidneys of small animals.[7]

Lymphosarcoma can occur as a discrete nodule or a diffuse enlargement of the kidneys.[8] Involvement is usually bilateral.[8] Aspirates may yield large numbers of lymphoid cells that are primarily lymphoblasts. Many inflammatory processes cause accumulation of mature lymphocytes; therefore, recognizing the differences between lymphocytes and lymphoblasts is very important. With lymphosarcoma, the disease is often advanced by the time it is clinically recognized, and aspirates typically yield a large number of lymphoblasts, with scattered or no renal tubular epithelial cells (Plate 7).

Malignant epithelial-cell tumors are carcinomas (Plate 6). While identification of exact tumor type is usually not possible, the presence of large epithelial cells with malignant changes suggests a general diagnosis of carcinoma, which is often sufficient information for handling the case. Carcinoma cells may show anisocytosis, anisonucleosis, a variable nucleus:cytoplasm ratio and large, angular, variably sized nucleoli. When there is evidence of inflammation, caution must be used in evaluating atypical cells.[4] Inflammation alone can cause dysplastic changes that are often indistinguishable from neoplastic changes.

Malignant tumors of mesenchymal origin are sarcomas. They occur less commonly in the kidney than carcinomas. Mesenchymal cells are usually tapered to some degree of one or both ends (spindle cells). Again, extreme caution should be used when evaluating malignant criteria if inflammation is present. Fibroblasts normally involved in repair processes display marked atypia that may be indistinguishable from malignant changes.

See Chapter 1 for a discussion of the evaluation of lesions for malignant potential.

References

1. Nguyen: Percutaneous fine-needle aspiration biopsy cytology of the kidney and adrenal. *Pathol Ann* 1:163-191, 1987.

2. Murphy *et al*: Aspiration biopsy of the kidney: simultaneous collection of cytologic and histologic specimens. *Cancer* 56:200-205, 1985.

3. Pillotti *et al*: The role of fine-needle aspiration in the assessment of renal masses. *Acta Cytol* 32:1-10, 1988.

4. Juul *et al*: Ultrasonically guided fine-needle aspiration biopsy of renal masses. *J Urol* 133:579-581, 1985.

5. Hidvegi: Percutaneous transperitoneal aspiration of renal adenocarcinoma guided by ultrasound. *Acta Cytol* 23:467-470, 1979.

6. Pettersson *et al*: Diagnostic value of lipid content in renal cyst fluid. *Proc 1st Intl Sympos Kidney Tumors*, 1982. pp 433-434.

7. Goldsschmidt, in Bovee: *Canine Nephrology*. Harwal Publishing, Media, PA, 1984. pp 687-705.

8. Madewell and Theilen: *Veterinary Cancer Medicine*. 2nd ed. Lea & Febiger, Philadelphia, 1987. pp 567-582.

9. Maxie, in Jubb *et al*: *Pathology of Domestic Animals*. 3rd ed. Academic Press, Orlando, FL, 1985. pp 343-400.

19

Urinary Sediment

J.G. Zinkl and B.F. Feldman

Indications for Cytologic Examination of Urine

Clinical signs of cystitis and neoplasia of the urinary bladder are similar, and include stranguria, pollakiuria, hematuria, urine dribbling, and incontinence.[1] Observation of unusual cells in unstained urine sediment examined under either reduced illumination or phase contrast is the most frequent reason a Wright's-stained smear is examined for cytologic evaluation. Occasionally, radiographic evidence of a mass in the bladder prompts clinicians to request cytologic examination of urine or of material obtained from the bladder by fine-needle aspiration.

Preparation of Slides from Urine

Many factors may affect cytologic findings in urine samples. Significant variables that must be considered include the following:

Collection Period

Though morning urine may be considered ideal for certain urologic analyses, it is the least desirable for cytologic purposes. Because urine has cytotoxic effects on exfoliated urothelium and other cells, samples that have been in contact with urine for some time (ie, overnight) are not recommended for cytologic evaluation. Random, voided urine or urine obtained by antepubic cystocentesis from well-hydrated patients is recommended for cytologic evaluation of suspected urologic disease.[2]

Collection Techniques

Collecting urine samples at voiding and by cystocentesis, because of their simplicity and atraumatic effect on the bladder, are the best methods of specimen collection. Bladder catheterization is not favored primarily because it is an invasive procedure that can cause traumatic exfoliation of urothelium. Such cells add to the inherent diagnostic difficulties, especially in cytodiagnosis of low-grade urothelial malignancies. Catheterization, however, has great potential in investigating lesions of the urethra and prostate. Bladder irrigation produces large volumes of cellular material in an excellent state of preservation and, therefore, may be useful in special situations.[3]

Specimen Preservation

Fresh, unfixed, voided urine is the specimen of choice for cytologic evaluation. When a sample cannot be examined immediately, a slide should be prepared as soon as possible. Preservation with acid, formaldehyde, alcohol, freezing and other methods is not recommended because of toxic effects on cells or interference with staining. Short-term preservation can be achieved by refrigeration.

Specimen Preparation

Two methods of specimen preparation are commonly used for urine cytodiagnosis. The simpler technique is to make smears of urine sediment obtained by centrifugation. Cell morphology is preserved by adding a drop of albumin or autologous serum to the sediment before making the smear. This procedure generally produces excellent results. Cytocentrifugation is especially useful when dealing with small volumes of urine and when cellularity is low. Cytocentrifuged preparations usually have excellent cellular morphology.

A membrane-filtration technique is also available.[3] This technique produces suitable results with some staining methods but is less useful with Wright's-stained preparations because some types of membranes are difficult to clear.

Cytologic Evaluation

Normal Urine

Normal urine sediment contains few cells. A few urothelial cells may be found; they are usually single and are large and round to oval. Their cytoplasm stains pale basophilic to pale acidophilic and in well-preserved cells may be finely vacuolated. Nuclei of urothelial cells are centrally located and have fine granular chromatin. Small, circular nucleoli with smooth outlines may be seen (Fig 1). Urothelial cells are occasionally shed in tightly molded clusters; these should be interpreted with caution. In voided urine, cell clusters may indicate neoplasia, but they also may be found in association with inflammation, catheterization and urolithiasis. Mild anaplasia of urothelial cells, probably due to hyperplasia, may be seen in urolithiasis and with some toxic agents. Finding atypical urothelial cells is complicated by the fact that degenerative changes are frequently associated with cells that have been in urine for some time.[2] Degenerative cellular changes with poorly preserved nuclear chromatin patterns dictate conservative cytologic interpretation. It cannot be overemphasized that cytologic diagnosis of neoplasia is reserved for cytologic characteristics matching the numerous criteria of malignancy.

Squamous epithelial cells may also be found in voided urine. In males they may represent contamination from the terminal urethra. In females, vaginal and vulvar squamous contaminants are also common in voided urine. In both males and females, squamous metaplasia of the urothelium may occur due to chronic irritation. Though not a common occurrence, squamous-cell carcinoma of the genital or urinary tracts may shed large numbers of well-differentiated, keratinized squamous cells into the urine. Finding large numbers of squamous cells necessitates a search for malignant features and further clinical examination (see below).

Cystitis

Urine from normal dogs and cats is virtually free of inflammatory cells, though an occasional neutrophil may be found. The presence of many neutrophils indicates inflammation somewhere in the urinary tract. Inflammatory cells are abundant in urine specimens in acute cystitis. Bacteria may accompany the inflammatory cells (Fig 2).

In chronic inflammation, neutrophils are the predominant cell type, but macrophages and lymphocytes are often present in moderate numbers, together with an occasional plasma cell. Macrophages have cytoplasm that is usually finely vacuolated, with round, oval or bean-shaped central or eccentric nuclei. Macrophages may contain erythrocytes, cellular debris, bacteria and sperm. Squamous metaplasia of the bladder epithelium may

Figure 1. A group of variably sized urothelial cells from a normal dog. Small round nucleoli are visible in some cells. Cytoplasmic vacuolation (hydropic change) is present, likely due to delay in processing the sample. Cells were concentrated by the cytospin method. (160X) (Courtesy of Dr. R.L. Cowell, Oklahoma State University)

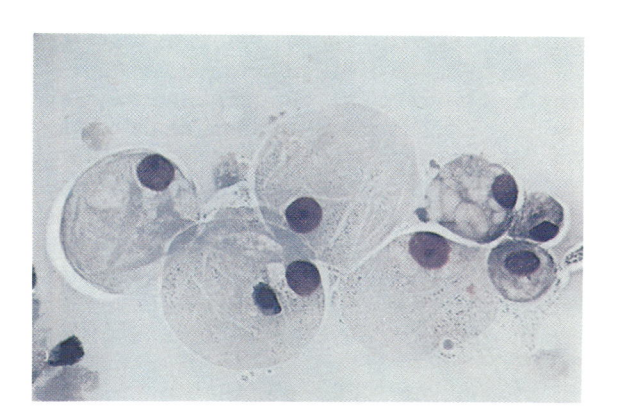

Figure 2. Infectious cystitis with many neutrophils, a bladder epithelial cell and bacilli. Cells were concentrated by the cytospin method. (400X)

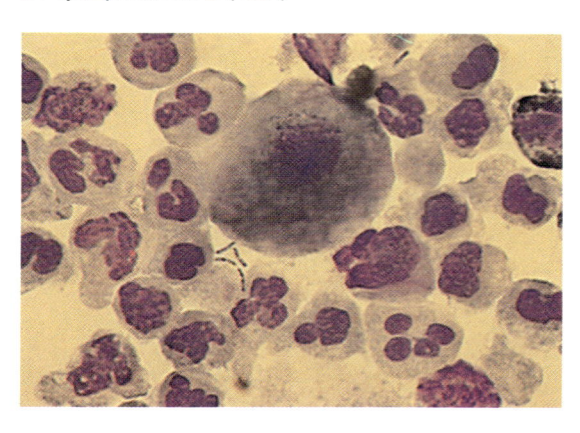

result from chronic inflammation or irritation. Exfoliated squamous cells resemble intermediate or superficial squamous cells found in other locations.

Erythrocytes are not normally found in urine and often accompany inflammatory cells with infection. They may also be seen with severe glomerular disease, urinary tract neoplasia, bladder lesions caused by chemotherapeutic drugs, and inflammatory and neoplastic disease of the genital tract.

Effects of Chemotherapy on the Urinary Bladder

A number of chemotherapeutic agents adversely affect the urothelium. The alkylating agents cyclophosphamide and busulfan inhibit DNA replication by binding to nucleic acids. These drugs are concentrated in the urine. Patients receiving these drugs exfoliate abnormal cells from the urothelium (Fig 3).[3,4] Resultant cytologic changes include nuclear and cytoplasmic enlargement. Nuclei are large, with a reticulated chromatin pattern, and may have nucleoli. Multinucleated cells may be found. The cytoplasm is basophilic and often vacuolated. Cellular debris with inflammation and hemorrhage is common.

If cytologic changes are sufficiently severe, it may not be possible to differentiate changes induced by alkylating agents from those induced by urothelial carcinoma. Secondary, new malignancies of the urinary bladder have been reported in people receiving cyclophosphamide.[4]

Figure 3. A population of moderately pleomorphic epithelial cells from a dog with cyclophosphamide-induced hyperplastic cystitis. Cells vary in size and staining. Cells were concentrated by the cytospin method. (40X) (Courtesy of Dr. L. O'Rourke, Louisiana State University)

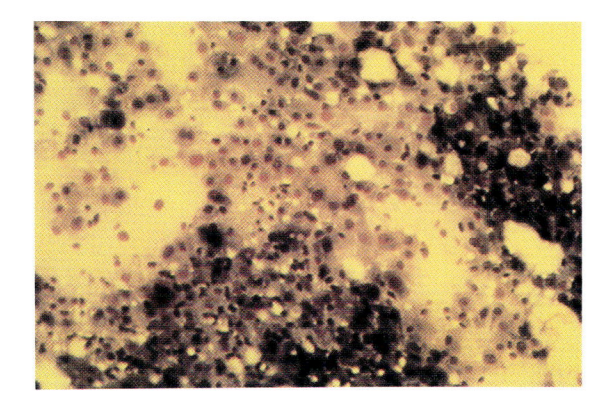

Figure 4. A cluster of very pleomorphic epithelial cells from a dog with urothelial carcinoma. Cells vary markedly in size and staining. Cell crowding has caused cellular and nuclear molding. Cells were concentrated by the cytospin method. (100X)

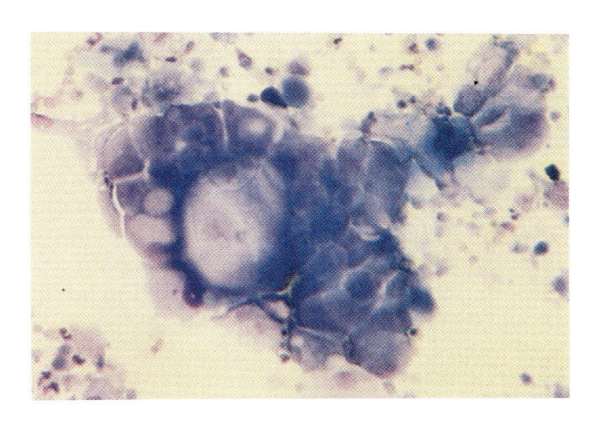

Neoplasms of the Urinary Tract

Traditionally, neoplasms arising from bladder epithelium or urothelium have been called transitional-cell carcinomas, though the term urothelial carcinoma is also used. These are characterized by various cell types and growth patterns. A papilloma is a benign neoplasm growing into the lumen of the bladder, composed of urothelium indistinguishable from normal urothelium.[5]

Transitional-cell carcinomas may have papillary, nonpapillary or invasive growth patterns.[5] The most common site is the bladder trigone, but other areas of the bladder and the tubular system may also be sites of transitional-cell carcinomas. Clinical signs and sequelae depend on the tumor's location.

Transitional-cell carcinomas exfoliate isolated cells and cell clusters. Very large clusters of cells with marked pleomorphism (based on variation in staining and variations in cell size) are frequently found. Their cytoplasm is often deeply basophilic. Within clusters, cell borders are usually not distinct. Cell crowding is evidenced by cellular and nuclear molding. The nucleus:cytoplasm ratio is distinctly increased in many cells, but there are usually a few very large cells with abundant cytoplasm and, concomitantly, a low nucleus:cytoplasm ratio.

Some cells have large, relatively light-staining vacuoles, indicating they are undergoing hydropic degeneration. This degeneration may be induced by the toxic effects of urine. Nuclear chromatin is finely to coarsely reticulated. Large, indistinct nucleoli are occasionally found. Mitotic cells may be present but are not essential for diagnosis (Figs 4-6).

Some transitional-cell carcinomas contain foci of squamous-cell carcinoma or adenocarcinoma. Squamous-cell carcinomas and adenocarcinomas have also been found in the urinary bladder, but these tumors may, in large part, represent metaplasia associated with neoplasia of the transitional epithelium.[4,5] Features of squamous-cell carcinomas and adenocarcinomas are difficult to recognize cytologically, especially when these tumors are associated with transitional-cell carcinomas, though cells similar to squamous cells are frequently found in cytologic preparations of transitional-cell carcinomas. Cytologic features of urinary adenocarcinomas have not been described. Perhaps tumors histologically classified as adenocarcinomas do not exfoliate clusters of cells with the more subtle features, such as acinus formation, that are used to diagnose adenocarcinomas in other locations.

Figure 5. A population of pleomorphic urothelial cells that are variable in size and staining quality from a dog with urothelial carcinoma. Some cells have large vacuoles in their cytoplasm as a result of hydropic change. Cells were concentrated by the cytospin method. (160X)

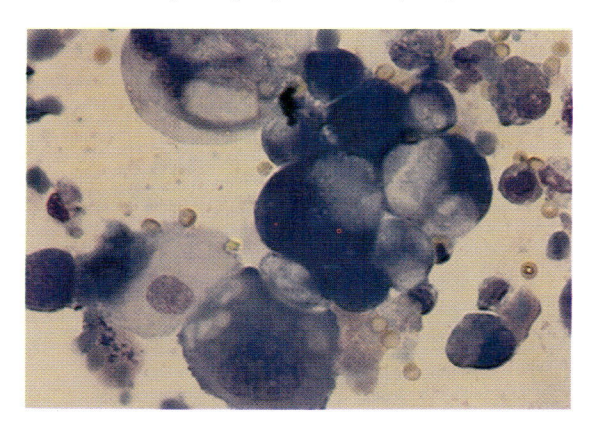

Figure 6. A large, basophilic cell containing 2 nuclei from a urothelial carcinoma. Cells were concentrated by the cytospin method. (400X)

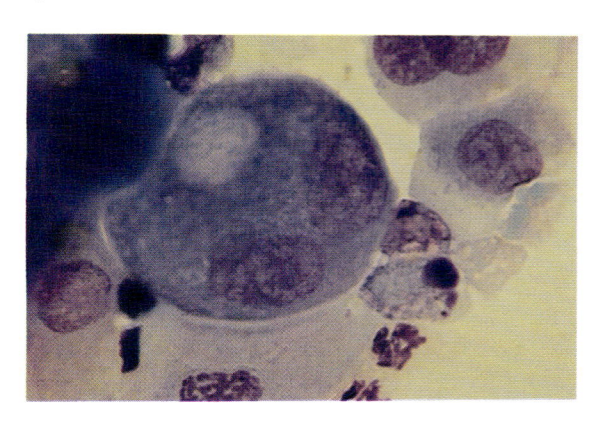

References

1. Bojrab *et al*: Transitional cell carcinomas of the canine bladder: Diagnosis and management. *Comp Cont Ed Pract Vet* 8:495-500, 1986.

2. Perman *et al*: *Cytology of the Dog and Cat.* American Animal Hospital Association, Denver, CO, 1979. pp 22-23.

3. Holmquist, in Weid: *Monographs of Clinical Cytology.* Vol 6. S. Karger, New York, 1977. pp 69-76.

4. Theilen and Madewell: *Veterinary Cancer Medicine.* Lea & Febiger, Philadelphia, 1987. pp 183-196.

5. Moulton: *Tumors of Domestic Animals.* 2nd ed. Univ California Press, Berkeley, 1978. pp 294-308.

20

The Male Reproductive Tract:
Prostate, Testes, Semen

J.G. Zinkl and B.F. Feldman

THE PROSTATE GLAND

Collecting and Preparing Samples

The general indication for aspiration and cytologic evaluation of the prostate gland is enlargement. Clinical signs suggesting prostatic enlargement include difficult defecation or, less frequently, difficult micturition. Infrequently, urine may be red-tinged from blood, or blood or pus may drip from the penis. Rectal palpation of the prostate may reveal symmetric enlargement, unilateral enlargement or focal irregularities.[1,2]

Material from the prostate can be obtained by digital massage while aspirating through a urinary catheter passed to the level of the gland.[3] More prostatic material can be obtained by washing the urethra in the area of the prostate with a small amount of saline. Gentle injection and aspiration is used while gently massaging the prostate. Fluid with low cellularity should be concentrated by centrifugation to prepare slides with sufficient material to evaluate properly.

Direct fine-needle aspiration of the prostate yields enough material to make 1-2 slides. One method is to pass the needle through the skin in the perineal area and guide it into the prostate along a finger placed in the rectum. Alternatively, the dog is placed on its back and the prostate is elevated with rectal digital palpation to a location lateral to the penis. The needle is passed into the visible bulge produced by the prostate in the caudoventral abdomen.

Especially with the perirectal technique, local anesthesia of the skin is necessary to prevent discomfort and to assure easy guidance of the needle. Gentle aspiration of the gland is performed while moving the needle within the prostate.[4] Only a small amount of material is usually obtained with this method, but it is usually adequate for making 1-2 direct smears.

Material may also be obtained from the prostate by inducing ejaculation.[2] The prostate is gently massaged during the process to increase the amount of material of prostatic origin. This method may produces samples that contain contaminant substances from other parts of the reproductive tract. The first part of the ejaculate contains material primarily derived from the prostate gland.[2] The sample is usually large and has a moderate concentration of cells. In addition to prostatic epithelial cells, samples may contain numerous spermatozoa and cells of other structures of the reproductive tract and urethra. Collection of a urethral wash specimen and a urine sample by antepubic cystocentesis can alleviate some of the problems in interpreting cytologic and microbiologic findings.

Preparation and staining of slides of prostatic material are similar to that for other samples. Samples with few cells require concentration techniques.

Cytologic Evaluation

When specimens without prostatic epithelium or adequate numbers of cells are obtained,

Chapter 20

results are reported as "not diagnostic," with a comment indicating the problem and a recommendation for additional sampling.

Normal Prostate

Cytologic findings of the normal prostate vary, depending upon the method by which materials are obtained. Differences are in cellularity and types of contaminating cells found. Epithelial cells of the normal prostate are found in small to medium-sized clusters. Their nuclei are central and have a homogeneous to fine reticular pattern. Their cytoplasm stains slightly acidophilic and has a fine granular appearance (Figs 1,2).

Certain cells of nonprostatic origin may be encountered relatively frequently. These include:

Spermatozoa: Characteristically, sperm heads stain blue-green by Wright's method. Spermatozoa often adhere to other cells, and many may be attached to a single epithelial cell. They are most frequently found in ejaculated material, but can also be found in massage or wash samples (Fig 3).

Squamous Cells: Squamous cells are large cells with a flattened, floppy appearance. More differentiated squamous cells have pyknotic or karyorrhectic nuclei. Immature squamous cells are difficult to differentiate from urothelial cells and prostatic epithelial cells. They may originate from the distal urethra or external genitalia. They may also be found with squamous metaplasia of the prostate.

Figure 1. Epithelial cells from a normal prostate. The cells are in large clusters, and have mildly acidophilic cytoplasm and relatively large nuclei. (Prostatic massage slightly concentrated by centrifugation, 160X)

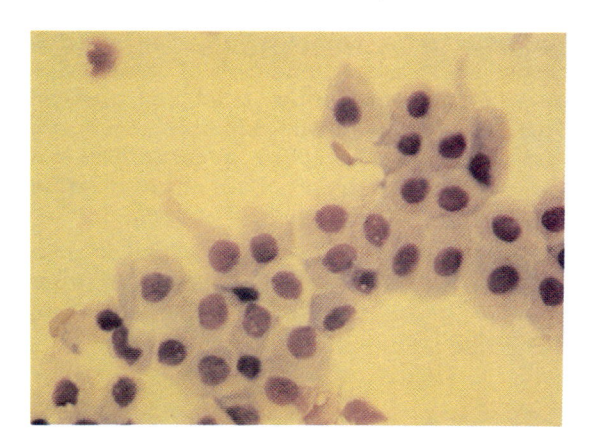

Figure 2. Epithelial cells from a normal prostate. The cytoplasm is grainy and acidophilic. The nuclei are central and have a moderately reticular chromatin network. (Prostatic massage slightly concentrated by centrifugation, 400X)

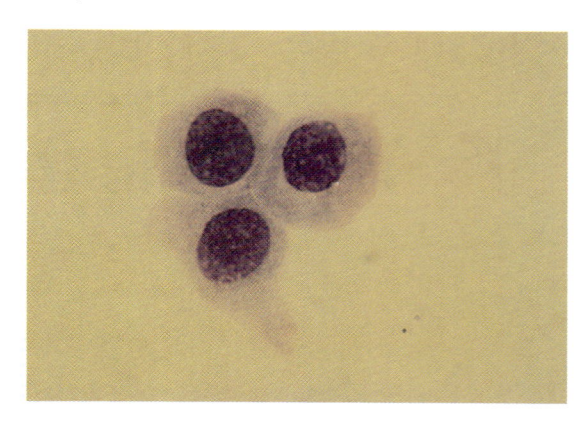

Urothelial Cells: Urothelial cells (transitional epithelial cells) usually are single or in small clusters. They are larger than prostatic epithelial cells, and have lower nucleus:cytoplasm ratios and less grainy cytoplasm (Fig 1, Chapter 19).

Other Epithelial Cells: Cells of the ductus deferens and epididymis are difficult to distinguish from prostatic cells.

Prostatic Cysts

Usually aspiration techniques are necessary to obtain samples adequate for examination because it is difficult to obtain material from prostatic cysts by massage. Cytologically, prostatic cysts are quite variable. Some cysts may contain poorly cellular fluid that, even when concentrated, contains only a few epithelial cells, rare neutrophils and some debris. Sometimes moderate numbers of normal or slightly hyperplastic (basophilic) epithelial cells are found. Rarely are squamous cells obtained.

Prostatitis

Cellular material with some clusters of cells of various sizes may be obtained by aspiration or massage of an inflamed prostate. Neutrophils are the most common inflammatory cells, but macrophages are often present. Bacteria are frequently found.[3] It is necessary to determine if the bacteria are actually the cause of inflammation, or if they are contaminants from other locations in the genital or urinary tract. When bacteria are found in neutrophils, they are considered to be involved in the etiology of the prostatitis (Fig 4).

Prostatic abscesses are focal areas of severe inflammation containing degenerated neutrophils. Digital palpation usually is necessary to guide a needle to the site of the abscess to be certain the abscess has been sampled. Abscesses may be large, single accumulations of pus or they can be small and multiple. Karyolytic neutrophils with a background of cellular debris are found. Prostatic cells are often single or in small clusters. Hyperplasia may accompany both generalized prostatic inflammation and prostatic abscesses. Squamous metaplasia may also be found (see below).

Prostatic Hyperplasia

Prostatic hyperplasia is found most frequently in older dogs and is considered to be caused by sex hormone imbalance.[5] Cellularity of cytologic material is sparse to moderate, and cells are often found in sheets of variable size. In cell sheets, acinus formation may be found but is unusual. In cell clusters, cytoplasmic borders are often indistinct. The cytoplasm is basophilic and slightly granular. Nuclei are round to oval and may be eccentric. Chromatin patterns are fine, and nucleoli are unusual. The nucleus:cytoplasm ratio is increased as compared to the ratio in normal prostatic cells (Fig 5). Occasionally neutrophils, lymphocytes and macrophages may be found. These cells suggest that hyperplasia is a sequel to inflammation. Hyperplasia may be a preneoplastic change as well.[6]

Figure 3. A prostatic epithelial cell, neutrophil, macrophage and many spermatozoa from a dog with mild prostatitis. The background contains proteinaceous material that is probably the product of prostatic epithelial cells. Spermatozoa characteristically stain aqua with Wright's stain. (Prostatic ejaculate slightly concentrated by centrifugation, 400X)

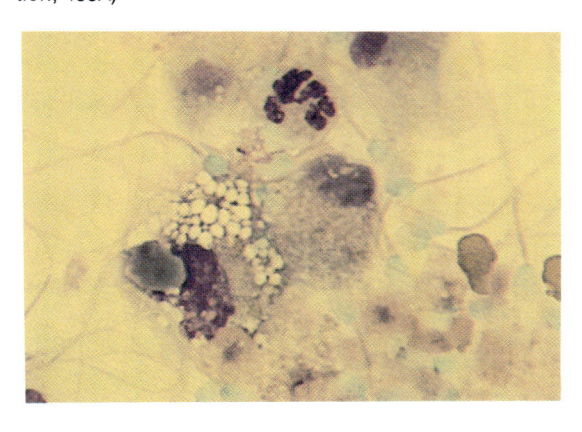

Figure 4. Neutrophils and prostatic epithelial cells from a dog with acute prostatitis. Bacilli are in some neutrophils showing mild degeneration with acidophilic, foamy cytoplasm and minimal nuclear degeneration. (Prostatic massage slightly concentrated by centrifugation, 400X)

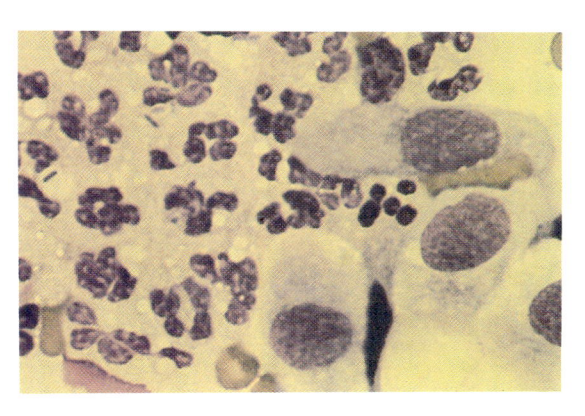

Squamous Metaplasia

Under the influence of estrogen-like hormone activity, such as occurs in Sertoli-cell tumors, the prostatic epithelium may undergo metaplasia to squamous-like epithelium. Squamous metaplasia may also occur as a sequel to chronic irritation or inflammation, but the most prominent squamous metaplastic changes are found in dogs with Sertoli-cell tumors or dogs treated with exogenous estrogens.[3,7] Aspirates are moderately cellular. Clusters of slightly basophilic to slightly

Figure 5. Hyperplasia of prostatic epithelium from a dog with prostatitis. The cells are basophilic and have an increased nucleus:cytoplasm ratio. Pleomorphism is minimal and a suggestion of differentiation can be appreciated along the edges of the cell clusters. (Prostate massage slightly concentrated by centrifugation, 160X)

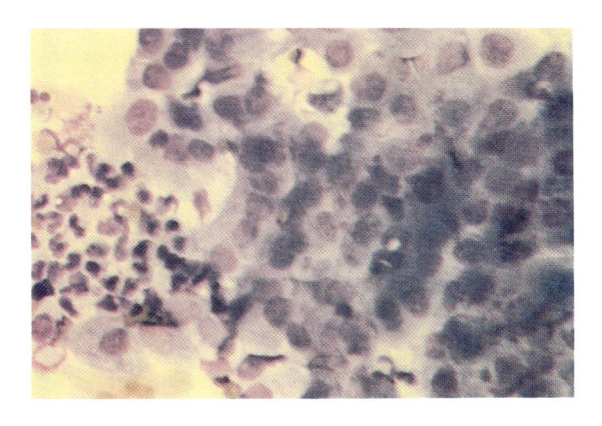

acidophilic cells are found. These cells are very large and have a flattened, floppy appearance. An occasional cell contains a pyknotic or karyorrhectic nucleus. Inflammatory cells and hyperplastic cells can be found occasionally (Fig 6).

Adenocarcinoma

Prostatomegaly and its accompanying signs occur in dogs with prostatic adenocarcinoma. On palpation, the prostate may be very large, irregular and asymmetric.[1,6] Prostatic adenocarcinomas metastasize to the iliac lymph nodes.[1,6] Cytologic examination of these nodes is suggested in suspected cases of prostatic adenocarcinoma.

Typically, prostatic aspirates or massage samples are moderately to markedly cellular. Anisokaryosis, nuclear enlargement, nuclear irregularity and an increased nucleus:cytoplasm ratio are often evident. Nucleoli are often present. Usually nucleoli are small, single and uniform, but large and sometimes irregular forms may be present. Cell membranes may be distinct in well-differentiated neoplasms, but in poorly differentiated tumors the cell membranes are indistinct. Cohesion of cells is often apparent and, occasionally, acinus formation may be suggested within some cell clusters (Figs 7,8).

THE TESTIS

Obtaining Testicular Samples

Enlargement, either unilaterally or bilaterally, is the major indication for fine-needle aspiration biopsy and cytologic evaluation of the testis.[8] If the epididymis is enlarged, fine-

Figure 6. Squamous metaplasia of prostatic epithelium in a dog with a Sertoli-cell tumor. The cells are large and light-staining. Some cells contain karyorrhectic nuclei. (Prostatic massage slightly concentrated by centrifugation, 160X)

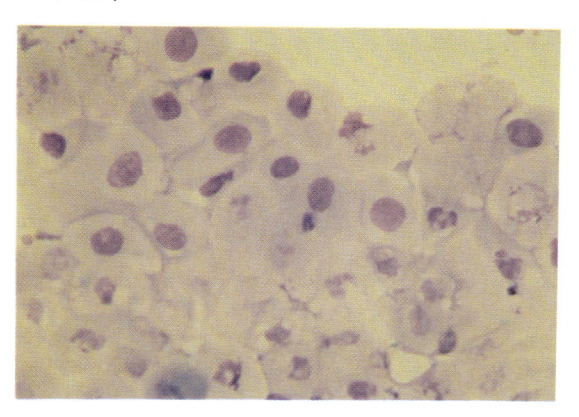

Figure 7. Crowded neoplastic prostatic epithelial cells show cellular and nuclear molding. The cytoplasm is granular, suggesting differentiation toward a secretory-type cell. (Prostatic massage slightly concentrated by centrifugation, 400X)

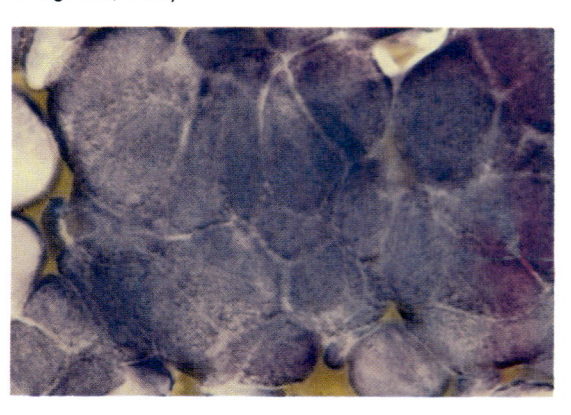

needle aspiration of the epididymis can be performed. Decreased size with increased firmness of the testes suggests atrophy. Fine-needle aspiration of atrophic testes usually does not yield a sample adequate for cytologic evaluation; biopsy and histopathologic evaluation may be required for an informed diagnosis. Semen evaluation may also provide information on testicular lesions, though its main values are for determining sperm quantity and quality.

Cytologic Evaluation

Normal Testis

Few cells can be obtained from normal testes. Occasional spermatozoa or their precursors and round cells, such as Sertoli cells and interstitial cells, may be found. Often material obtained from normal testes is contaminated with blood.

Orchitis and Epididymitis

The cytologic characteristics of orchitis and epididymitis are similar to those of inflammation of other tissues. Neutrophils are the predominant cells, but large numbers of other inflammatory cells may be found, depending upon the duration of the lesion. Occasionally the etiology of the lesion may be determined by cytologic or microbiologic methods. *Blastomyces dermatitidis* organisms may be observed in testicular aspirates in some cases of blastomycosis (Plate 4), but *Brucella canis* is rarely seen in cases of brucellosis-associated orchitis and epididymitis.[7,9,10] In both blastomycosis and brucellosis of the testis, macrophages and even giant cells may be present.

Figure 8. A group of neoplastic prostatic epithelial cells, some of which contain distinct nucleoli. Cell borders are indistinct, and modest cell crowding is evident. (Prostatic massage slightly concentrated by centrifugation, 400X)

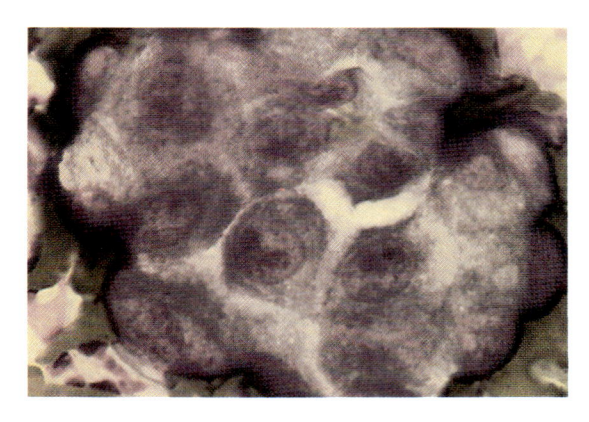

Figure 10. A group of cells aspirated from a Sertoli-cell tumor. The cells have abundant cytoplasm. Several large vacuoles are seen in some cells. The chromatin is coarsely reticular, and a large, somewhat irregular nucleolus is present at the top center. (400X)

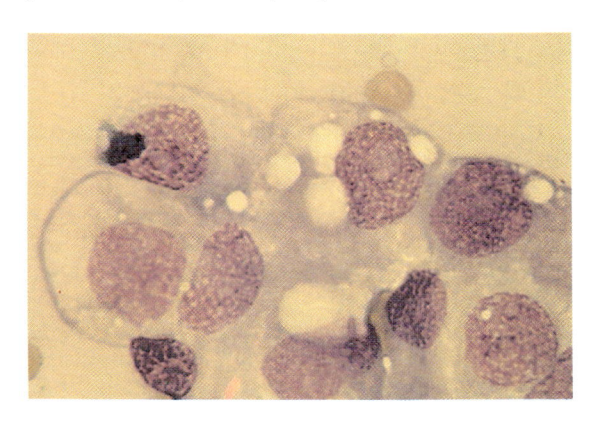

Neoplasia

There are 3 major tumors of the canine testis: seminomas, Sertoli-cell tumors and interstitial-cell tumors. They are difficult to differentiate on a cytologic basis, but when evaluated along with clinical signs and history, a clinical diagnosis is usually possible. Differentiation of testicular neoplasia from inflammation, the other major cause of testicular enlargement, is relatively simple.

Sertoli-Cell Tumor: Sertoli-cell tumors commonly occur in testes of older dogs or in undescended testes of cryptorchid dogs. Many affected dogs show feminization that, among many other signs, results in atrophy of the contralateral testis. It may be difficult to obtain material from intraabdominal Sertoli-cell tumors, but inguinal cryptorchid testes are easily aspirated.

Figure 9. A group of vacuolated cells aspirated from a Sertoli-cell tumor. The cells have abundant cytoplasm, with moderate-sized, clear vacuoles. Nuclear chromatin patterns are coarse, and there is a mitotic figure at the top. (400X)

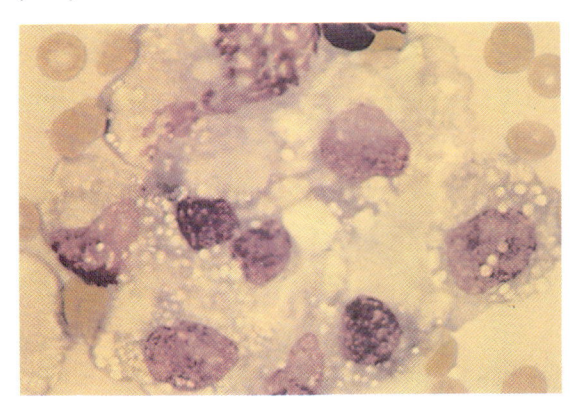

Aspirates of Sertoli-cell tumors have many cells. The cells vary in size and amount of cytoplasm. Mitotic figures may be found. The nuclear chromatin is reticulated, and small to large nucleoli may be present. The most unique feature is light-staining, vacuolated cytoplasm. Vacuoles are variable in size and very distinct (Figs 9, 10). Rarely, spindle-shaped cells with abundant cytoplasm may be found.

Seminoma: Clinical signs are minimal in dogs with seminomas, except if there is a coexisting Sertoli-cell tumor (a moderately common occurrence). Cryptorchidism is a predisposing factor, and undescended testes have an increased risk of seminoma development. Some affected dogs show feminization. Prostatitis, prostatic hyperplasia and perianal adenomas may be seen concomitantly. The major feature is testicular enlargement, which is usually unilateral but occasionally bilateral.

Figure 11. A large cell from a seminoma shows a high nucleus:cytoplasm ratio, finely reticular chromatin pattern and an irregular nucleolus. (400X)

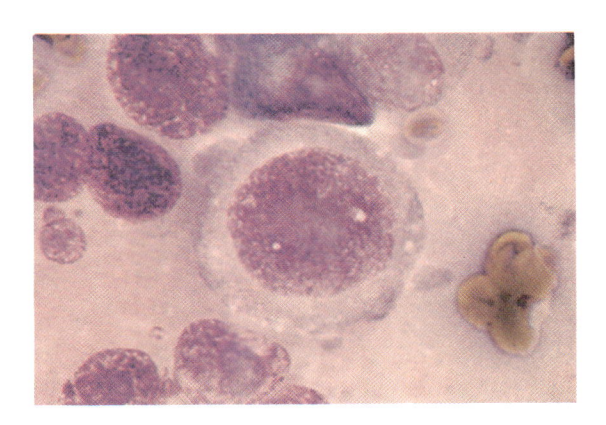

Aspiration usually yields moderate to large numbers of cells. The cells vary in size and amount of cytoplasm, though usually the amount of cytoplasm is sparse to moderate (Fig 11). Nuclei are homogeneous to finely reticular, and may be multiple (Figs 11, 12). Relatively large nucleoli are found (Fig 11). Mitotic figures are common (Fig 13).

Interstitial-Cell Tumor: Clinical signs are unusual in dogs with interstitial-cell tumors. Aspirates of these tumors often yield few cells. Cell clusters frequently surround an endothelium-lined capillary (Fig 14). Cells are variable in size but usually have abundant cytoplasm. The nucleus:cytoplasm ratio is usually low. Nuclei are small to medium sized, with a fine reticular or homogeneous chromatin pattern, and may contain small nucleoli. The cytoplasm is usually abundant and lightly basophilic. Many cells contain small vacuoles, but this is not a consistent feature (Fig 15). Small black granules occasionally are seen in a few cells (Fig 16).

Transmissible Venereal Tumor: Transmissible venereal tumor (TVT) usually occurs on the external genitalia of dogs. It may also be found in the nasal cavity, mouth and pharynx (especially near the tonsils), and on nongenital skin. Occasionally a TVT may metastasize to other locations. Impression smears or smears of aspirated material are usually quite cellular. The tumor cells have distinctive characteristics. They are intermediate in size with a moderate amount of cytoplasm. Their nucleus:cytoplasm ratio is moderately increased. The nuclei are immature, with homogeneous to finely reticulated chromatin patterns.

Figure 12. A multinucleated cell and several other cells from a seminoma. The cells have a moderate to high nucleus:cytoplasm ratio and finely reticular chromatin pattern. (400X)

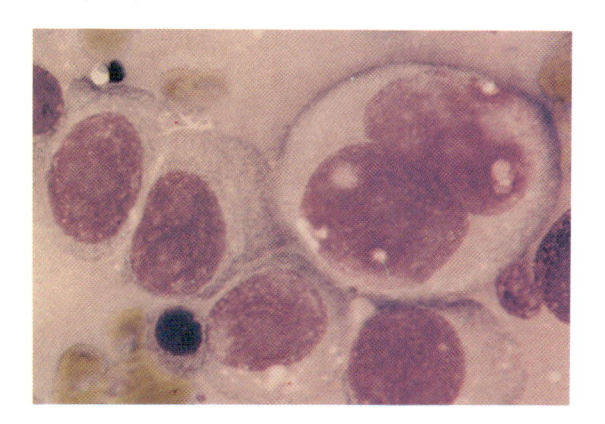

Figure 13. A mitotic figure from a seminoma. (400X)

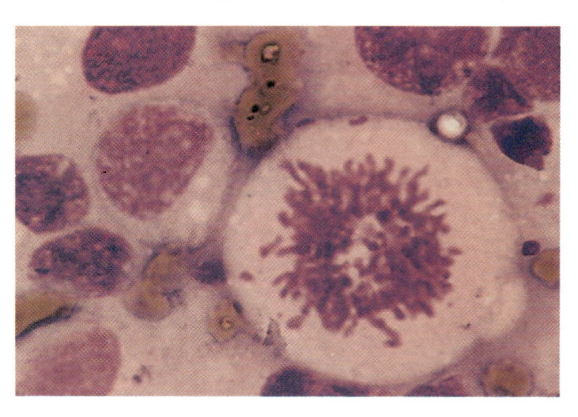

Large, round nucleoli can be found in a few cells. Cytoplasmic staining varies from lightly to heavily basophilic. Most cells contain distinct, small (1-2 μ diameter), punctate vacuoles. Mitotic cells are frequently found.

Other cells may be seen in cytologic preparations of TVTs. During the regressive stage, many lymphocytes are present, and a few neutrophils and macrophages may be found. Impression smears made from the surface of ulcerated tumors may contain bacteria, neutrophils and epithelial cells (Plate 7).

SEMEN

Semen is usually evaluated to determine its quality in infertile or subfertile males or as part of a routine breeding soundness examination.[11] Semen examination can also provide information on lesions in the genital tract of

Figure 14. Impression smear of an interstitial-cell tumor. Round to polygonal cells are free and surround an endothelium-lined capillary. (Diff-Quik stain, 25X) (Courtesy of Dr. R.L. Cowell, Oklahoma State University)

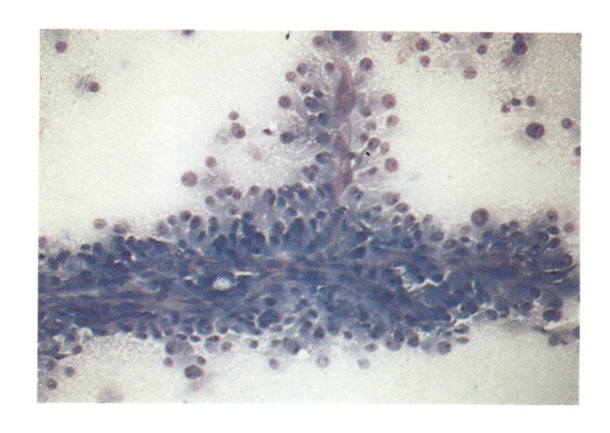

male dogs. Semen contains material derived from the testis and the remainder of the reproductive tract, including the prostate gland. Thus, semen may be examined for breeding purposes, as well as for diagnosis of some inflammatory or neoplastic lesions of the reproductive tract.

Semen Collection

Semen is often collected into an artificial vagina while masturbating the penis in the presence of a teaser bitch. Interest of the male can be enhanced by applying a solution of a 1:100 dilution of p-hydroxybenzoate methyl ester to the perineum of the teaser bitch. The technique is more fully described elsewhere.[11,12] Semen may be collected from tom cats by using an artificial vagina or by electroejaculation.[13]

Semen Evaluation

The gross characteristics of semen, including color, consistency and volume, should be assessed immediately after collection. Normal semen is milky and moderately viscous. A red color indicates blood in the sample, while yellow discoloration suggests the presence of urine. Serous, greenish or grayish semen indicates inflammation, especially when small flecks of material are seen in the thinner areas of the collection tube.

Dogs produce 1-40 ml of semen per ejaculate.[11] Cats produce up to 0.5 ml.[13]

The number of spermatozoa per ejaculate is the most important criterion for evaluating the breeding potential of a male dog.[11] Sperm concentration is determined using a hemacytometer after appropriate semen dilution. A portion of the ejaculate is diluted 1:100 with saline or a red cell Unopette (Becton-Dickinson), and the total number of sperm in the central primary square is determined. The total sperm count is calculated by multiplying the count by 1 million (10^6) and the volume of ejaculate. In samples with few sperm, the sample should be diluted less, or a greater area of the hemacytometer should be used for counting. Appropriate adjustments of the multiplication factor must be made for calculating the total sperm count.

Sperm motility should be evaluated immediately after semen collection. The sample should be maintained at body temperature or warmed to body temperature in an incubator. A drop of semen is placed on a warm slide and immediately covered with a coverslip. Samples with a high concentration of spermatozoa may be diluted 1:1 with warm physiologic saline or 2.9% sodium citrate.

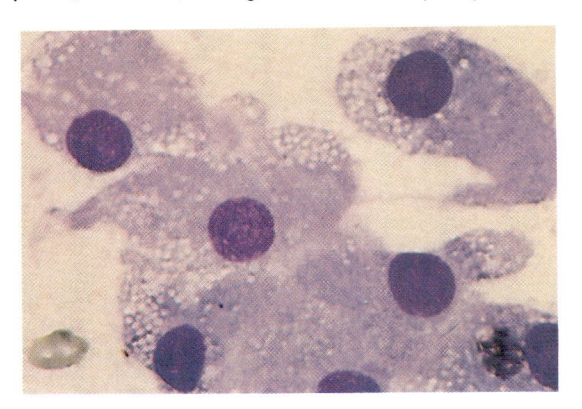

Figure 16. Fine-needle aspirate of an interstitial-cell tumor. The cells and their nuclei vary in size and show prominent vacuolization. Some cells contain blue-black cytoplasmic granules. (Diff-Quik stain, 100X) (Courtesy of Dr. R.L. Cowell, Oklahoma State University)

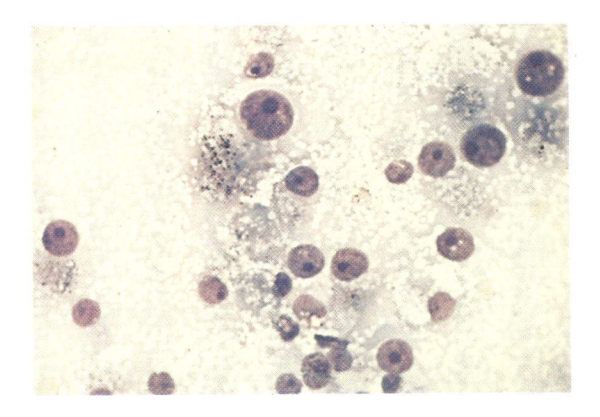

Figure 15. Cells in an aspirate of an interstitial-cell tumor are variable in shape, with moderately basophilic cytoplasm, and small, homogeneous nucleoli. (400X)

Progressive forward motility of individual sperm is estimated at high-dry magnification. Such movement is thought to reflect viability and ability to fertilize the ovum. Spermatozoa may have side-to-side motion without forward progression, may move in small circles, or may be immotile or hypomotile. A normal semen sample should have greater than 70% motility. Sperm motility may be decreased in semen contaminated with urine or exposed to pus. Overall sperm motility of the first ejaculate after a long period of sexual inactivity is decreased because of an increased percentage of old and dead sperm.[11]

Sperm morphology is assessed in a stained smear or by phase-contrast microscopy (Fig 17). A smear is mounted in a drop of new methylene blue.[14] Two hundred sperm are classified as follows: normal sperm; abnormal sperm; abnormal midpiece; coiled tail; head only; protoplasmic droplet; and abnormal head attachment (Fig 17).

Nearly all the spermatozoa in high-quality semen are morphologically normal. An increased percentage of abnormalities may indicate poor semen quality and poor breeding potential. However, correlations between the percentage of sperm abnormalities and conception rate have not been determined in dogs.[11]

Semen should be examined after Wright's staining when inflammation or neoplasia is suspected. Neutrophils indicate inflammation in the reproductive tract. However, when abnormal cells are found, one must rule out contamination from the external surface of the penis, and inflammation of the urethra or bladder. Ejaculates, especially the first portion, occasionally contain cells from the prostate gland. A diagnosis of prostatic inflammation or neoplasia may be suggested from such observations. Evaluation of the prostate gland is indicated with these findings.

Figure 17. A. Normal spermatozoa. B. Sperm with a protoplasmic droplet. C. Detached sperm head. D. Sperm with abnormally attached head. E. Sperm with double tail. F. Sperm with coiled tail.

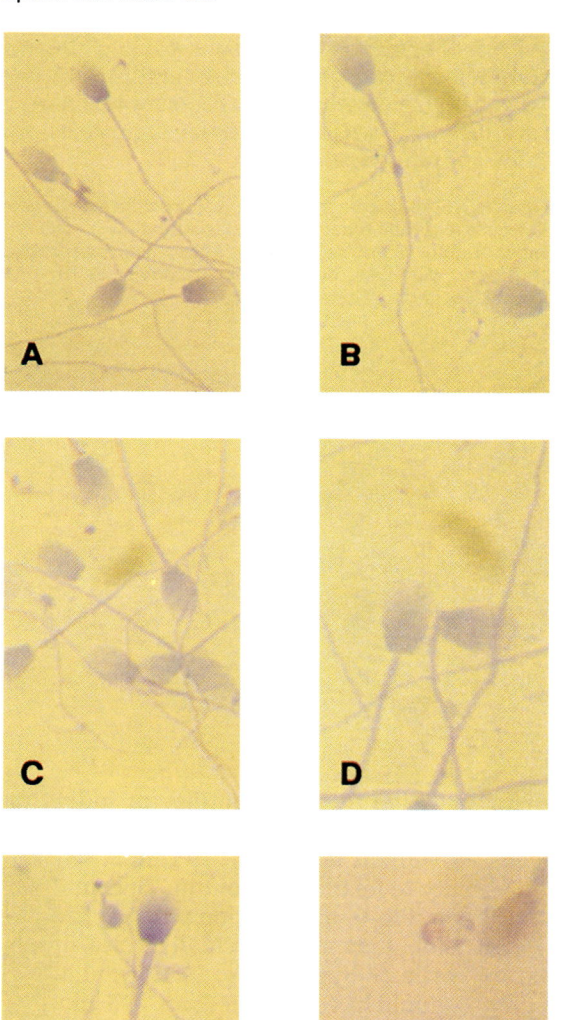

References

1. Greiner and Johnson, in Ettinger: *Textbook of Veterinary Internal Medicine.* 2nd ed. Saunders, Philadelphia, 1983. pp 1459-1492.

2. Ling *et al*: Canine prostatic fluid: Techniques of collection, quantitative bacterial culture, and interpretation of results. *JAVMA* 183:201-206, 1983.

3. Thrall *et al*: Cytologic diagnosis of canine prostatic disease. *JAAHA* 21:95-102, 1985.

4. Finco: Prostate gland biopsy. *Vet Clin No Am* 4:367-375, 1974.

5. Rogers *et al*: Diagnostic evaluation of the canine prostate. *Comp Cont Ed Pract Vet* 8:799-811, 1986.

6. Madewell and Theilen: *Veterinary Cancer Medicine.* 2nd ed. Lea & Febiger, Philadelphia, 1987. pp 583-600.

7. DeNicola *et al*: *Cytology of the Canine Male Urogenital Tract.* Ralston Purina, St. Louis.

8. Larsen: *Testicular biopsy in the dog. Vet Clin No Am* 7:747-755, 1977.

9. Barsanti, in Greene: *Clinical Microbiology and Infectious Diseases of the Dog and Cat.* Saunders, Philadelphia, 1984. pp 675-686.

10. Greene and George, in Greene: *Clinical Microbiology and Infectious Diseases of the Dog and Cat.* Saunders, Philadelphia, 1984. pp 646-662.

11. Feldman and Nelson: *Canine and Feline Endocrinology and Reproduction.* Saunders, Philadelphia, 1987. pp 481-524.

12. Seager, in Kirk: *Current Veterinary Therapy VI.* Saunders, Philadelphia, 1977. pp 1245-1251.

13. Seager, in Kirk: *Current Veterinary Therapy VI.* Saunders, Philadelphia, 1977. pp 1252-1254.

14. Jain: *Schalm's Veterinary Hematology.* Lea & Febiger, Philadelphia, 1986. pp 20-86.

21

The Vagina

M.A. Thrall and P.N. Olson

Examination of exfoliated cells from the vagina is a simple technique that can be used to accurately monitor the progression of proestrus and estrus in dogs and cats.[1-3] The vaginal epithelium, a target tissue for ovarian hormones, changes from 2-4 layers in thickness into a multilayered epithelium during estrus, resulting in exfoliation of large numbers of superficial epithelial cells. Cytologic examination of vaginal smears is also useful in detecting inflammation and neoplasia in the female reproductive tract.[4]

Collecting Vaginal Samples

Cells are obtained by passing a cotton-tipped swab into the caudal vagina (Figs 1,2). A narrow spreading speculum may be used to allow unimpeded swab passage. The swab should be directed craniodorsad when entering the vaginal vault. Once cranial to the urethral orifice, the swab is rubbed against the vaginal wall. The vestibule and clitoral fossa should be avoided, as superficial cells from these areas might alter cytologic interpretation (Fig 3). The cells are then transferred to a glass slide by gently rolling the swab. The film is allowed to air dry and stained with a hematologic stain. Most Wright's-type stains result in good-quality preparations. Diff-Quik (Harleco) is a rapid and convenient modified Wright's-Giemsa stain. New methylene blue is satisfactory but provides only temporary staining, so cytologic preparations cannot be filed for examination at a later time.

Classifying Vaginal Cells

Vaginal epithelial cells are described beginning with the deepest layer near the basement membrane and progressing superficially to the layer nearest the vaginal lumen (Fig 4).

Figure 1. The labia are carefully parted to allow unimpeded passage of the swab.[1] (Courtesy of Kal Kan Forum)

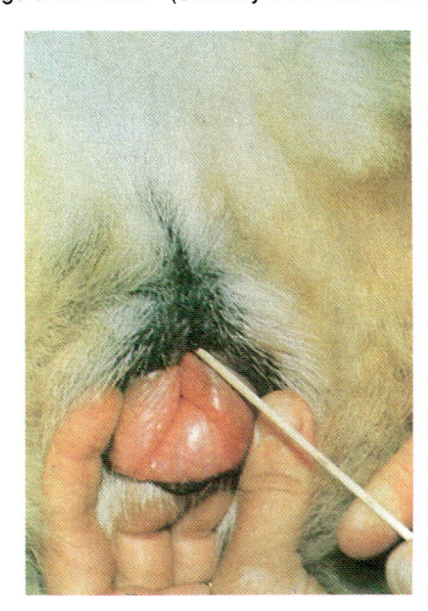

Figure 2. The swab is directed craniodorsad to avoid entering the clitoral fossa. (Courtesy of Kal Kan Forum)

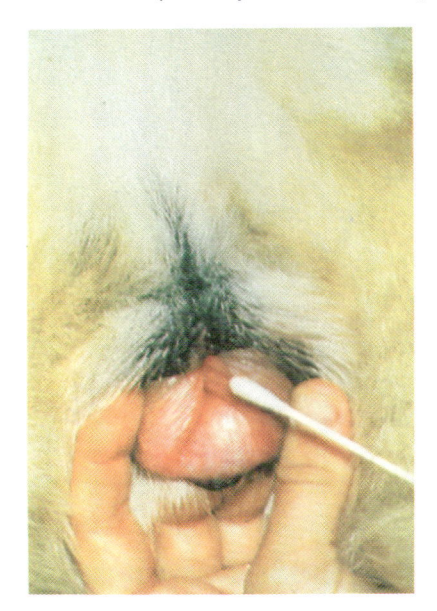

Chapter 21

Figure 3. Epithelial cells obtained from the clitoral fossa.

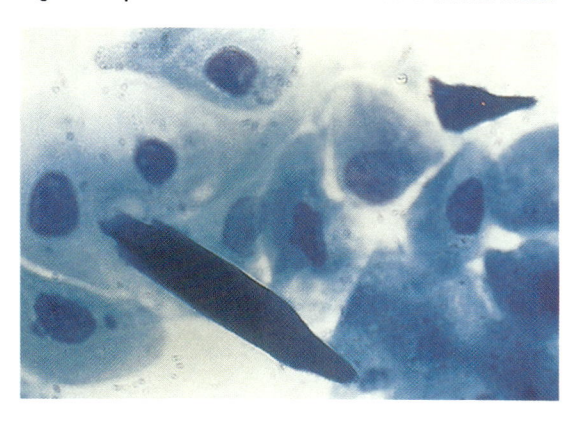

Basal Cells

Basal cells give rise to all epithelial cell types observed in a vaginal smear. They are small cells, with a small amount of cytoplasm. They are rarely observed in vaginal smears.

Parabasal Cells

Parabasal cells are small round cells with round nuclei and a small amount of cytoplasm (Fig 5). Large numbers of parabasal cells may exfoliate when the vagina of a prepubertal animal is swabbed. These cells are usually quite uniform in size and shape.

Intermediate Cells

Intermediate cells may be small or large, depending on the amount of cytoplasm pres-

Figure 4A-E. Diagrams of cells from the canine vagina. A. Parabasal epithelial cell. (Courtesy of Kal Kan Forum)

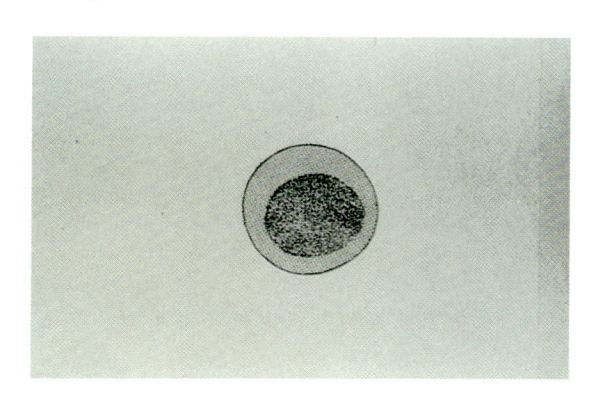

Figure 4C. Large intermediate cell. (Courtesy of Kal Kan Forum)

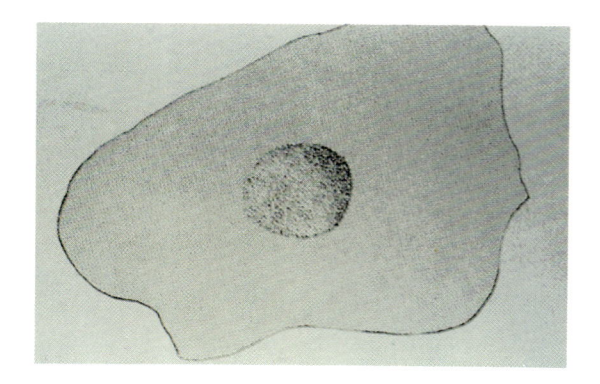

Figure 4B. Small intermediate cell. (Courtesy of Kal Kan Forum)

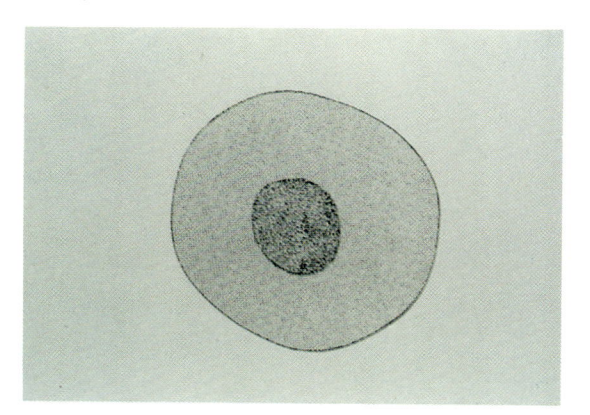

Figure 4D. Superficial cell with pyknotic nucleus. (Courtesy of Kal Kan Forum)

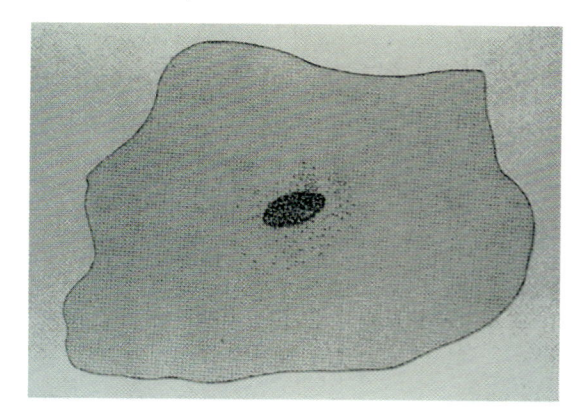

The Vagina

Figure 4E. An anuclear superficial cell.[1] (Courtesy of Kal Kan Forum)

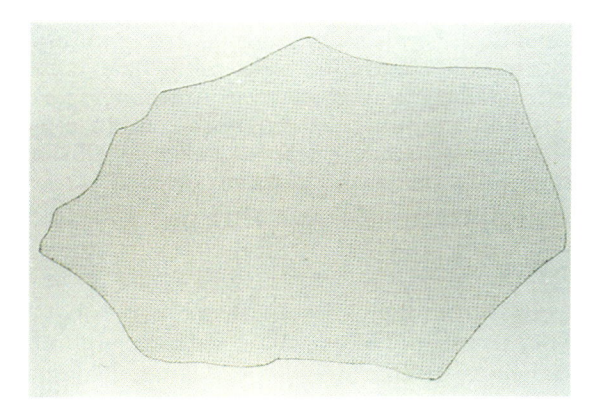

Figure 5. Parabasal epithelial cells. (Wright's stain, 400X)

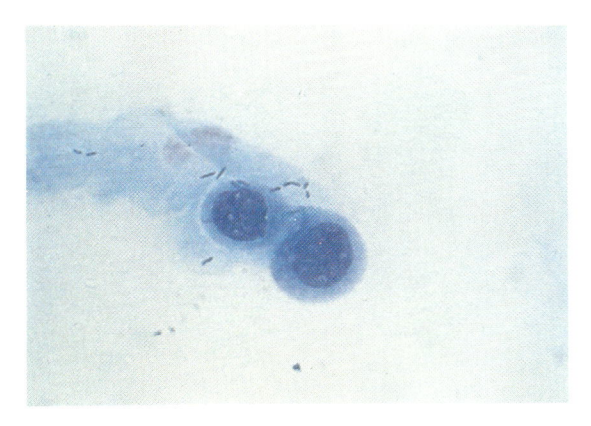

Figure 6. Small intermediate epithelial cells. (Wright's stain, 400X)

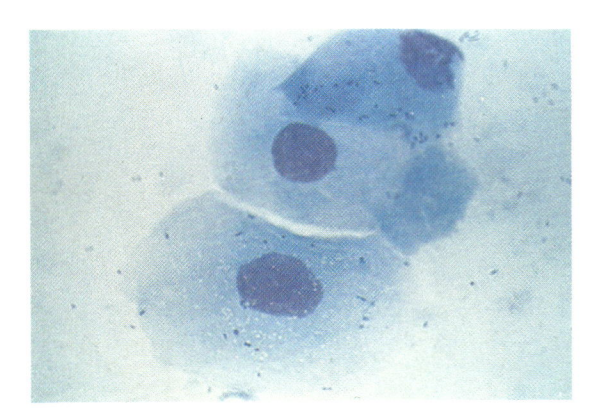

Figure 7. Large intermediate epithelial cells. (Wright's stain, 400X)

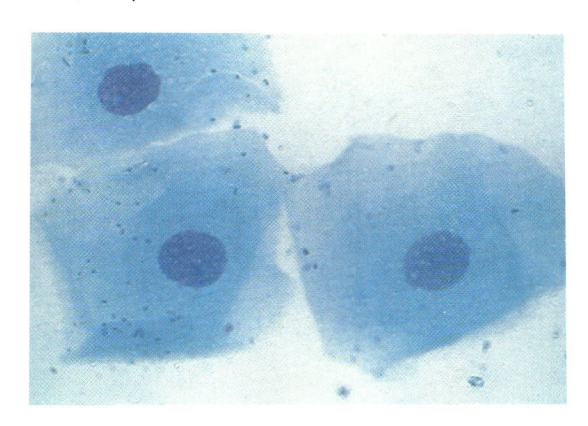

Figure 8. Superficial epithelial cell with nucleus becoming pyknotic, and folded angular cytoplasm. (Wright's stain, 400X)

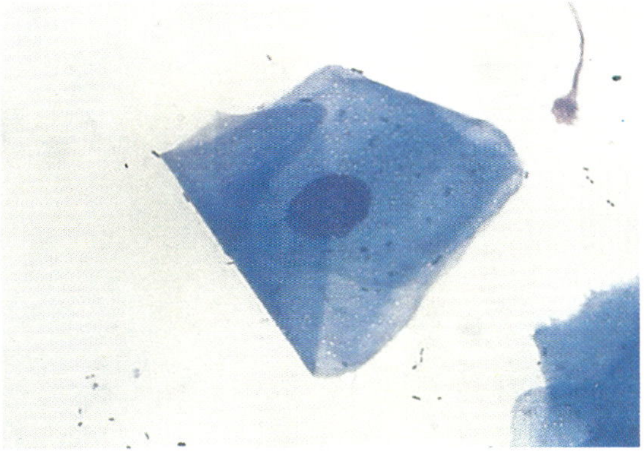

ent. While the nuclei of both small and large intermediate cells are similar in size to parabasal cell nuclei, intermediate cells are about twice the size of parabasal cells (Figs 6,7). As intermediate cells increase in size, their cytoplasm becomes irregular, folded and angular, similar to the cytoplasm of superficial cells. Large intermediate cells are sometimes termed superficial intermediate or transitional intermediate cells.

Superficial Cells

Superficial cells are the largest epithelial cells seen in vaginal smears (Fig 8). As they age and degenerate, their nuclei become pyknotic and then faded, and occasionally they disappear (Fig 9). Their cytoplasm is abundant, angular and folded. As the cells degenerate, the cytoplasm may contain small vacu-

227

Figure 9. Anuclear superficial epithelial cells.[1] (Wright's stain, 400X) (Courtesy of Kal Kan Forum)

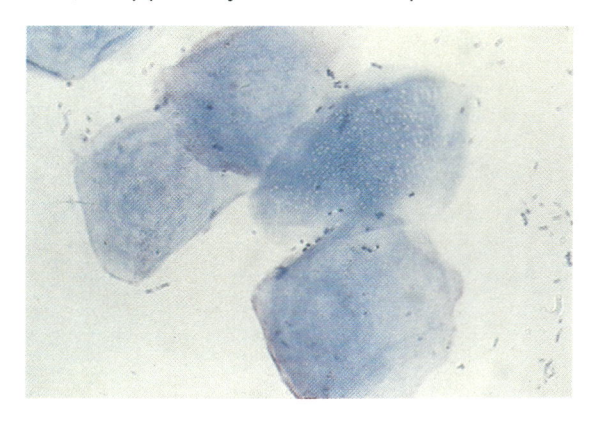

Figure 10. Degenerating superficial epithelial cell with vacuolated cytoplasm. (Wright's stain, 400X)

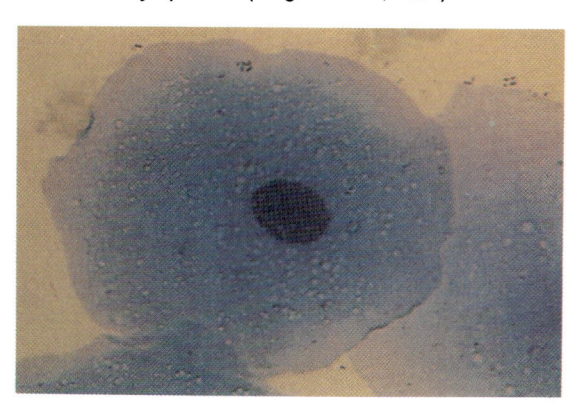

Figure 11. Vaginal smear made at proestrus. Intermediate epithelial cells predominate. Note the RBC and a few neutrophils. (Wright's stain, 100X)

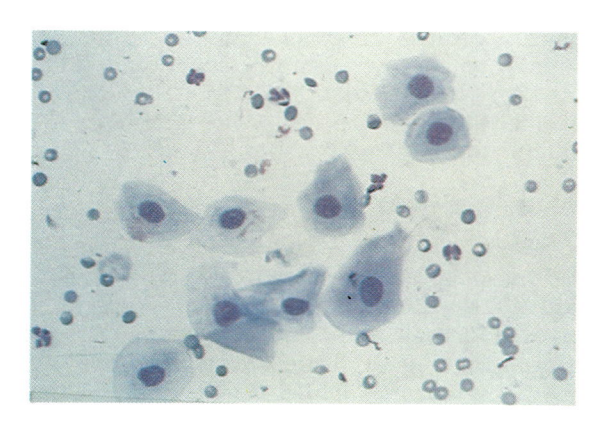

oles (Fig 10). The degeneration process of stratified squamous epithelial cells into large flat dead cells is referred to as cornification; superficial epithelial cells are commonly referred to as cornified cells. Superficial cells with small pyknotic nuclei and anuclear superficial epithelial cells have the same significance, since most bitches never reach the stage with exclusively anuclear cells.

Staging the Canine Estrous Cycle

Proestrus

As ovarian follicles mature and serum concentrations of estradiol increase, vaginal epithelium proliferates and RBC pass through uterine capillaries. These changes result in the typical appearance of vaginal cytologic preparations made during proestrus (Fig 11). Cytologic specimens obtained in early and

Figure 12. A superficial cell (arrow) and 2 intermediate cells. Note the abundant bacteria on the surface of the epithelial cells. (Wright's stain, 400X)

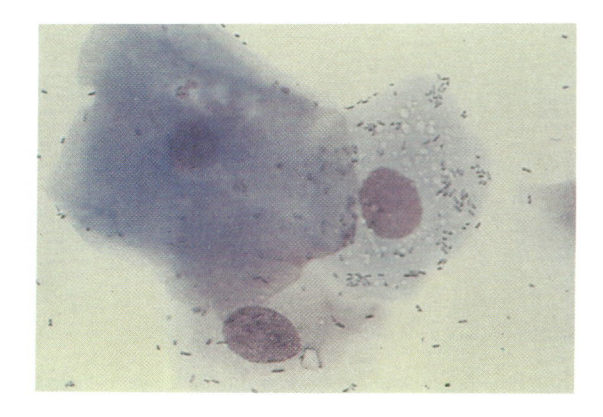

Figure 13. Vaginal smear made during estrus. Superficial epithelial cells with pyknotic nuclei. (Wright's stain, 100X)

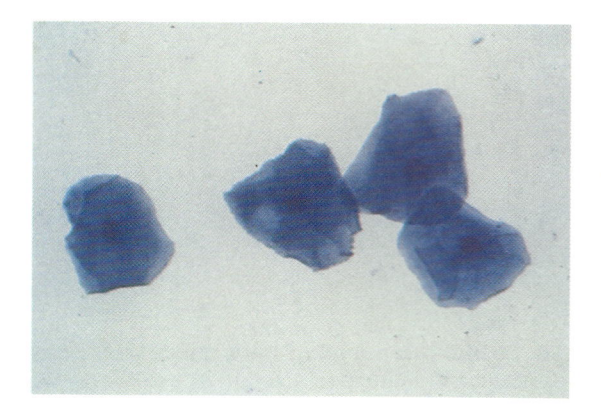

The Vagina

Figure 14. Vaginal smear made during diestrus. Note the numerous neutrophils and intermediate cells. (Wright's stain, 100X)

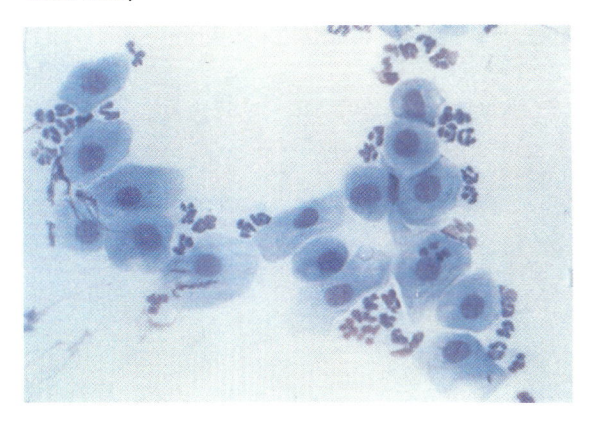

Figure 15. Neutrophils within the cytoplasm of an epithelial cell. These cells have been termed metestrous cells but may be seen at any time during the cycle. (Wright's stain, 400X)

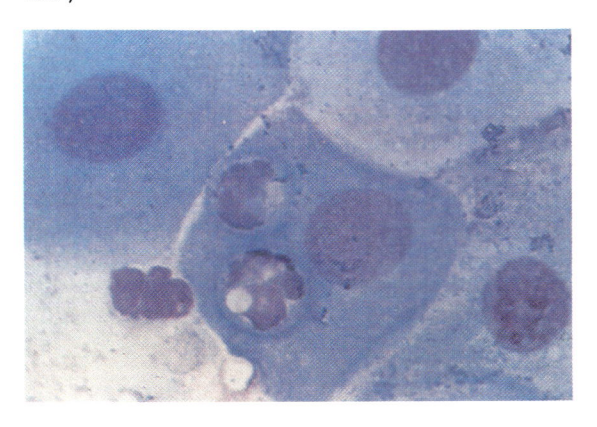

Figure 16. Vaginal smear made during diestrus may contain very few neutrophils. (Wright's stain, 100X)

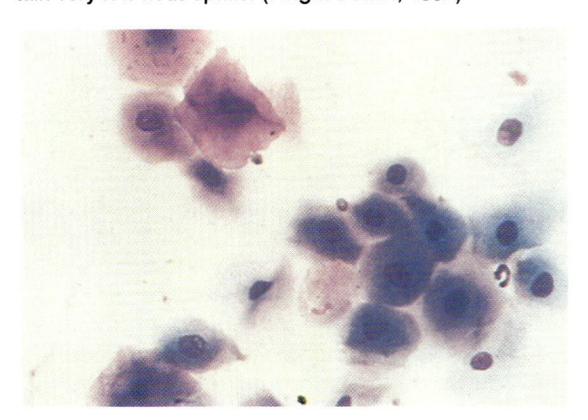

mid-proestrus are characterized by a mixture of epithelial cells, including parabasal, small and large intermediates, and superficial cells (Fig 12). Neutrophils and RBC usually are also present. By late proestrus, neutrophils usually decrease in number, and large intermediate and superficial cells predominate. Parabasal and small intermediate cells are no longer seen on smears about 4 days before the luteinizing hormone (LH) peak.[3] In proestrus, RBC may be abundant or absent. Bacteria are often present in large numbers, both free and on the surface of epithelial cells (Fig 12). The mean duration of proestrus in mature bitches is 9 days, though a range of 2-15 days is seen in normal dogs.[1]

Estrus

More than 90% of epithelial cells exfoliated during estrus are superficial cells. Most commonly, estrual cytologic preparations contain almost all superficial cells with small pyknotic nuclei (Fig 13). However, samples from some bitches contain nearly 100% anuclear cells; in other bitches, large intermediate cells are retained. The time of maximum cornification is variable and may range from as early as 6 days before the LH peak to 3 days following the LH peak. Ovulation usually occurs 1-3 days after the LH peak. This variation precludes predicting the LH peak and time of ovulation with great accuracy. Cytologic preparations made during estrus do not contain neutrophils and may or may not contain RBC. Large numbers of bacteria are commonly observed on and around superficial epithelial cells. The average duration of estrus is

Figure 17. Parabasal cells in a vaginal smear made during anestrus. (Wright's stain, 400X)

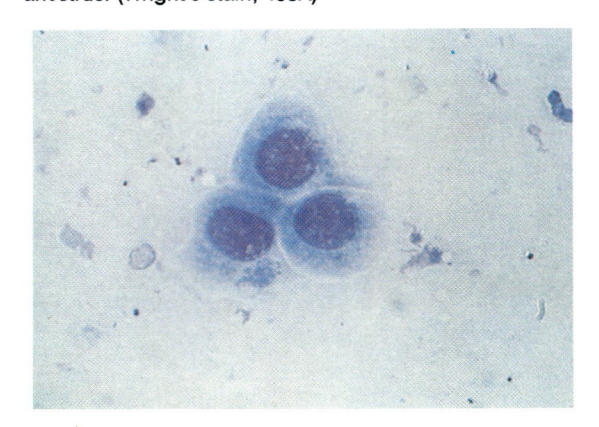

Figure 18. Spermatozoa and a superficial epithelial cell in a vaginal smear from a bitch several hours after mating. (Wright's stain, 400X)

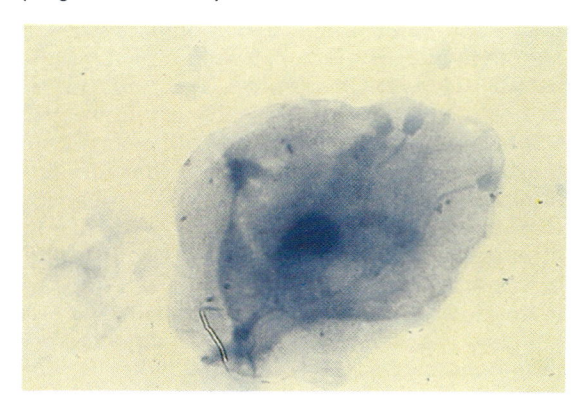

Figure 20. Vaginal smear from a cat in estrus. Anuclear superficial epithelial cells with folded angular cytoplasm. (Wright's stain, 400X)

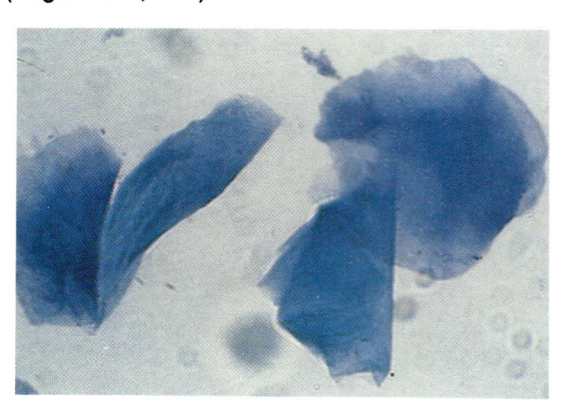

9 days for mature bitches, but a range of 3-21 days has been reported.[1]

Diestrus

Diestrus occurs about 8 days (range 6-10 days) after the LH peak in most cycles and is cytologically characterized by an abrupt change in relative numbers of superficial epithelial cells. Superficial cell numbers decrease by at least 20%; numbers of parabasal and intermediate cells, which were absent or comprised <5% of the total, increase to >10% and often to >50%. Neutrophils appear in variable numbers and usually coincide with increased numbers of parabasal and intermediate cells (Fig 14). Neutrophils may be seen within the cytoplasm of epithelial cells (Fig 15). Some

Figure 19. Cells that appear to be uterine glandular epithelial cells in a vaginal smear from a bitch with subinvolution of placental sites after whelping. (Wright's stain, 400X)

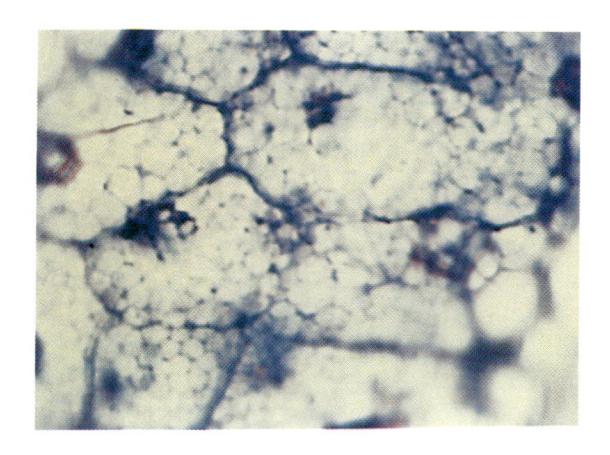

bitches have few or no neutrophils in cytologic preparations made during diestrus (Fig 16). Red blood cells may or may not be present.

Individual cytologic preparations made during the transition period from late estrus to early diestrus, without benefit of prior preparations, can appear very similar to smears made in early or mid-proestrus. At both times there can be a similar mixture of superficial and nonsuperficial cells, and both RBC and neutrophils may be present. Vaginoscopy, vulvar examination and the animal's behavior are usually helpful in making the differentiation.

Anestrus

Parabasal and intermediate cells predominate during anestrus (Fig 17). If present, neutrophils and bacteria are few in number.

Management of Breeding

Optimum breeding times can be more accurately determined with cytologic examination. The duration of proestrus and estrus may be quite short in some bitches, particularly young ones. Some bitches have no discernible behavioral proestrus or estrus, yet they ovulate normally. Bitches should be bred every fourth day throughout the period when >90% of vaginal epithelial cells are superficial. Since canine spermatozoa can survive for at least 4-6 days in the uterus of bitches in estrus, mating may be successful from shortly before the time of ovulation to about 4 days after ovulation. Once diestrus occurs, fertility rapidly declines. Breedings are unlikely to be successful if

Figure 21. Large numbers of neutrophils and intermediate epithelial cells from a puppy with vaginitis.[4] (Wright's stain, 100X)

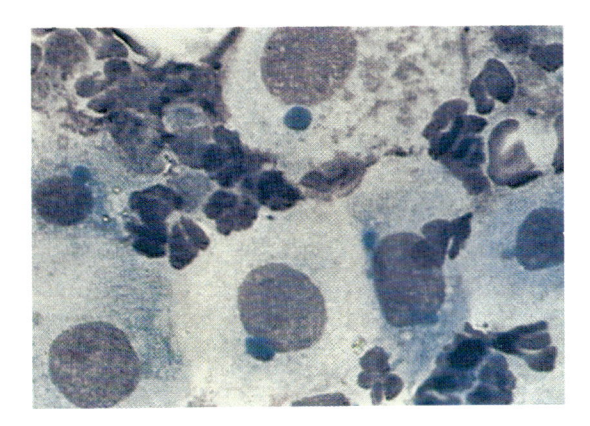

Figure 24. Neutrophils and streptococci in a vaginal smear from a bitch with metritis. (Wright's stain, 400X)

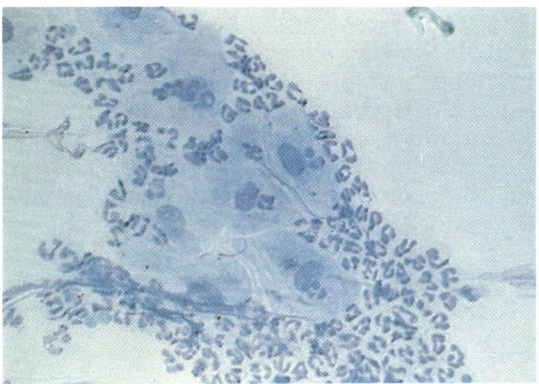

Figure 22. Mucus in a vaginal smear from a bitch with a chronic vulvar discharge. (Wright's stain, 400X)

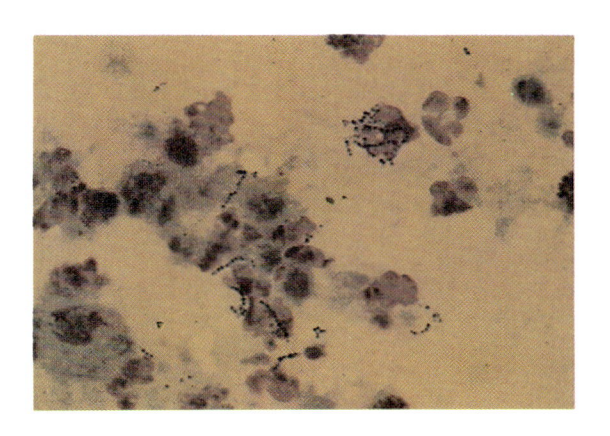

Figure 25. Neutrophils and muscle fibers from decomposing puppies in a vaginal smear from a bitch with a herniated uterus and metritis. (Wright's stain, 400X)

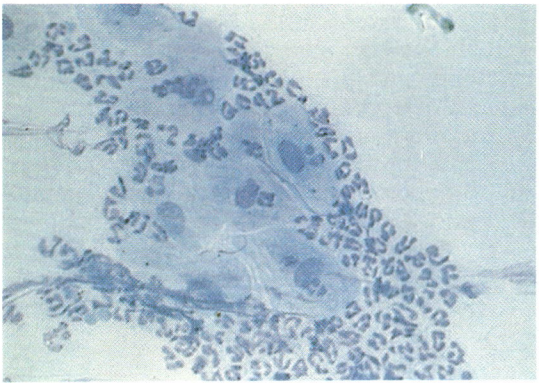

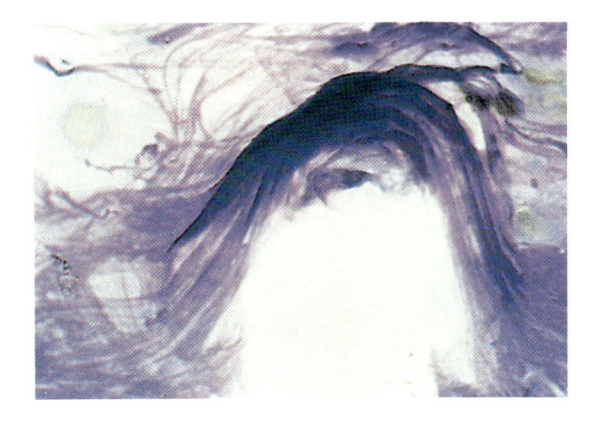

Figure 23. Basophilic intracytoplasmic inclusions in epithelial cells in a vaginal smear from a bitch with vaginitis.[4] (Wright's stain, 400X)

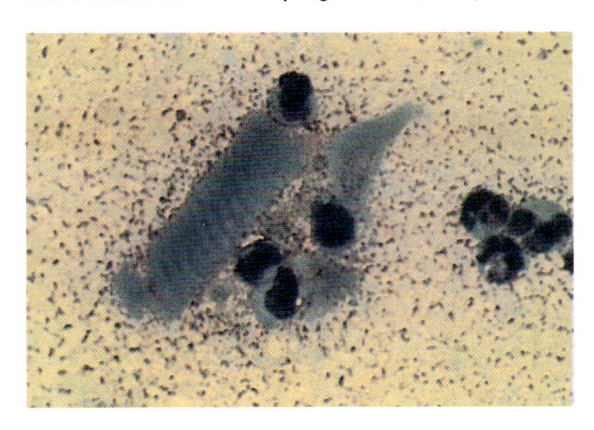

Figure 26. Transitional-cell carcinoma cells and neutrophils in a vaginal smear from a bitch with transitional-cell carcinoma invading the vagina. (Wright's stain, 1000X)

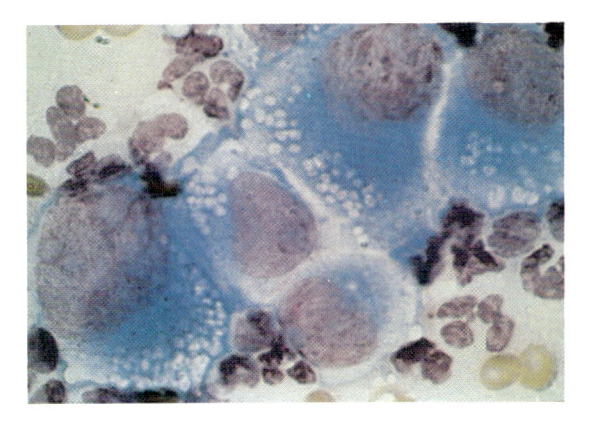

delayed more than 24 hours after the onset of cytologic diestrus.

Spermatozoa are sometimes observed in vaginal cytologic preparations from mated bitches (Fig 18). The period during which they are present is variable. The presence of spermatozoa confirms a mating, but their absence does not ensure that a bitch was not bred. We have observed intact spermatozoa or sperm heads in about 65% of vaginal smears made 24 hours after a natural mating and in 50% of smears made 48 hours after mating. Cells that appear to be uterine glandular epithelial cells occasionally may be observed in vaginal cytologic preparations, particularly several weeks after whelping in bitches with suspected subinvolution of placental sites (Fig 19).

Staging the Feline Estrous Cycle

Female cats (queens) are seasonally polyestrus. Coitus is necessary for ovulation, and in the absence of ovulation, successive estrous periods occur. The mean duration of estrus is about 8 days (range 3-16 days). The average interval between estrous periods is 9 days (range 4-22 days) if ovulation does not occur. Ovulation and the subsequent pseudopregnancy delay the return to estrus for about 45 days. Vaginal smears may be examined to accurately detect estrus in cats.[5-9] Rarely, ovulation may be induced while obtaining cells for vaginal cytologic preparations.

Vaginal cytologic characteristics of the queen are similar to those of the bitch. However, RBC are not usually seen in proestrus, and neutrophils are an inconsistent finding during diestrus. Between estrual periods, epithelial cell types are mixed. Intermediate cells predominate, and parabasal cells and anuclear superficial cells are present in small numbers. Vaginal epithelial cells become progressively cornified as serum estradiol concentrations increase. The proportion of anuclear superficial cells increases to >10% on the first day of estrus. On the fourth day of estrus, about 40% of the cells are anuclear superficial cells (Fig 20).[5] Numbers of anuclear superficial cells remain relatively constant during estrus, ranging from 40 to 60% of the total. Intermediate cell numbers decrease to <10% during the first 4 days of estrus. Neutrophils and parabasal cells are absent during estrus. In early pregnancy or pseudopregnancy, parabasal cells reappear and intermediate cell numbers increase. A few neutrophils may be seen at the end of estrus and in early pseudopregnancy.

Cytologic Characteristics of Vaginitis and Metritis

Cytologic samples obtained from animals with inflammation of the vagina or uterus are characterized by many neutrophils (Fig 21). Cytologic samples from bitches in early diestrus also contain many neutrophils and can resemble those from bitches with vaginal or uterine inflammation. However, the number of neutrophils in smears from normal bitches in diestrus markedly decreases by 1 week postestrus. Mucus and a few macrophages and lymphocytes may also be present (Fig 22).

Vaginitis is often caused by noninfectious factors, such as vaginal anomalies, clitoral hypertrophy, foreign bodies or vaginal immaturity. If bacteria are contributing to the inflammation, they are usually seen within the cytoplasm of neutrophils. Epithelial intracytoplasmic inclusions that are morphologically similar to *Chlamydia* or *Mycoplasma* have been observed in bitches with vaginitis (Fig 23). Their significance is unknown. Neutrophils may appear degenerate or nondegenerate. Degenerate neutrophils are usually associated with bacteria.

Vaginal smears from animals with pyometra or metritis usually contain large numbers of very degenerate neutrophils. Bacteria also are frequently observed (Fig 24). Rarely, muscle fibers from decomposing fetuses may be seen in bitches with metritis secondary to dystocia (Fig 25).

Cytologic Characteristics of Neoplasia

Neoplasia of the urinary and reproductive tracts can occasionally be diagnosed by cytologic examination of vaginal smears. Transitional-cell carcinomas that have invaded the vagina (Fig 26), transmissible venereal tumors (Plate 7) and squamous-cell carcinomas (Plate 6) are the more common types of cytologically diagnosed tumors. Vaginal lymphosarcoma also may be diagnosed (Plate 7). The cytologic criteria of malignancy have been discussed elsewhere and apply to the reproductive tract.

References

1. Olson *et al*: Vaginal Cytology. Part I. A useful tool for staging the canine estrous cycle. *Comp Cont Ed Pract Vet* 6:288-298, 1984.

2. Linde and Karlsson: The correlation between the cytology of the vaginal smear and the time of ovulation in the bitch. *J Small Anim Pract* 25:77-82, 1984.

3. Concannon, in Kirk: *Current Veterinary Therapy IX.* Saunders, Philadelphia, 1986. pp 1214-1224.

4. Olson *et al*: Vaginal cytology. Part II. Its use in diagnosing canine reproductive disorders. *Comp Cont Ed Pract Vet* 6:385-390, 1984.

5. Shille *et al*: Follicular function in the domestic cat as determined by estradiol-17β concentrations in plasma: Relation to estrus behavior and cornification of exfoliated vaginal epithelium. *Biology Repro* 21:953-963, 1979.

6. Lofstedt: The estrous cycle of the domestic cat. *Comp Cont Ed Pract Vet* 4:52-58, 1982.

7. Cline *et al*: Analysis of the feline vaginal epithelial cycle. *Feline Practice* 10(6):47-49, 1980.

8. Mowrer *et al*: Vaginal cytology: an approach to improvement of cat breeding. *VM/SAC* 70:691-696, 1975.

9. Herron: Feline vaginal cytologic examination. *Feline Practice* 7(3):36-39, 1977.

22

Rectal Mucosal Scrapings

P.M. Rakich and K.S. Latimer

Indications

Rectal scrapings are indicated with signs of large intestinal disease. These signs typically include tenesmus and small amounts of liquid to semiliquid feces with abundant mucus. If blood is present, it is undigested and, therefore, bright red (hematochezia). Digital rectal examination in large bowel disease reveals a uniformly or irregularly thickened mucosa, with mucus and/or blood on the glove when the finger is withdrawn.

Generally, rectal scrapings are most productive when the disease is one that diffusely infiltrates the lamina propria of the mucosa. Often, the small intestine is involved also; however, rectal scraping is invariably unrewarding if the diarrhea is strictly of small intestinal origin. Rectal mucosal scrapings are more commonly and easily performed on dogs because of their larger size and less fractious temperaments but may be performed on cats also.

Technique

The object of rectal mucosal scrapings is to remove the covering epithelium and obtain a sample of lamina propria. Microscopic examination of this sample may reveal infiltrating tumor or inflammatory cells or infectious agents responsible for the large bowel disease. Rectal mucosal scraping is performed with a rigid instrument, such as a chemistry spatula, conjunctival scraper or ear curet (Fig 1). Cotton swabs usually do not produce diagnostic samples because they are not abrasive enough to get a subepithelial sample.

The rectum is first cleaned of feces so a sample of mucosa, rather than adherent feces, is obtained. The instrument is guided into the rectum using a gloved finger as for performing a digital rectal examination. Lubricant is avoided or used only sparingly because it stains intensely and can obscure cytologic structures on the stained smear. The instrument must be inserted far enough craniad to avoid the anus and reach the rectum. The instrument is drawn along the mucosa several times in a firm stroking motion. The scraping must be done firmly enough to remove the epithelium and collect material in the lamina propria but not vigorously enough to perforate the rectum. Perforation is especially a consideration in animals with chronic ulcerative colitis, in which the colon may be very friable.

The scraper is removed from the rectum with the finger protecting the surface of the instrument so the sample is not lost. The material is then placed on a glass slide and

Figure 1. Various instruments used to perform rectal mucosal scrapings include (from top to bottom) a conjunctival scraper, an ear curet and 2 blunt chemistry spatulas.

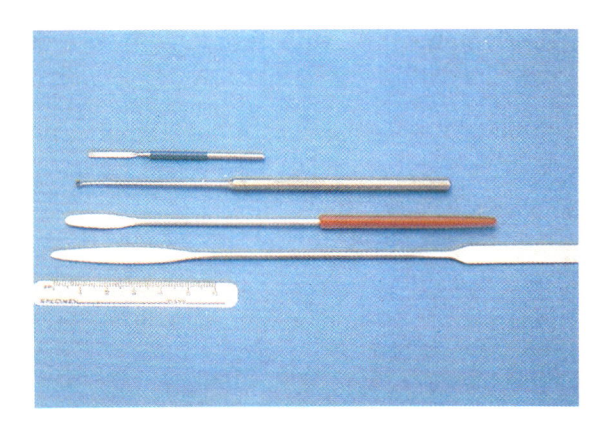

Figure 2. A cluster of columnar epithelial cells and a mixed population of bacteria obtained from normal canine rectal mucosa. (650X)

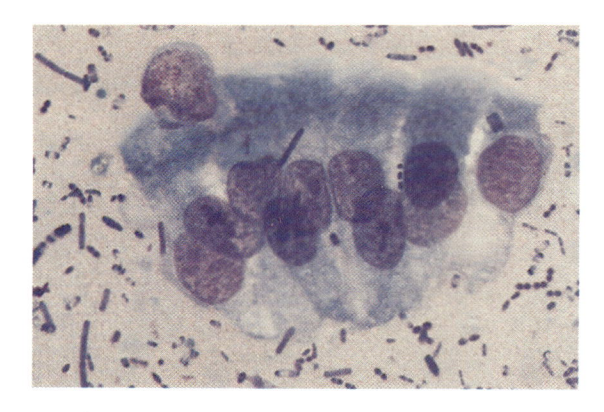

smeared with the scraping instrument or gently pressed with a second slide to make a smear consisting of a single layer of cells. (See Chapter 1 for a detailed discussion of slide preparation.)

Smears can be stained with such commonly used stains as Wright's, rapid Wright's or new methylene blue. When measurement of cells or organisms is necessary as an aid in their identification, size can be approximated by comparing the structures in question to RBC (6-7 μ in diameter in dogs and cats) and neutrophils (12-14 μ in diameter in dogs and cats).

Normal Rectal Mucosal Scrapings

A normal rectal scraping consists of clusters of columnar epithelial cells, a mixed bacterial population of rods and cocci of varying size, a small amount of mucus, and amorphous debris

Figure 3. Two squamous epithelial cells, 2 neutrophils, scattered RBC and a mixed population of bacteria. Squamous epithelial cells are obtained from the terminal rectal and anal areas. (650X)

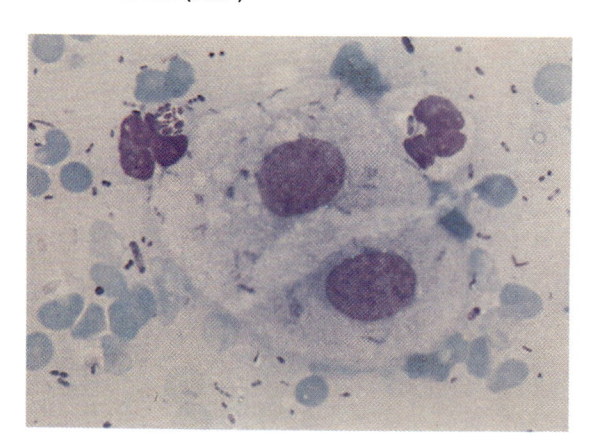

(Fig 2). The amount of debris is minimal when feces are removed before scraping. Squamous epithelial cells indicate that the anus rather than the rectum was scraped and the procedure may have to be repeated (Fig 3). Inflammatory cells are rare in healthy animals and consist of lymphocytes, plasma cells and mast cells (Plates 1 and 2). These may be in the lamina propria in small numbers. Neutrophils and RBC may be derived from the small amount of bleeding induced by the procedure, in which case they occur in an approximate WBC:RBC ratio of 1:500-1000.

When lubricant jelly is used, the smear contains varying amounts of bright pink amor-

Figure 4. A cluster of columnar and 2 squamous epithelial cells. Morphology of the squamous epithelial cells is partially obscured by bright pink-staining surgical lubricant. (650X)

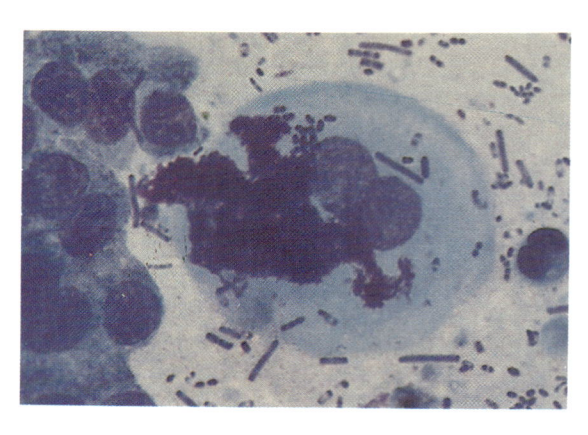

phous granular or fibrillar material (Fig 4). If a large amount of this material is present on a smear, it can obscure diagnostic structures. Occasionally, a section of mucosa containing a normal lymphoid follicle is scraped (Fig 5). This can be differentiated from lymphosarcoma by the presence of a heterogeneous population of lymphocytes consisting primarily of small lymphocytes, with fewer medium and large lymphocytes as well as plasma cells. (See Chapter 8 on lymph node cytology for a more complete discussion of differentiating lymphosarcoma from reactive lymphoid tissue.)

Inflammation

Eosinophilic Inflammation

Eosinophilic colitis may occur as a primary disease of the colon or rectum or may be part of a more extensive syndrome, eosinophilic gastroenteritis.[1] Cocker Spaniels and German Shepherds appear predisposed to this condition.[1] Rectal scrapings yield moderate to large numbers of eosinophils (Fig 6). Because ulceration occurs in this disease, numerous RBC may also be seen.

Purulent Inflammation

Predominance of neutrophils on a smear from a rectal scraping is a nonspecific finding because colitis due to any cause produces a layer of fibrin and neutrophils covering denuded areas (Plate 3). In some types of deep lesions that may cause extensive tissue necrosis, such as various malignant tumors, the mucosa is frequently ulcerated and infiltrated with neutrophils. For this reason, a scraping performed in any animal with ulcerative colitis is likely to yield numerous neutrophils and fibrin. Fibrin is not seen on smears stained with any Wright's-type stains but appears as pale granular or fibrillar ma-terial on new methylene blue-stained smears.

Fungal Infection

Histoplasmosis: Disseminated histoplasmosis in dogs frequently causes chronic large intestinal diarrhea as well as signs referable to other affected organ systems.[2] Definitive diagnosis can be made by rectal scraping. *Histoplasma capsulatum* organisms are seen as round to oval yeasts measuring 2-4 μ in diameter (Plate 4). They consist of a basophilic center surrounded by a thin clear halo. The yeasts are usually multiple within macrophages; a few organisms may be scattered extracellularly. Macrophages devoid of organisms, neutrophils and a few lymphocytes and plasma cells are also usually present.

Figure 5. Cytologic appearance of cells from a lymphoid follicle. A heterogeneous population of small, medium and large lymphocytes is present. The bacteria represent normal colonic flora. (650X)

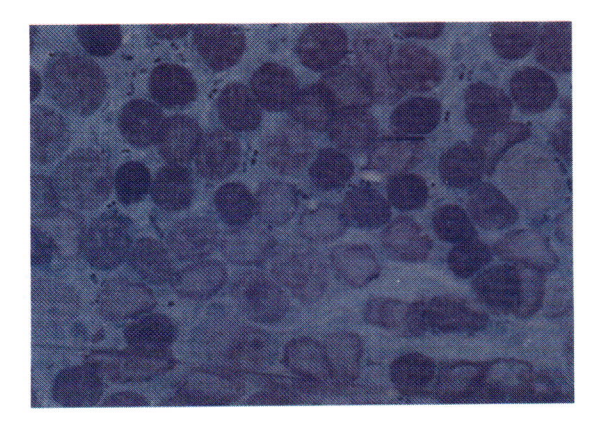

Figure 6. A mixture of eosinophils, neutrophils and macrophages in a rectal scraping from a dog with eosinophilic colitis. Eosinophil granules in cytologic tissue specimens often stain a muddy red-brown color in contrast to the bright red-orange granules in blood eosinophils. (650X)

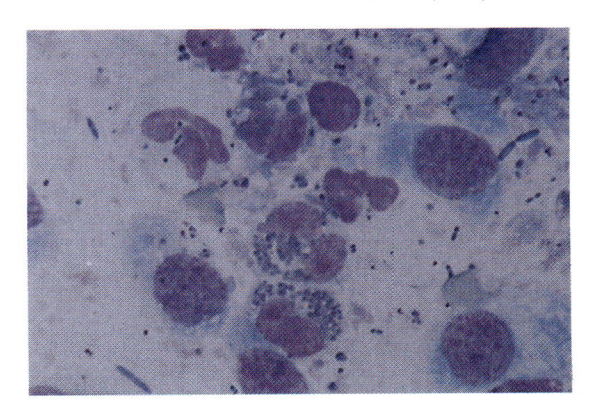

Cryptococcosis: *Cryptococcus neoformans* infects many tissues but intestinal infection is uncommon.[3] Large bowel involvement rarely occurs in dogs with disseminated cryptococcosis. The organisms are seen on smears as extracellular round to oval basophilic yeasts 3.5-7μ in diameter, with a clear capsule of variable thickness (1-30 μ) (Plate 4).[3] Only rarely are *Cryptococcus* organisms seen within macrophages.

Protothecosis: *Prototheca* is a colorless alga that is ubiquitous in the environment and only rarely causes disease.[1] In dogs, a disproportionate number of cases have been reported in Collies.[4] In cats, only the cutaneous form of the disease has been reported.[1] Protothecosis in dogs frequently causes intermittent and protracted bloody diarrhea, though the organism is usually widely disseminated throughout the body.[4]

Definitive diagnosis of protothecosis often can be made by rectal scraping. The organisms are round to oval, 1.3-13.4 μ wide, and 1.3-16.1 μ long. They have granular basophilic cytoplasm and a clear cell wall about 0.5 μ thick.[4] A small nucleus is present in all but the small immature forms. Frequently a single organism consists of 2, 4 or more endospores (Fig 7 and Plate 5). The organisms are predominantly extracellular but small forms may be seen in macrophages and/or neutrophils. Usually numerous organisms are present along with a mixed population of inflammatory cells and blood.

Protozoal Infection

Occasionally, protozoa are found in rectal scrapings. Not all protozoa in the intestinal tract are considered pathogenic, however. The tendency to produce disease depends on the virulence of the organism and host factors.[5]

Pentatrichomonas hominis is a pyriform flagellate that inhabits the large intestine of people, dogs, cats, monkeys and some rodents. The pathogenicity of this organism is uncertain; it may be an opportunist pathogen.[5] Trichomoniasis is reported infrequently in dogs. The trophozoites measure 6-14 μ by 4-6.5 μ, and usually have 5 anterior flagella.[5] Trichomonads have an undulating membrane that on cytologic smears appears as an unstained curvilinear structure coursing the long axis of the organism. The organisms have a dark nucleus and basophilic cytoplasm that may have small clear vacuoles (Fig 8).

Balantidium coli is the largest protozoan capable of infecting dogs.[5] This ciliated protozoan can colonize the human and canine colon.[1] Balantidiasis has not been reported in cats.[5] The pig is the definitive host and dogs become infected by eating pig feces.[1] Canine balantidiasis may be complicated by concurrent trichuriasis. Damage to the colonic mucosa caused by whipworms may predispose to infection with *B coli*.[5]

Balantidiasis can be diagnosed by fecal flotation, direct fecal smear or rectal scraping. The organism may be seen in smears in 2 forms. Trophozoites are oval and usually 40-80 μ by 25-45 μ but may be as large as 30-300 μ by 30-100 μ.[5] They have spirally arranged longitudinal rows of cilia and a large oval nucleus (Fig 9). Round to oval cysts that measure up to 40-60 μ in diameter may also be seen. In each stage of the organism, diagnosis

Figure 7. Six protothecal organisms and a cluster of columnar epithelial cells. *Prototheca* spp vary in size and have granular basophilic cytoplasm and a thin, clear cell wall. The 2 larger organisms are composed of several endospores. (650X)

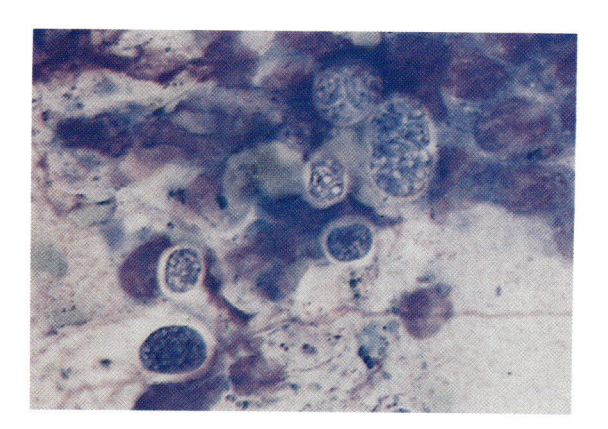

Figure 8. Two *Pentatrichomonas hominis* organisms and mixed bacterial flora in a rectal mucosal scraping from a dog with large bowel diarrhea. A nucleus and vacuoles are present in each organism. In addition, a curvilinear structure representing the undulating membrane is present within one trichomonad. (650X)

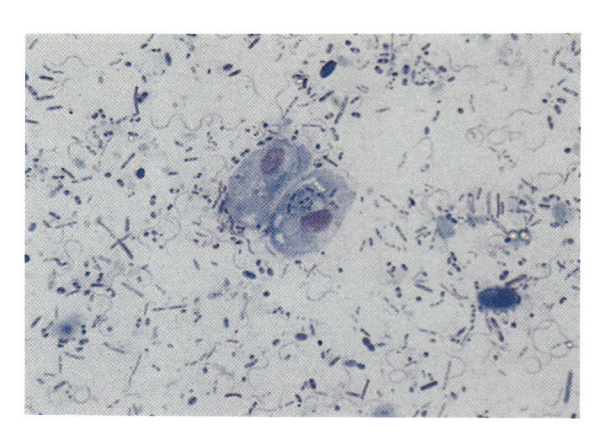

of balantidiasis is facilitated by the large size and prominent oval nucleus of the ciliate.

Entamoeba histolytica is an ameba that can occur as a commensal organism in the lumen of the colon or as a pathogen that invades the intestinal wall.[1] It is primarily a parasite of people but can also invade the large intestine of dogs and cats.[5] Infection with this organism is uncommon.[5] Trophozoites invade the mucosa by their lytic action and produce colonic ulceration and inflammation, with bloody mucoid diarrhea.[1,5] Trophozoites measure 12-50 μ in diameter and cysts measure 10-20 μ in diameter. Trophozoites have a dark nucleus and basophilic cytoplasm that may contain clear vacuoles. The presence of ingested RBC distinguishes *Entamoeba histolytica* from nonpathogenic amebae.[5] Because of the cytoplasmic vacuoles and ingested RBC, *E histolytica* trophozoites may be mistaken for macrophages and overlooked if only a cursory examination of the smear is done (Fig 10).

Neoplasia

Lymphosarcoma in dogs is the neoplasm most commonly diagnosed by rectal scraping. In contrast, intestinal lymphosarcoma in cats usually involves small intestine only, and rectal scraping is not diagnostic. Despite extensive involvement of the colon in dogs, lymphosarcoma usually does not cause ulceration and thus no hematochezia occurs.[1] As with lymphosarcoma involving other tissues, the lymphoid population is monomorphic. The lymphocytes can vary from 8-15 μ in diameter in small-cell neoplasms to 10-24 μ in diameter in

Figure 9. *Balantidium coli* cyst characterized by a smooth wall, large size and prominent curved nucleus. (650X)

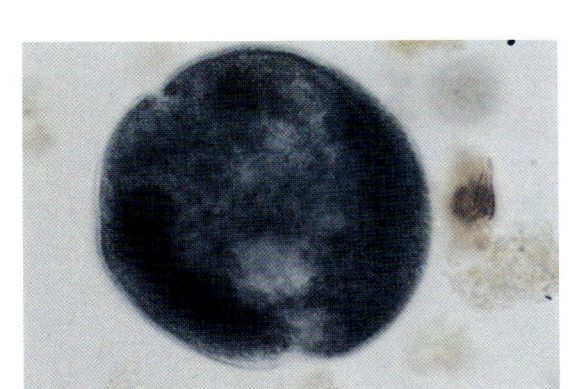

Figure 10. *Entamoeba histolytica* trophozoite adjacent to a whipworm egg. (650X)

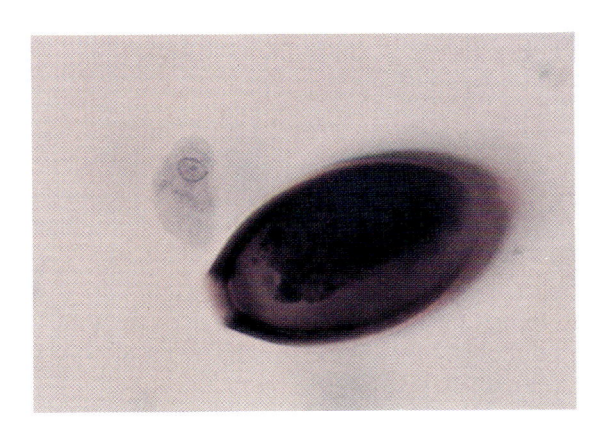

large-cell neoplasms but most lymphocytes are very similar in size in any single neoplasm (Plate 7). Nuclei can be round, indented or cleaved. Chromatin clumping is variable but nucleoli are usually prominent. Mitotic figures may be very few to frequent. Cytoplasm is scant to moderate in amount and stains intensely blue. Occasionally small clear vacuoles are present in the cytoplasm. Cytoplasmic projections, cytoplasmic fragments and lysed or smudged cells may be numerous in some smears. (See Chapter 8 on lymph node cytology for further discussion of lymphosarcoma.)

Though other tumors, such as leiomyomas, leiomyosarcomas and adenocarcinomas, occur in the large intestine, rectal scraping is usually not diagnostic. Generally, these tumors either originate within or penetrate the muscularis mucosa and involve the lamina propria only minimally. Likewise, scrapings of discrete masses that protrude into the intestinal lumen (such as polyps and adenomas) may also be nondiagnostic. This is because material obtained by scraping the surface of such tumors is not necessarily representative of the entire mass. In such instances, biopsy of the lesion is a more appropriate diagnostic technique.

References

1. Lorenz, in Ettinger: *Textbook of Veterinary Internal Medicine.* Saunders, Philadelphia, 1983. pp 1346-1372.

2. Barsanti, in Greene: *Clinical Microbiology and Infectious Diseases of the Dog and Cat.* Saunders, Philadelphia, 1984. pp 687-699.

3. Barsanti, in Greene: *Clinical Microbiology and Infectious Diseases of the Dog and Cat.* Saunders, Philadelphia, 1984. pp 700-709.

4. Tyler, in Greene: *Clinical Microbiology and Infectious Diseases of the Dog and Cat.* Saunders, Philadelphia, 1984. pp 747-756.

5. Kirkpatrick, in Greene: *Clinical Microbiology and Infectious Diseases of the Dog and Cat.* Saunders, Philadelphia, 1984. pp 806-823.

Plate 1

Figure 1. Nondegenerate neutrophils. Note the tightly clumped, dark-staining (basophilic) nuclear chromatin. (Wright's stain, original maginification 250X)

Figure 2. A hypersegmented neutrophil. Hypersegmentation is an age-related change. (Wright's stain, original magnification 250X)

Figure 3. A toxic band neutrophil (arrow) and a reactive lymphocyte. Toxic changes develop in neutrophils during their production in the bone marrow, and are caused by inflammation. (Wright's stain, original magnification 250X)

Figure 4. Neutrophils showing hydropic degeneration (degenerate neutrophils). Hydropic degeneration develops in neutrophils after they have migrated from the blood into an area of inflammation. It is caused by toxins such as endotoxin. Note that the nuclear chromatin is spread out, fills up more of the cytoplasm and stains more eosinophilic than that of the nondegenerate neutrophil. Bacterial rods (arrows) are present within the cytoplasm of some neutrophils on the side. A pyknotic cell with round, somewhat eosinophilic spheres of nuclear chromatin is also present (double arrow). (Wright's stain, original magnification 250X)

Figure 5. Plasma cells (arrows), characterized by an eccentric round nucleus with abundant deep blue cytoplasm and a prominent clear Golgi apparatus, and small lymphocytes. (Wright's stain, original magnification 250X).

Figure 6. Several lymphoblasts, characterized by their moderate amount of bluish cytoplasm and finely stippled nuclear chromatin and prominent nucleolus. (Wright's stain, original magnification 250X)

Figure 7. A reactive lymphocyte, characterized by an increased amount of bluish cytoplasm. (Wright's stain, original magnification 250X)

Figure 8. A reactive lymphocyte. (Wright's stain, original magnification 250X)

Plate 1

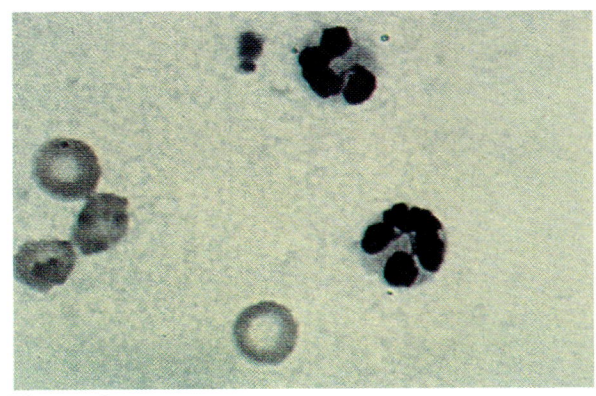

Figure 1

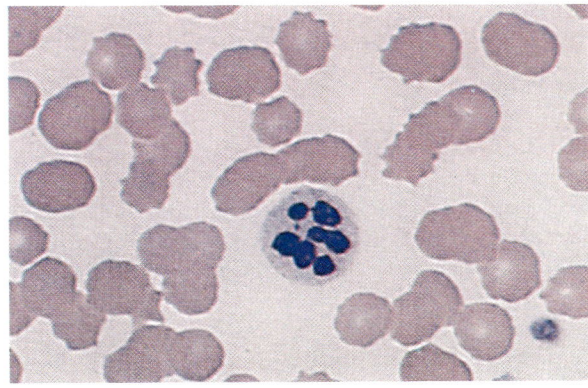

Figure 2

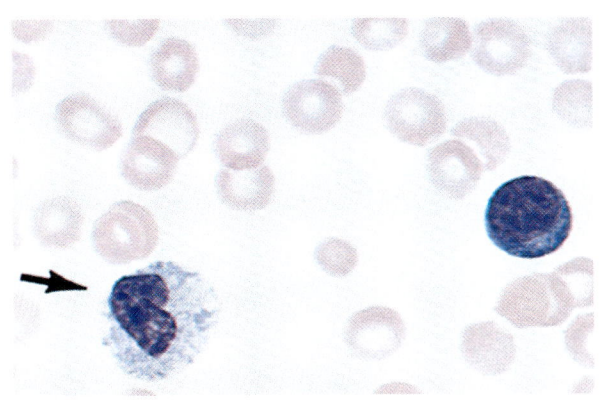

Figure 3

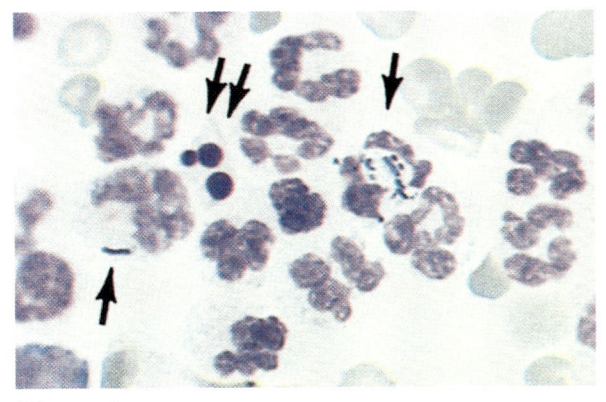

Figure 4

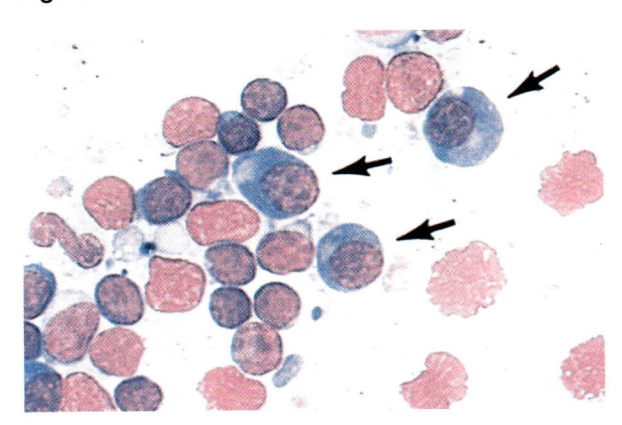

Figure 5

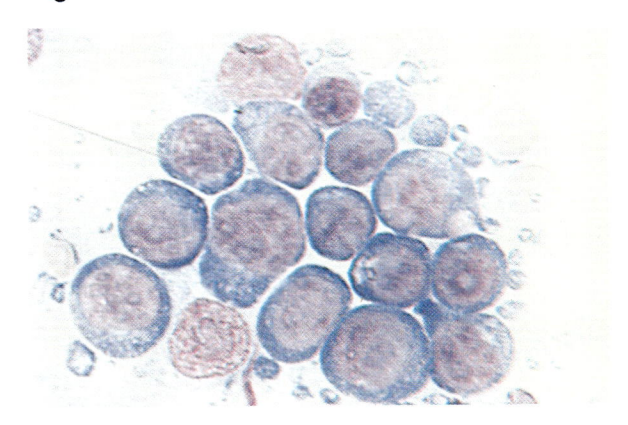

Figure 6

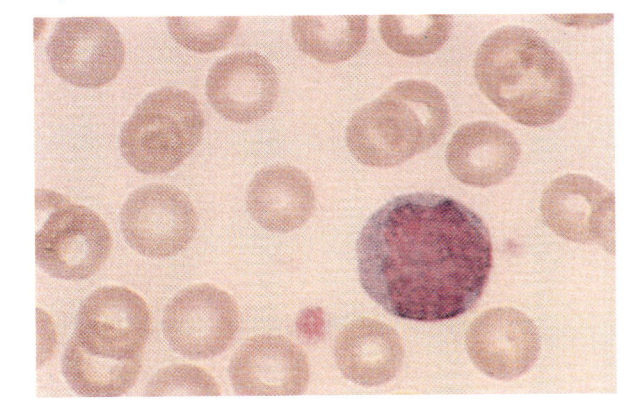

Figure 7

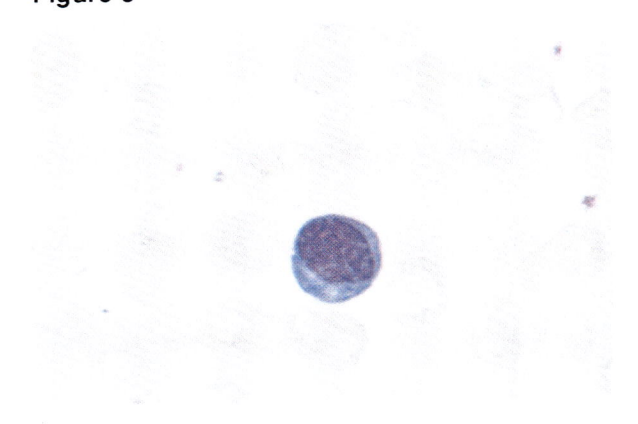

Figure 8

Plate 2

Figure 1. Large foamy macrophages with intracytoplasmic golden hematoidin crystals. Hematoidin is a product of erythrocyte breakdown and is often referred to as tissue bilirubin. It indicates intratissue or intracavity hemorrhage. (Wright's stain, original magnification 250X)

Figure 2. A macrophage showing erythrophagocytosis. (Wright's stain, original magnification 250X) (Courtesy of Oklahoma State University)

Figure 3. An epithelioid macrophage. (Wright's stain, original magnification 250X)

Figure 4. Three foamy macrophages from peritoneal fluid. (Wright's stain, original magnification 100X)

Figure 5. *Left insert:* A canine eosinophil, characterized by variably sized, round, eosinophilic intracytoplasmic granules. (Wright's stain, original magnification 250X)

Right insert: A feline eosinophil, characterized by rod-shaped eosinophilic granules. A dysplastic fibroblast is also present. (Wright's stain, original magnification 250X)

Figure 6. A feline basophil, characterized by numerous, round, lavender, intracytoplasmic granules. (Diff-Quik stain, original magnification 250X)

Figure 7. A canine basophil, characterized by scattered, round, red-purple, intracytoplasmic granules. (Diff-Quik stain, original magnification 250X)

Figure 8. *Left insert:* Cutaneous mast cells, characterized by round to oval nuclei and numerous red-purple granules. In some mast-cell tumors, granules may be sparse. Sometimes Diff-Quik does not stain mast-cell granules. Eosinophils are also present. (Wright's stain, original magnification 250X)

Right insert: Two mast cells and an eosinophil in peritoneal fluid. Mast cells in fluids frequently "pole" their granules to one side. Occasionally, the nucleus fails to take stain or stains only poorly. (Wright's stain, original magnification 100X)

Plate 2

Figure 1

Figure 2

Figure 3

Figure 4

Figure 5

Figure 6

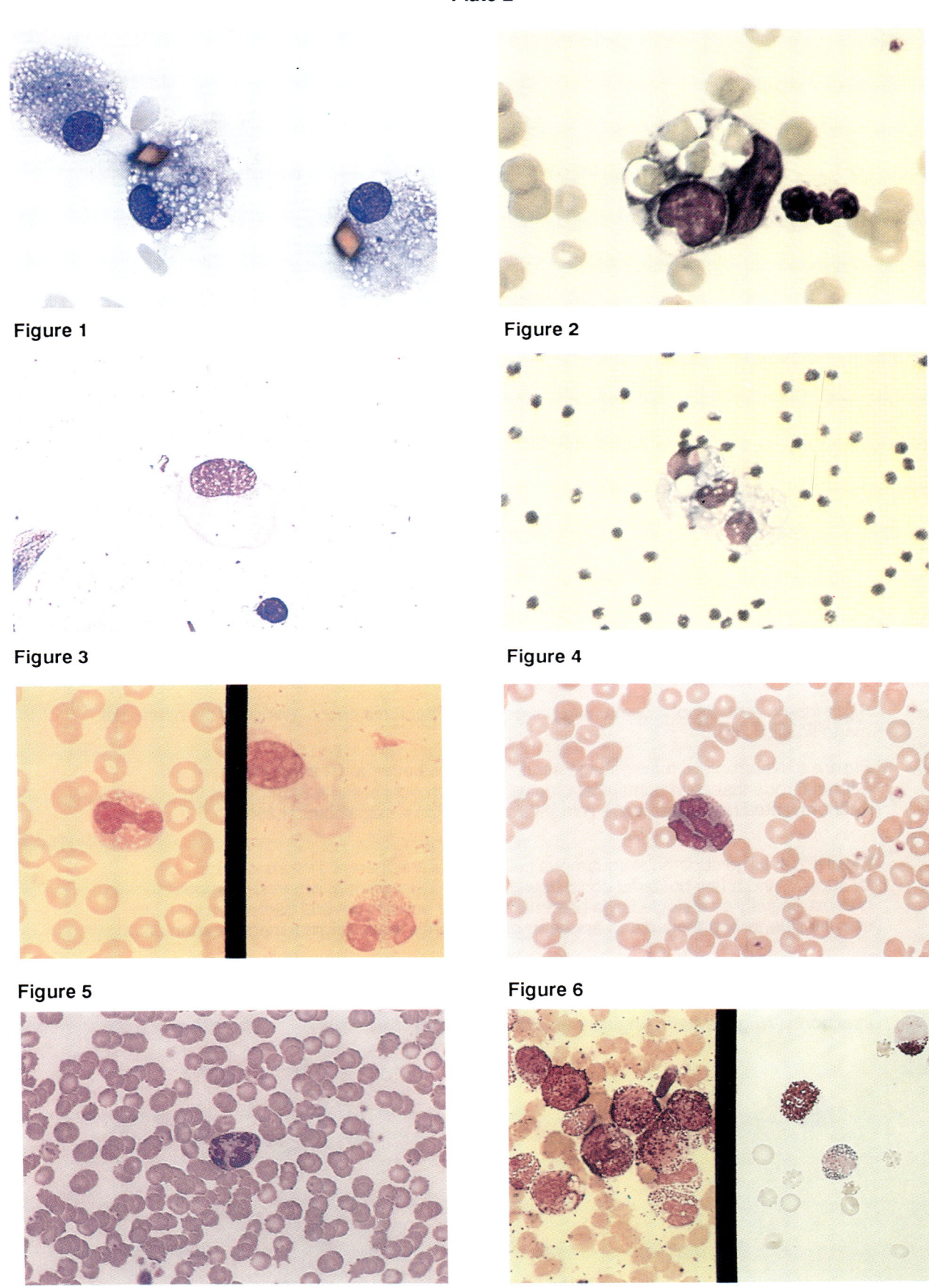

Figure 7

Figure 8

243

Plate 3

Figure 1. Purulent inflammation is characterized by the predominance of neutrophils. Many of the neutrophils in this slide are degenerate. (Wright's stain, original magnification 100X)

Figure 2. Pyogranulomatous inflammation from a dog with blastomycosis. A *Blastomyces dermatitidis* organism (arrow) is in the center of the field. Neutrophils, macrophages and an inflammatory giant cell are present. (Wright's stain, original magnification 100X)

Figure 3. Eosinophilic inflammation is characterized by large numbers of eosinophils. The eosinophils in this slide are readily recognized by their intracytoplasmic round eosinophilc granules. (Wright's stain, original magnification 250X)

Figure 4. *Left insert:* Numerous small, bipolar bacterial rods are present extracellularly. (Wright's stain, original magnification 250X)

Right insert: Several degenerate neutrophils. One neutrophil contains phagocytized bacterial rods. (Wright's stain, original magnification 330X)

Figure 5. *Left insert:* Many bacterial cocci are present extracellularly. (Wright's stain, original magnification 250X)

Right insert: A neutrophil containing phagocytized bacterial cocci. (Wright's stain, original magnification 250X)

Figure 6. Neutrophils, macrophages and numerous bacteria. The long filamentous bacterial rods that stain somewhat blue with reddish dots are characteristic of the Actinomycetes family (arrows). (Wright's stain, original magnification 250X)

Figure 7. A large superficial squamous cell with many adherent *Simonsiella* bacteria on its surface and a few bacterial cocci (lower center). *Simonsiella* organisms appear microscopically as a single large bacterium but are actually several bacterial rods lying side by side, giving the striated appearance. (Wright's stain, original magnification 250X)

Figure 8. A neutrophil containing a phagocytized spore-forming bacillus. The spore is recognized as a clear area in the bacterium. This slide is from a dog with a clostridial infection. (Wright's stain, original magnification 250X)

Plate 3

Figure 1

Figure 2

Figure 3

Figure 4

Figure 5

Figure 6

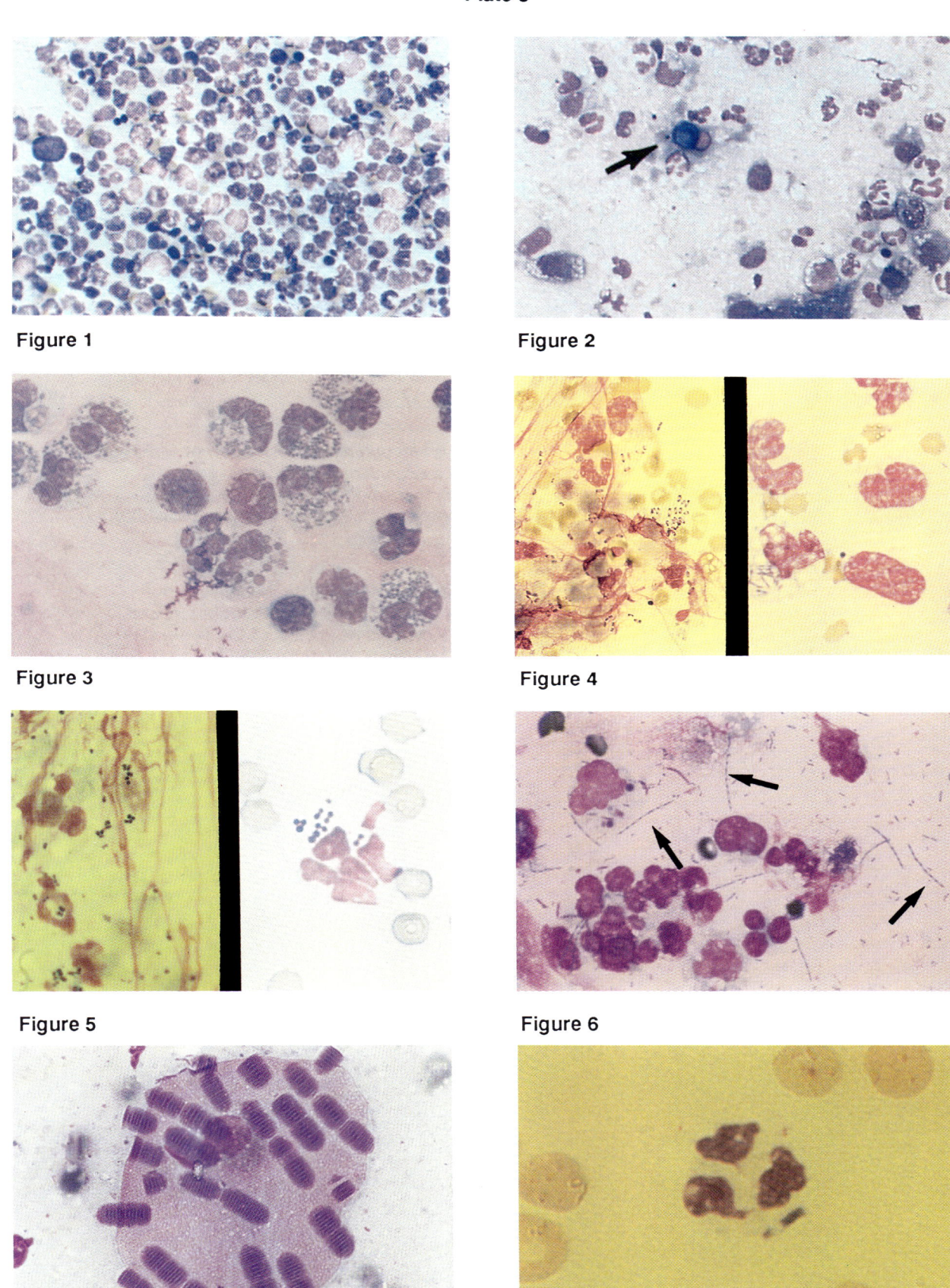

Figure 7

Figure 8

245

Plate 4

Figure 1. Fine-needle aspirate of a consolidated pulmonary mass. An alveolar macrophage containing nonstaining bacterial rods identified as clear streaks through the cell (arrow) is suggestive of a *Mycobacterium* infection. Numerous neutrophils are also present. (Wright's stain, original magnification 400X)

Figure 2. Acid-fast stain from the same dog as in Figure 1, showing the reddish filamentous *Mycobacterium* organisms (arrows). (Acid-fast stain, original magnification 300X)

Figure 3. A large macrophage containing numerous *Histoplasma capsulatum* organisms is in the center of the field. *Histoplasma capsulatum* organisms are small (1-4 μ in diameter), round to oval, yeast-like organisms. They have a dark blue/purple-staining nucleus surrounded by a very thin, clear halo. (Wright's stain, original magnification 330X) (Courtesy of Oklahoma State University)

Figure 4. A neutrophil containing numerous *Sporothrix schenckii* organisms in the center of the field. *Sporothrix schenckii* organisms are small (1-4 μ in diameter), round to oval, with a thin, clear halo. *Sporothrix schenckii* organisms are about the same size as *Histoplasma capsulatum* organisms. They can be differentiated by identifying the oval or oblong (cigar) shape that some, but not all, of the organisms have. (Wright's stain, original magnification 250X)

Figure 5. *Blastomyces dermatitidis* (arrows) is a bluish, spherical, thick-walled, yeast-like organism in Romanowsky-stained smears. The organisms are 8-20 μ in diameter. Occasionally, a single broad-based bud may be present. (Wright's stain, original magnification 250X)

Figure 6. *Blastomyces dermatitidis* organisms (arrows). (Wright's stain, original magnification 250X)

Figure 7. A budding *Blastomyces dermatitidis* organism (arrow). (Wright's stain, original magnification 100X)

Figure 8. *Cryptococcus neoformans* is a spherical, yeast-like organism that frequently has a thick, clear-staining, mucoid capsule. The organism with its capsule ranges in size from 8 to 40 μ. Occasionally, a single narrow-based bud may be present. Numerous budding and nonbudding *Cryptococcus neoformans* organisms with prominent nonstaining capsules are shown. (Wright's stain, original magnification 250X)

Plate 4

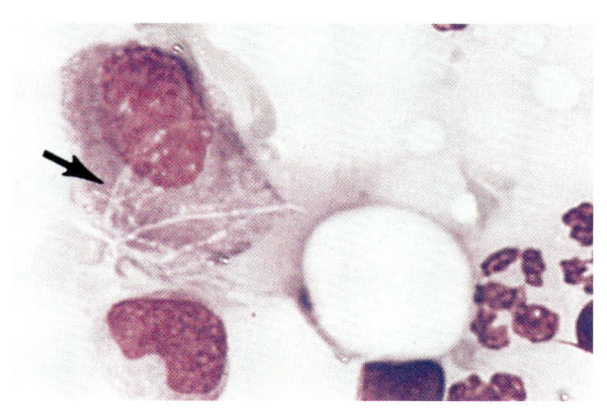

Figure 1

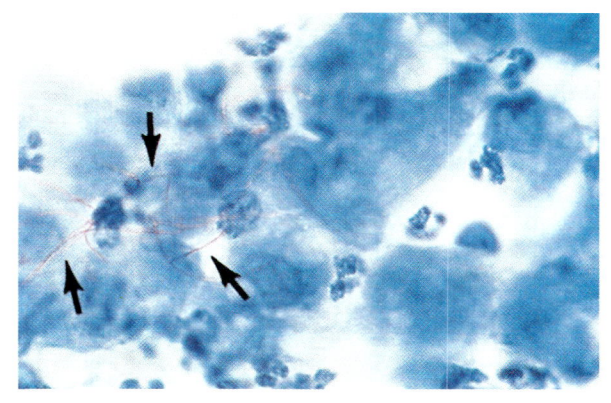

Figure 2

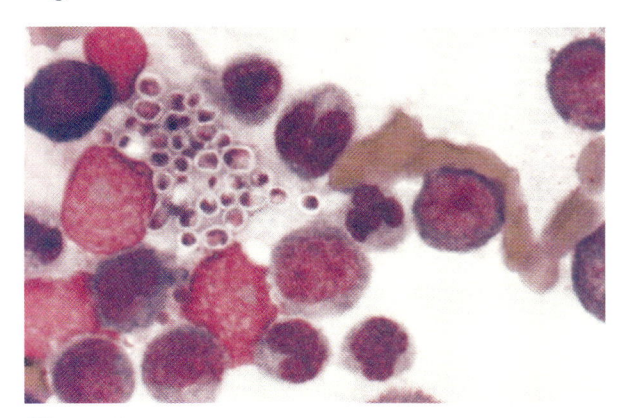

Figure 3

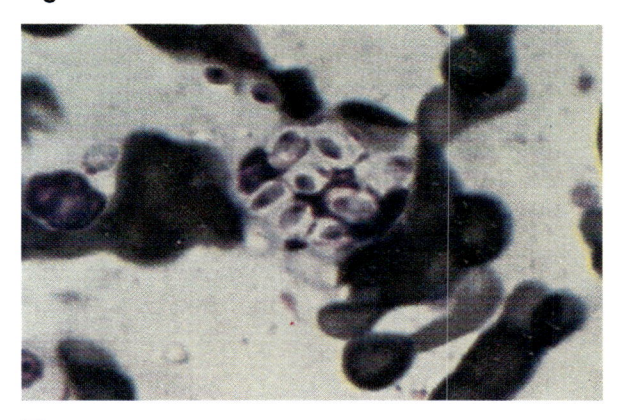

Figure 4

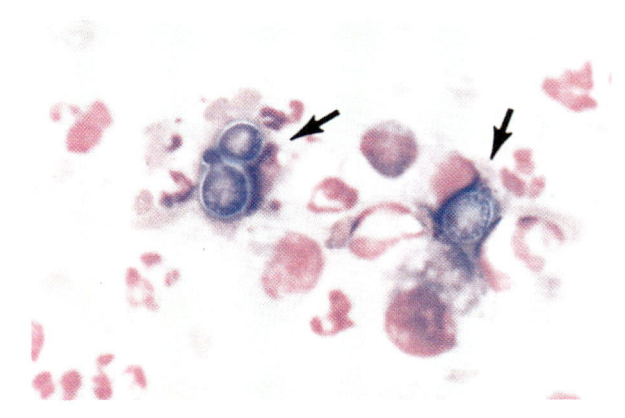

Figure 5

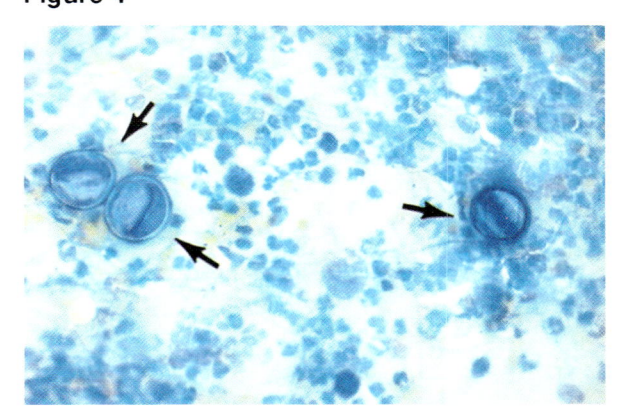

Figure 6

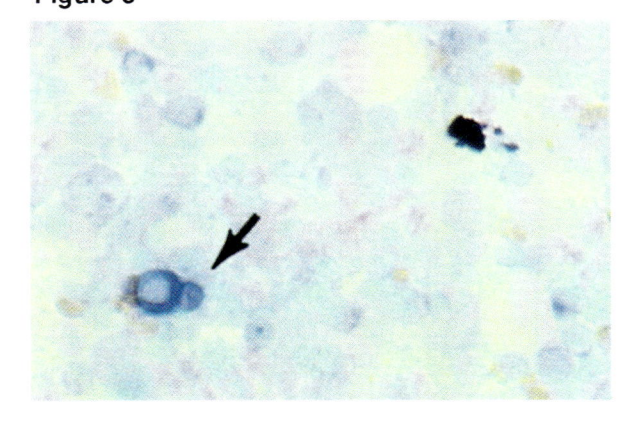

Figure 7

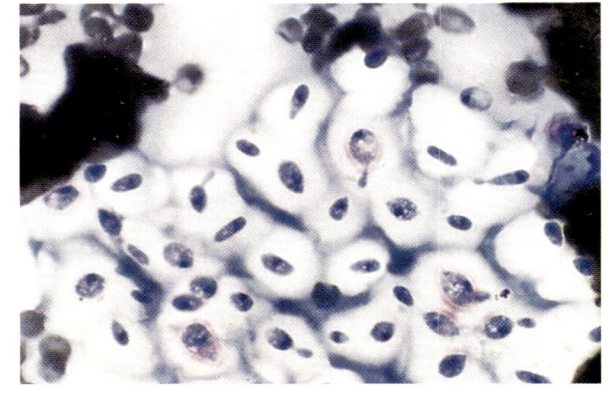

Figure 8

# Plate 5

Figure 1. Transtracheal wash from a dog with coccidioidomycosis. *Coccidioides immitis* organisms are large, double-contoured, blue-staining, spherical bodies (10-100 μ in diameter). Occasionally, endospores varying from 2 to 5 μ in diameter may be seen within some of the larger spherules.

Left insert: A large *Coccidioides immitis* spherule with a thick, deeply stained wall surrounded by neutrophils. The wall is out of focus becuase the rigid nature of the wall causes it to be out of the focal plane of the camera when the inflammatory cells are in focus. (Wright's stain, original magnification 400X)

Right insert: Same as the left insert except the wall of the organism is in focus and the neutrophils in the background are out of focus. (Wright's stain, original magnification 400X) (Courtesy of Dr. Zinkl, University of California)

Figure 2. *Prototheca* organisms (arrows) are round to oval, 1.3-13.4 μ wide and 1.3-16.1 μ long. They have granular basophilic cytoplasms and a clear cell wall. (Wright's stain, original magnification 250X)

Figure 3. Numerous fungal hyphae. The many macrophages and neutrophils indicate a pyogranulomatous response. (Wright's stain, original magnification 250X)

Figure 4. The negative image of a nonstaining fungal hyphae can be seen in the background of inflammatory cells. Some fungi do not stain with the routine Romanowsky stains. However, most stain with new methylene blue. (Wright's stain, original magnification 50X) (Courtesy of Dr. Latimer, University of Georgia)

Figure 5. Two huge mononuclear cells with abundant cytoplasm, an eccentric nucleus and prominent nucleolus. These cells contain many developing *Cytauxzoon* merozoites, which appear as either small, dark-staining bodies or larger irregularly defined clusters. (Wright's stain, original magnification 250X) (Courtesy of Dr. French, Cornell University)

Figure 6. *Toxoplasma gondii* tachyzoites appear as small, crescent-shaped bodies. The cytoplasm is generally light blue. A dark-staining pericentral nucleus is present.

Left insert: A *Toxoplasma gondii* organism (arrow) in a transtracheal wash from a dog. (Wright's stain, original magnification 250X)

Right insert: A cluster of *Toxoplasma gondii* organisms in a lung impression from a cat. (Wright's stain, original magnification 300X)

Figure 7. Numerous *Leishmania donovani* organisms within a mononuclear phagocyte and extracellularly. *Leishmania donovani* organisms are small and round to oval. They have clear to very light blue cytoplasm, an oval nucleus, and a small, dark, ventral kinetoplast. (Wright's stain, original magnification 300X)

Figure 8. Lung imprint. A *Pneumocystis carinii* cyst (arrow) is in the center. *Pneumocystis carinii* cysts are 5-10 μ in diameter and usually contain 4-8 intracystic bodies 1-2 μ in diameter. With Romanowsky stains, intact cysts are distinctive in appearance, but the free trophozoites are difficult to differentiate from debris. (Wright's stain, original magnification 250X)

Plate 5

Figure 1

Figure 2

Figure 3

Figure 4

Figure 5

Figure 6

Figure 7

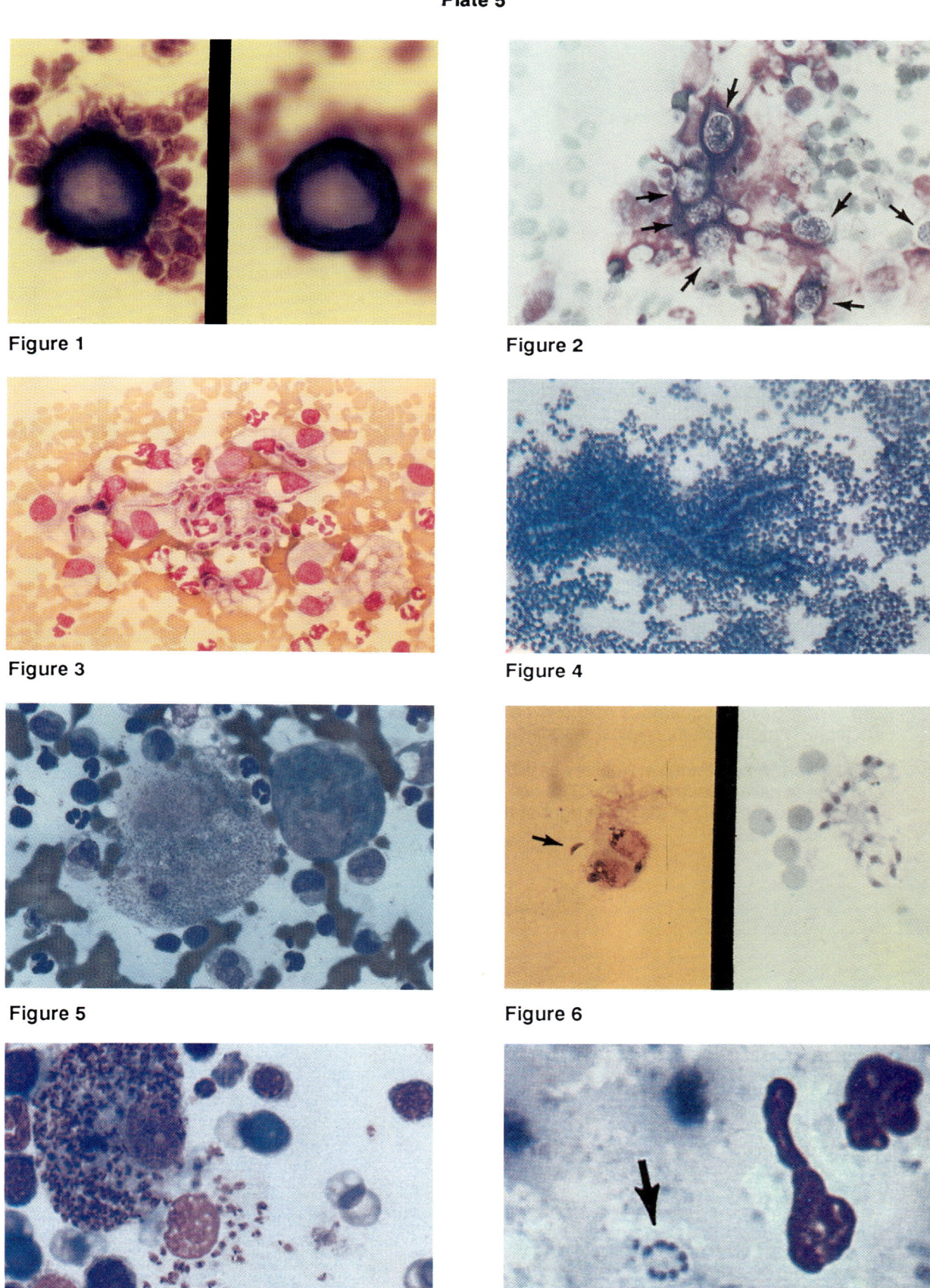

Figure 8

249

Plate 6

Figure 1. Lung imprint. Two cells contain *Ehrlichia canis* morulae (arrows). (Wright's stain, original magnification 330X)

Figure 2. Aspirate from a lymph node with metastatic carcinoma. Several carcinoma cells and neutrophils are present. (Courtesy of Dr. Duncan, University of Georgia)

Figure 3. Aspirate from a sebaceous adenoma. A cluster or acinus of sebaceous cells is shown. (Wright's stain, original magnification 250X)

Figure 4. Aspirate of a bronchoalveolar adenocarcinoma in a dog. A cluster of malignant glandular epithelial cells is shown. Note the large clear vacuole in one of the cells, suggesting glandular origin. Also notice the coarse chromatin pattern, anisocytosis, anisokaryosis and prominent large nucleoli. One of the cells has a nucleolus that is larger than the RBC present (arrow). (Wright's stain, original magnification 250X)

Figure 5. Four basal squamous cells and 3 mature superficial squamous cells. (Wright's stain, original magnification 100X) (Courtesy of Dr. Andreasen, University of Georgia)

Figure 6. Aspirate from a squamous-cell carcinoma in a dog.

Left insert: Several squamous epithelial cells with perinuclear vacuolation and prominent nucleoli. (Wright's stain, original magnification 100X)

Right insert: A squamous epithelial cell with a tail of cytoplasm. These cells are sometimes called "tadpole" cells. The cell has a nucleolus that is larger than $10\,\mu$ (compare to the RBC at the lower right of the photograph). (Wright's stain, original magnification 250X)

Plate 6

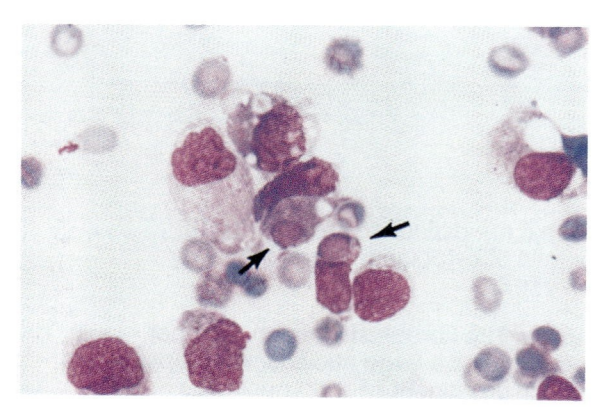

Figure 1

Figure 2

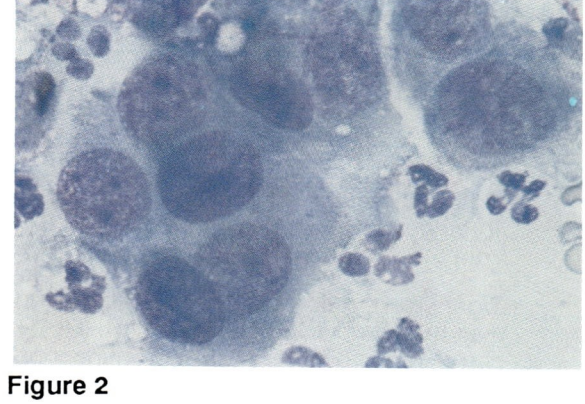

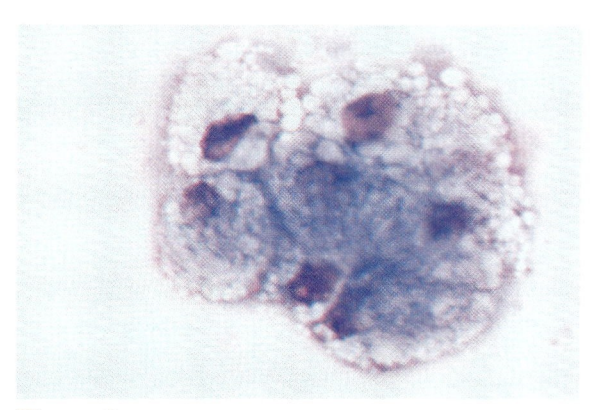

Figure 3

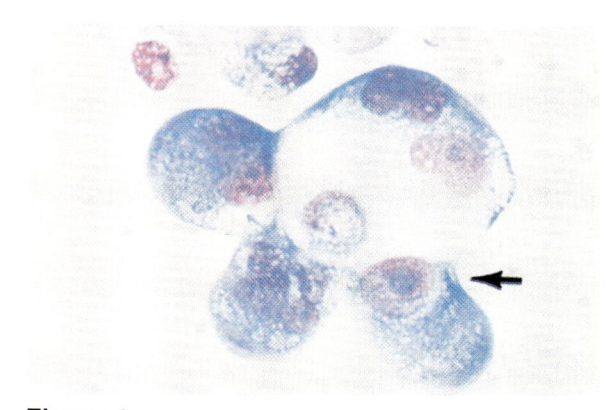

Figure 4

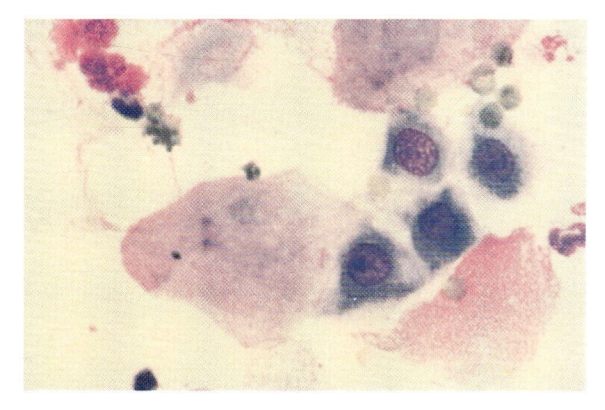

Figure 5

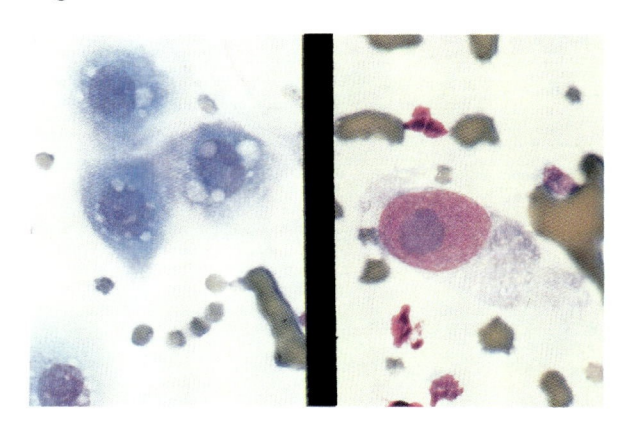

Figure 6

Plate 7

Figure 1. *Left insert:* Two fibrocytes and several cells that are difficult to identify. The 2 fibrocytes have long slender nuclei, with long slender tails of cytoplasm streaming away from the nuclei. (Wright's stain, original magnification 250X)

Right insert: A fibroblast, 3 eosinophils and 2 neutrophils. The fibroblast is much plumper than the fibrocytes in the left insert. It is dysplastic and contains a large nucleus, with ropy chromatin and either 2 large prominent nucleoli or 1 large prominent bilobed nucleolus. This is an aspirate from an eosinophilic granuloma in a cat. (Wright's stain, original magnification 250X)

Figure 2. *Left insert:* Aspirate from a hemangiopericytoma in a dog. Numerous spindle-shaped cells are present along with many RBCs. (Wright's stain, original magnification 250X)

Right insert: Aspirate from a hemangioma in a dog. Several spindle-shaped cells are present along with some blood components. Note how the nuclei of the hemangioma cells appear very thin and capable of folding over upon themselves. (Wright's stain, original magnification 250X)

Figure 3. Aspirate from a malignant spindle-cell tumor.

Left insert: Several spindle cells with criteria of malignancy including anisocytosis; coarse chromatin; large, prominent, variably sized and occasionally angular nucleoli; and increased nucleus:cytoplasm ratio. (Wright's stain, original magnification 250X)

Right insert: A higher magnification of cells from the same sarcoma showing large, prominent variably sized and angular nucleoli. (Wright's stain, original magnification 330X)

Figure 4. Aspirate from a highly granulated mast-cell tumor. The granules are so dense in some mast cells that they obscure the nucleus. Other mast cells contain nuclei that stain weakly because of the affinity of the cytoplasmic granules for the stain. Several eosinophils (arrows) are also present but are difficult to recognize because the light intensity required to photograph the mast cells was so great it did not allow the eosinophil granules to be visualized. (Wright's stain, original magnification 100X)

Figure 5. Aspirate from a poorly granulated mast-cell tumor. Numerous mast cells are present along with a few eosinophils. Many of the mast cells contain only a few red-purple granules in their cytoplasm, and some of the mast cells appear not to contain any granules. (Wright's stain, original magnification 100X)

Figure 6. Aspirate from a transmissible venereal tumor (TVT). Numerous TVT cells with coarse chromatin, 1-2 prominent large nucleoli, and smoky gray vacuolated cytoplasm are shown. (Wright's stain, original magnification 250X)

Figure 7. Aspirate from a lymphomatous lymph node in a dog. Over 50% of the lymphoid cells are lymphoblasts. They are larger than the small lymphocytes that are also present. (Wright's stain, original magnification 330X) (Courtesy of Oklahoma State University)

Plate 7

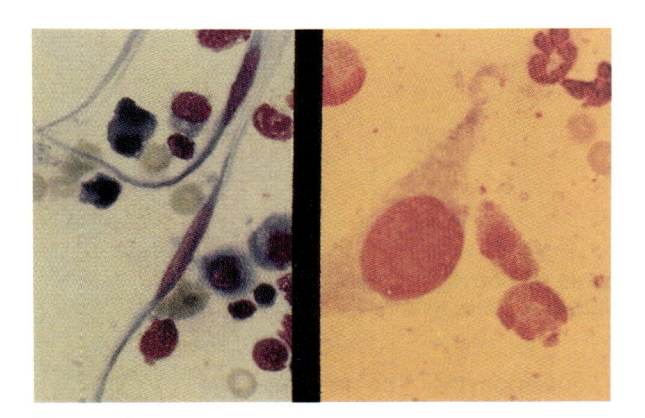

Figure 1

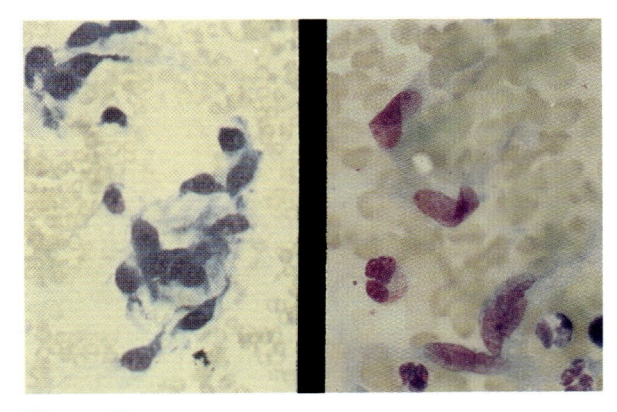

Figure 2

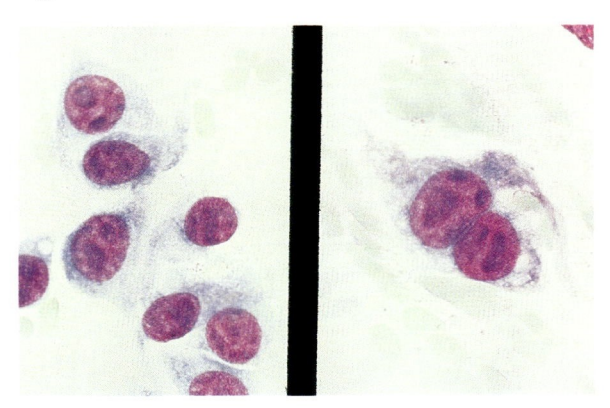

Figure 3

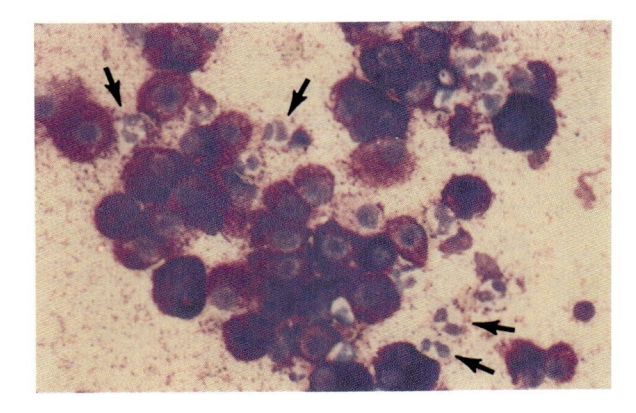

Figure 4

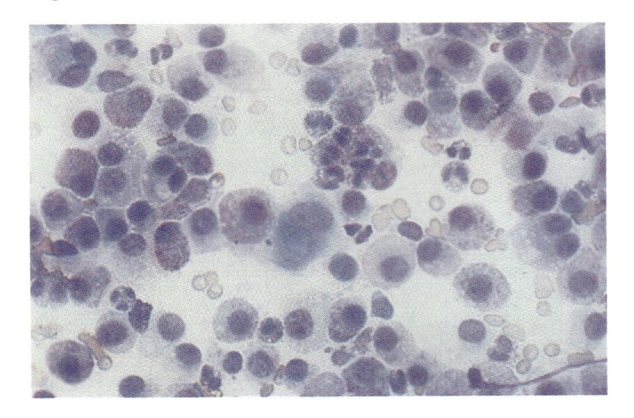

Figure 5

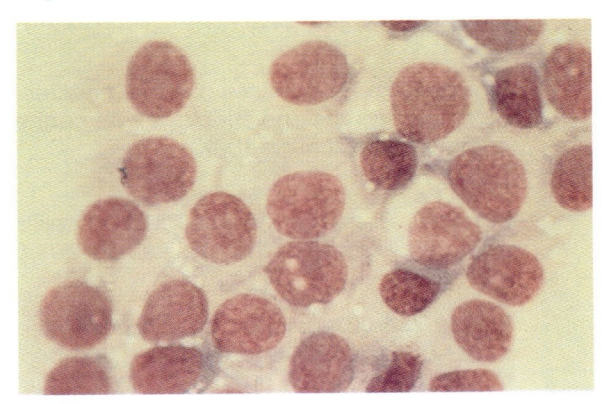

Figure 6

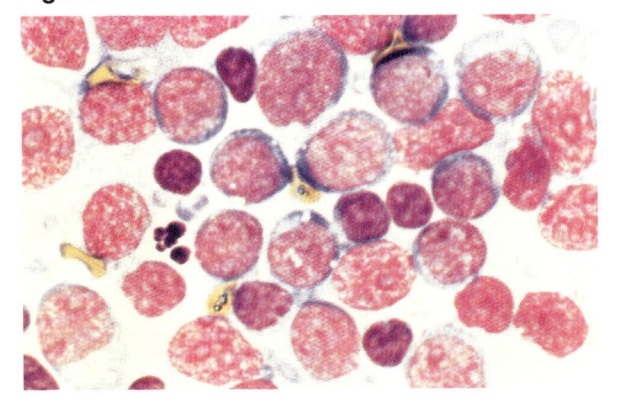

Figure 7

253

Plate 8

Figure 1. *Left insert:* Smear from a melanoma that was so heavily pigmented that most cellular and nuclear detail was obscured. This is often the case. (Wright's stain) (Courtesy of Dr. Prasse, University of Georgia)

Right insert: A melanophage (uppermost cell) and 2 melanocytes. The melanophage contains granules that are larger than those of the melanocytes. One of the melanocytes is more densely granulated than the other, but its granules are smaller than those of the melanophage. (Wright's stain, original magnification 250X)

Figure 2. Aspirate from a malignant melanoma. Several melanoma cells containing melanin pigment are present. Numerous criteria of malignancy are seen. These include anisocytosis; coarse chromatin; increased nucleus:cytoplasm ratio; and prominent, variably sized and often angular nucleoli. (Wright's stain, original magnification 250X)

Figure 3. A sheet of mesothelial cells obtained while attempting a hepatic aspirate in a dog. Mesothelial cells line the abdominal and thoracic cavities and can be accidentally collected while obtaining aspirates from organs or fluid in these cavities. (Wright's stain, original magnification 100X) (Courtesy of Dr. Meyer, University of Florida)

Figure 4. Aspirate from a lipoma in a dog. Numerous fat cells are present. They are large and round, with pyknotic nuclei and clear cytoplasm (though many have a pink cast). (Wright's stain, original magnification 25X)

Figure 5. Three granules of glove powder (arrows). Glove powder is a common artifact on cytologic smears and should not be confused with an organism cell. (Wright's stain, original magnification 100X)

Figure 6. Bone marrow aspirate. A capillary is shown stretching across the photomicrograph. (Wright's stain, original magnification 100X)

Figure 7. A cluster of hepatocytes with an interposed microfilaria. Microfilariae are occasionally seen secondary to blood contamination on cytologic smears from microfilaremic dogs. (Wright's stain, original magnification 100X) (Courtesy of Dr. Meyer, University of Florida)

Plate 8

Figure 1

Figure 2

Figure 3

Figure 4

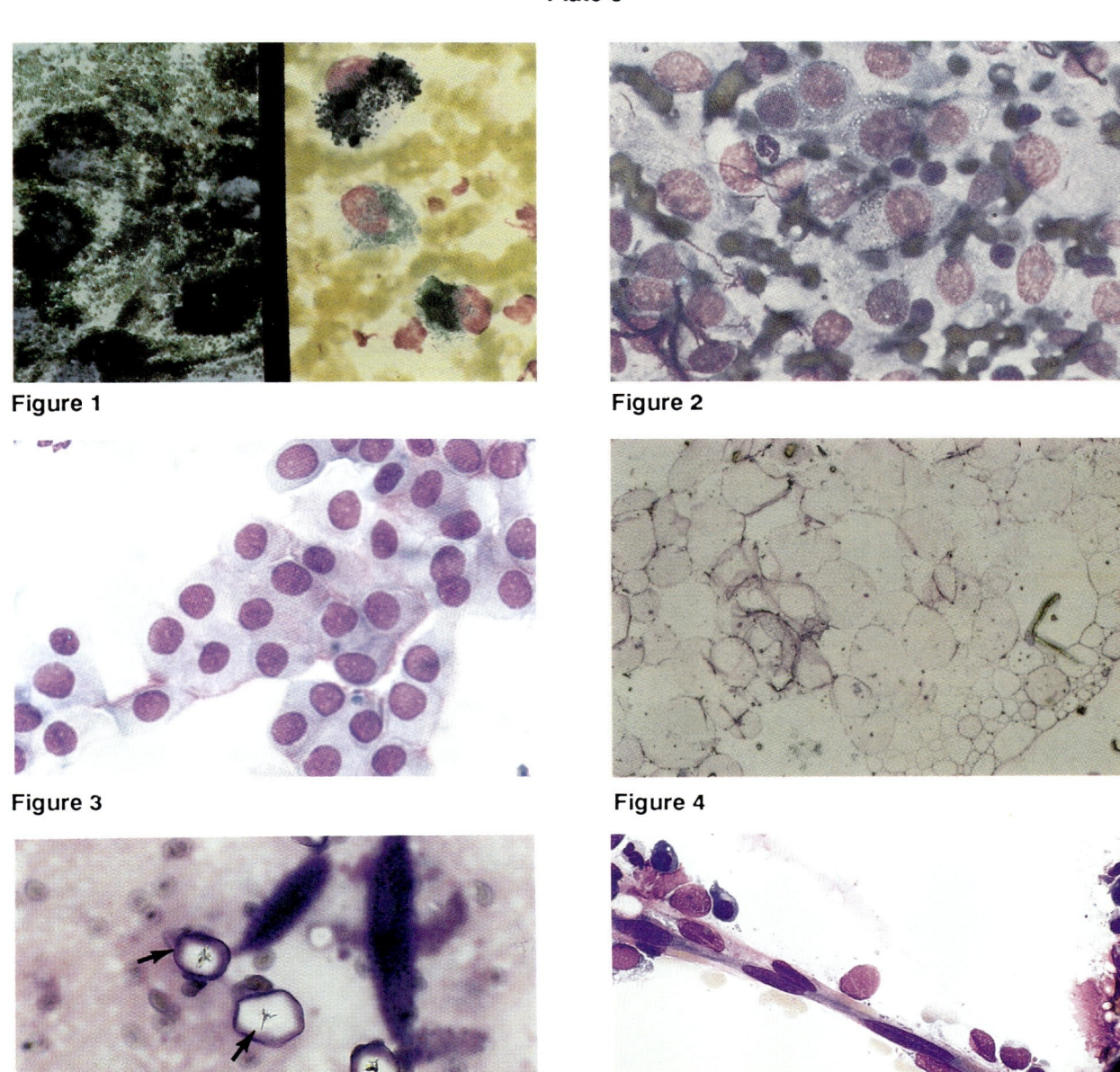

Figure 5

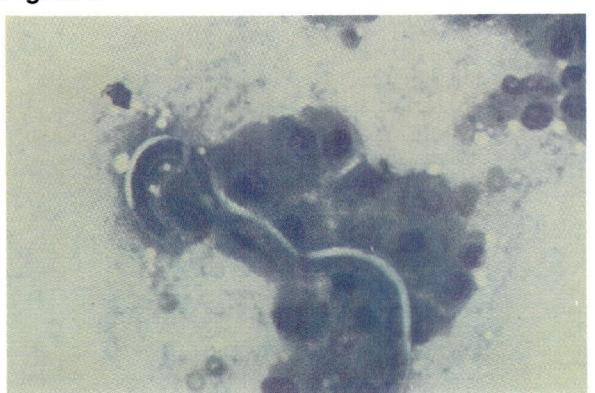

Figure 6

Figure 7

255

Index

A

Abdominal fluid, 151-166
    abdominocentesis, 152
    ascites, 163
    bile peritonitis, 163
    cell counts, 154
    cell types, 155-162
    culture, 154
    effusions, 155-166
    exudates, 160-162
    feline infectious peritonitis, 162, 163
    glove powder, 157
    hemoperitoneum, 165
    hemorrhagic effusion, 165
    mesothelial cells, 155, 156
    neoplastic effusions, 165, 166
    peritonitis, 162, 163
    protein content, 154
    sample collection, 152
    smear preparation, 152-154
    transudates, 158-160
    uroperitoneum, 163
Abdominocentesis, 152
Abscesses, 44, 45, 209, 210, 219
Acid-fast stain, 27, 246
Acinar-cell tumors, 88
Actinomyces, 27, 138, 155, 184, 244
Adenocarcinomas, 51, 59, 86, 88, 166, 177, 185, 186, 220, 250
Adenoma, 250
Aelurostrongylus abstrusus, 175
Allergic reactions, 30, 184
Allergic rhinitis, 52
Alveolar cells, 182
Amyloidosis, 195
Anaplasia, 2
Anemia, 112, 114
Anestrus, 230
Anthracotic pigment, 176
Anticancer therapy, 187
Aqueous flare, 72
Aqueous humor, 72
Arthritis, 129-133
Arthrocentesis, 121-123
Artifacts, staining, 10, 11
Ascites, 163
Aspergillus, 49, 71, 176, 185, 210
Aspiration, 4-9
    abdominal fluid, 152
    aqueous humor, 72
    bladder, 213
    bone marrow, 99-103
    cerebrospinal fluid, 143
    cutaneous, 21-23
    cystocentesis, 213
    hepatic, 189, 190
    joint, 121-123
    kidney, 207, 208
    liver, 189, 190
    lung, 179-181
    lymph nodes, 93
    masses, 4-9, 21-23
    orbit, 74
    peritoneal fluid, 152
    pleural fluid, 151, 152
    procedure, 4, 5
    prostate, 217
    renal, 207, 208
    skin, 21-23
    smear preparation, 5-9
    spleen, 199-201
    synovial fluid, 121-123
    testicular, 220
    thoracic fluid, 151, 152
    tracheal, 167-171
    urine, 213
    vitreous body, 73

B

Babesia, 199, 202
Bacilli, 27
Bacillus, 28
Bacteria, see Infectious agents
Balantidium coli, 238
Band cells, 106
Basal cells, 226
Basal-cell tumors, 37, 38
Basket cells, 108, 157
Basophils, 106, 242
Bile duct carcinoma, 193
Bile peritonitis, 163
Bile pigment, 191
Bladder, aspiration, 213
Blastomyces dermatitidis, 28, 29, 63, 72, 73, 96, 131, 138, 176, 185, 210, 220, 244, 246
Blepharitis, 63
Bone, cortical, 137-140, also see Bone marrow
    chondroid, 139
    neoplasia, 138-140
    osteoid, 138
    osteomyelitis, 137, 138
    sample collection, 137
    tumors, 138-140
Bone marrow, 99-119
    aspiration biopsy, 100
    cells, 103-108
    core biopsy, 103
    evaluation, 109-119
    Mott's cells, 107, 118
    myelofibrosis, 118
    myeloid:erythroid ratio, 112-117
    sample collection, 99-103
Breeding, time of, 230
Bronchial washes, see Tracheal washes
Brucella canis, 220

C

Candida, 71, 78, 210
Canine distemper, 66
Capillaria aerophila, 50, 175
Capillary, 254
Carcinomas, 72, 86, 90, 97, 166, 177, 192, 193, 209, 211, 250
Carcinosarcomas, 43
Cerebrospinal fluid, 141-149
    cell counts, 144
    characteristics, 144
    coagulation, 144
    color, 144
    cytologic examination, 144-146
    enzymes, 147, 148
    glucose, 148
    myelography, 146
    neoplasia, 146
    pleocytosis, 145, 146
    proteins, 146, 147
    sample collection, 143
    turbidity, 144
Chalazion, 64
Charcot-Leyden crystals, 175
Cherry eye, 69
Chlamydia psittaci, 66, 67, 232
Cholangitis, 194
Cholesterol clefts, 45
Cholesterol concentration, 164
Cholesterol crystals, 45, 90
Cholesterol:triglyceride ratio, 164
Chondrosarcoma, 52, 139
Chromatin patterns, 2, 3
Chylous effusions, pleural, 156, 160, 163-165
Cladosporium, 70
Clostridium, 28
Coccidioides immitis, 2, 28, 29, 131, 138, 176, 185, 210, 248
Colitis, eosinophilic, 236, 237
    fungal, 237
    protozoal, 237, 238
Collagen necrosis, 31
Colon, see Rectum
Columnar epithelial cells, 56, 171, 181
Conjunctivitis, 65-68
Cornea, 70, 71
Corynebacterium, 131
Crenosoma vulpis, 175
Criteria of malignancy, 16, 17, 252
Cryptococcus neoformans, 28, 29, 49, 73, 96, 131, 176, 185, 210, 237, 246
Crystal-induced arthritis, 132
CSF, see Cerebrospinal fluid
Cuboidal epithelial cells, 56, 171, 181
Cultures, 18, 19, 154, 155
Curschmann's spirals, 171
Cystitis, 214, 215
Cystocentesis, 213
Cytauxzoon felis, 96, 176, 185, 199, 202, 248

D

Dacryocystitis, 69
Dacryops, 69
Demodex canis, 80
Demodex folliculorum, 63
Dermatitis, 23-31
Dermatophilus congolensis, 2, 29, 30
Dermatophytes, 29
Diestrus, 230
Diff-Quik stain, 2, 9
Dipetalonema, 157
DipStat stain, 9
Dirofilaria immitis, 157, 177
Döhle bodies, 155
Dyscrasia, 2
Dysplasia, 1, 173, 183, 185

E

Ear, 77-81
    ear mites, 79, 80
    neoplasia, 77, 80, 81
    otitis externa, 77-81
    Otobius megnini, 77
    Otodectes cynotis, 79, 80
    sample collection, 78
    tumors, 77, 80, 81
Effusions, 155-166
Ehrlichia, 108, 109, 117, 131, 155, 203, 250
Endophthalmitis, 73
Endospores, 248
Entamoeba histolytica, 238
Eosinophilic colitis, 236, 237
Eosinophilic conjunctivitis, 68
Eosinophilic granuloma, 30, 57, 68
Eosinophilic keratitis, 71
Eosinophilic plaques, 30
Eosinophils, 57, 106, 156, 172, 175, 183, 184, 242

Epididymitis, 220, 221
Epistaxis, 47
Epithelial cells, 97, 214
Epithelial tumors, 15, 33-37, 59
Epithelioid cells, 96, 97, 137
Epulis, 59
Erysipelothrix, 131
Erythrocytes, 105, 157, 173, 182, 215
Erythroid cells, 104, 105, 112, 203
Erythrophagocytosis, 118, 165, 242
Estrous cycle stages, 228-232
Estrus, 229, 232
Exophthalmos, 74
Extramedullary hematopoiesis, 196, 200, 203
Exudates, 160-162
Eye, 63-75
    aqueous flare, 72
    aqueous humor, 72
    blepharitis, 63
    chalazion, 64
    cherry eye, 69
    chlamydial conjunctivitis, 66, 67
    chronic superficial keratitis, 71
    conjunctivitis, 65-68
    cornea, 70, 71
    dacryocystitis, 69
    dacryops, 69
    endophthalmitis, 73
    eosinophilic conjunctivitis, 68
    eosinophilic keratitis, 71
    epithelial inclusion cyst, 71
    exophthalmos, 74
    follicular conjunctivitis, 69
    hemorrhage, intraocular, 74
    hordeolum, 64
    hyphema, 72
    hypopyon, 72
    iris, 72
    keratitis, 70, 71
    lacrimal duct cyst, 69
    lymphocytic-plasmacytic conjunctivitis, 68
    mast-cell conjunctivitis, 68
    mycoplasmal conjunctivitis, 67, 68
    nictitans, 68, 69
    neoplasia, 64, 71, 72, 74, 75
    neutrophilic conjunctivitis, 65-68
    nodular episcleritis, 70
    orbit, 74, 75
    pannus, 71
    parotid transposition cysts, 69
    plasmoma, 69
    postenucleation orbital cyst, 75
    sclera, 69, 70
    tumors, 64, 71, 72, 74, 75
    ulcers, corneal, 70, 71
    uveitis, 72
    vitreous body, 73, 74
    zygomatic mucocele, 68

F

Fat cells, 108, 254
Fat necrosis, 31
Feline infectious peritonitis, 162, 163, 185
Fibroblasts, 56, 57, 242, 252
Fibrocytes, 56, 70, 252
Fibromas, 40
Fibrosarcomas, 40, 52, 59, 139, 140, 206
Filamentous rods, 27, 184
Filaroides, 175
Fistulous tracts, 23
Foam cells, 84, 86
Follicular conjunctivitis, 69
Foreign bodies, 30
Fungal colitis, 237

Fungal hyphae, 248
Fusobacterium, 27, 184

G

Giant cells, 137, 176, 183, 244
Giant-cell tumors, 43
Giemsa stain, 2, 9
Glove powder, 157, 174, 182, 254
Goblet cells, 172, 181
Goiter, 89, 90
Golgi apparatus, 240
Granulocytes, 105, 106, 112

H

Heart disease, 163
Heinz bodies, 203
Hemangiomas, 41, 42, 252
Hemangiopericytomas, 41, 252
Hemangiosarcomas, 42, 52, 139, 204, 206
Hemarthrosis, 123, 127-129
Hematogones, 108
Hematoidin crystals, 70, 88, 177, 242
Hematologic stains, 2
Hematomas, 45
Hematopoietic cells, 197
Hemobartonella, 199
Hemoperitoneum, 165
Hemorrhagic effusions, 165
Hemosiderin, 118, 177, 191
Hemothorax, 165
Hepatic lipidosis, 194
Hepatitis, 194-196
Hepatocytes, 254
Hepatomegaly, 189
Hepatopathy, glucocorticoid, 194
Herpes felis, 66
Histiocytomas, 32, 34, 43, 64, 70, 140
Histoplasma capsulatum, 28, 73, 96, 99, 107, 108, 117, 138, 176, 185, 202, 210, 237, 246
Hordeolum, 64
Hydronephrosis, 209
Hygromas, 45
Hyperplasia, 1, 183
Hypertrophy, 1
Hyphae, 248
Hyphema, 72
Hypopyon, 72

I

Immune-mediated skin lesions, 30
Imprints, 2, 21
Infectious agents, also see Parasitism
    Actinomyces, 27, 138, 155, 184
    Aspergillus, 49, 71, 176, 185, 210
    bacilli, 27
    Bacillus, 28
    bipolar rods, 244
    Blastomyces dermatitidis, 28, 29, 63, 72, 73, 96, 131, 138, 176, 185, 210, 220, 244, 246
    Brucella canis, 220
    Candida, 71, 78, 210
    Chlamydia psittaci, 66, 67, 232
    Cladosporium, 70
    Clostridium, 28, 244
    cocci, 244
    Coccidioides immitis, 2, 28, 29, 131, 138, 176, 185, 210, 248
    Corynebacterium, 131
    Cryptococcus neoformans, 28, 29, 49, 73, 96, 131, 176, 185, 210, 237, 246
    Dermatophilus congolensis, 2, 29, 30
    dermatophytes, 29

    Ehrlichia, 108, 109, 117, 131, 155, 203, 250
    Erysipelothrix, 131
    extracellular bacteria, 244
    filamentous rods, 27, 184, 244
    Fusobacterium, 27, 184
    Herpes felis, 66
    Histoplasma capsulatum, 28, 73, 96, 99, 107, 108, 117, 138, 176, 185, 202, 210, 237, 246
    large rods, 244
    Leishmania donovani, 29, 72, 96, 99, 107, 108, 117, 131, 203, 248
    Malassezia canis, 78, 79
    Microsporum, 29
    Mycobacterium, 27, 96, 184, 246
    Mycoplasma, 232
    Mycoplasma felis, 67
    Neorickettsia helminthoeca, 96
    Nocardia, 27, 138
    nonstaining rods, 246
    Pasteurella, 131
    Penicillium, 49
    Peptococcus, 26
    phagocytosed, 240, 244
    Phycomycetes, 29
    Pityrosporum pachydermatis, 78, 79
    Pneumocystis carinii, 176, 185
    Proteus mirabilis, 79
    Prototheca, 248
    Prototheca wickerhami, 29
    Prototheca zopfii, 29, 72, 73, 210, 237
    Pseudomonas, 70, 79
    Rhinosporidium seeberi, 26, 49, 50
    salmon disease, 96
    Salmonella, 131
    Simonsiella, 48, 56, 175, 244
    spore-forming bacteria, 244
    Sporothrix schenckii, 28, 131, 176, 185, 246
    Staphylococcus, 26, 49, 79, 84, 131, 138, 176, 184, 210
    Streptococcus, 26, 49, 79, 84, 131, 138, 176, 184, 210
    Streptopeptococcus, 26
    Trichophyton, 29
Inflammation, 12, 23, 25
    eosinophilic, 244
    purulent, 244
    pyogranulomatous, 244, 248
Inflammatory giant cell, 244
Insect bites, 31
Intermediate cells, 226
Interpretation, cytologic preparations, 10-17
Interstitial-cell tumor, 222
Iris, 72

J

Joints, see Synovial fluid

K

Keratitis, 71
Kidney, 207-212
    abscesses, 209, 210
    cysts, 209
    cytologic evaluation, 208-212
    hydronephrosis, 209
    inflammation, 210
    neoplasia, 211, 212
    pyelonephritis, 210
    sample collection, 207, 208
    tumors, 211, 212
Kinetoplast, 248

L

Leishmania donovani, 29, 72, 96, 99, 107, 108, 117, 131, 203, 248

Leukemia, 97, 192, 204
Leukemoid response, 112
Linguatula serrata, 50
Lipidosis, hepatic, 194
Lipocytes, 108, 254
Lipomas, 41, 140, 187, 254
Liposarcomas, 41
Liver, 189-197
    amyloidosis, 195
    bile pigment, 191
    cholangitis, 194
    cytologic evaluation, 190-197
    glucocorticoid hepatopathy, 194
    hematopoietic cells, 197
    hepatitis, 194-196
    hepatocytes, 254
    hepatomegaly, 189
    hyperplasia, 196
    lipidosis, 194
    neoplasia, 191-194
    sample collection, 189, 190
    tumors, 191-194
Lungs, 179-187
    allergic reactions, 184
    anticancer therapy, effect of, 187
    atelectatic lobe, 181
    bacterial infection, 184
    cell types, 181-187
    cytologic evaluation, 181-187
    dysplasia, 183, 185
    eosinophilic infiltrate, 183
    glove powder, 182
    granulomatous inflammation, 183, 184
    hyperplasia, 183
    hypersensitivity, 184
    inflammation, 184
    lipoma, 187
    macrophage infiltrate, 183
    metaplasia, 185
    mycotic infection, 185
    neoplasia, 182, 185-187
    neutrophilic infiltrate, 183
    protozoal infection, 185
    sample collection, 179-181
    thymoma, 187
    tumors, 182, 185-187
    viral infection, 185
Lupus erythematosus, 133
Lymph nodes, 93-98
    hyperplasia, 95
    lymphadenitis, 95, 96
    lymphoglandular bodies, 94, 95
    lymphosarcoma, 32, 52, 72, 96, 97, 165, 191, 192, 211, 212, 232, 238, 252
    neoplasia, 96-98
    Russell's bodies, 94, 95, 107, 118
    tumors, 96-98
Lymphadenitis, 95, 96
Lymphoblasts, 57, 93-98, 202, 209, 211, 240, 252
Lymphocytes, 57, 93-98, 107, 156, 172, 182, 202, 203, 209, 211, 240, 252
Lymphocytic-plasmacytic conjunctivitis, 68
Lymphoglandular bodies, 94, 95
Lymphoid cells, 56, 57, 93-98, 203, 209, 211
Lymphoproliferative disorders, 204
Lymphosarcomas, 32, 52, 60, 72, 96, 97, 165, 191, 192, 211, 212, 232, 238, 252

M

Macrophages, 57, 94-98, 107, 172, 182, 183, 208, 210, 214, 242, 246
Malassezia canis, 78, 79

Malignancy criteria, 16, 17, 252
Mammary glands, 83-87
    cysts, 84, 86
    foam cells, 84, 86
    mastitis, 84
    neoplasia, 86, 87
    tumors, 86, 87
Mast cells, 157, 172, 182, 242
Mast-cell conjunctivitis, 68
Mast-cell tumors, 32, 34, 64, 165, 192, 252
Mastitis, 84
Megakaryoblasts, 107
Megakaryocytes, 107, 110
Melanin pigment, 254
Melanocytes, 254
Melanomas, 42, 59, 64, 71, 72, 97, 254
Melanophage, 254
Mesenchymal tumors, 15, 40-43, 51, 59, 60, 87, 165, 212
Mesothelial cells, 155, 156, 254
Mesotheliomas, 165, 166
Metamyelocytes, 106
Metaplasia, 1, 173, 185, 219
Metarubricytes, 104, 203
Metritis, 232
Microfilariae, 73, 157, 254
Microscopic evaluation, 10-17
Microsporum, 29
Monocytes, 107
Mott's cells, 107, 116
Mouth, see Oropharynx
Mucin clot test, 122, 123, 125
Multiple myeloma, 118
Muscle, 137, 140
Mycobacterium, 27, 96, 184
Mycoplasma, 232
Mycoplasma felis, 67
Myeloblasts, 105
Myelocytes, 105
Myelography, 146
Myeloid:erythroid ratio, 112-117
Myelophthisis, 119
Myeloproliferative disorders, 204
Myxomas, 43
Myxosarcomas, 43

N

Nasal passages, 47-53
    allergic rhinitis, 52
    foreign bodies, 49, 50
    infectious agents, 48-50
    neoplasia, 51, 52
    parasites, 50
    tumors, 51, 52
Neoplasia, abdominal, 165, 166
    acinar-cell tumors, 88
    adenocarcinomas, 51, 59, 86, 88, 166, 177, 185, 186, 220, 250
    adenoma, 250
    basal-cell tumors, 37, 38
    bile duct carcinoma, 193
    bone, 138-140
    carcinomas, 72, 86, 90, 97, 166, 177, 192, 193, 209, 211
    carcinosarcomas, 43
    cell types, 12-17
    chondrosarcoma, 52, 139
    definition, 1
    ear, 77, 80, 81
    effusions, 165, 166
    epithelial tumors, 33-37, 59
    epulis, 59
    eye, 64, 71, 72, 74, 75
    fibromas, 40
    fibrosarcomas, 40, 52, 59, 139, 140, 206
    fibrous histiocytomas, 43

    giant-cell tumors, 43
    granulation tissue, 40, 41
    hemangiomas, 41, 42, 252
    hemangiopericytomas, 41, 252
    hemangiosarcomas, 42, 52, 139, 204, 206
    hepatic, 191-194
    histiocytomas, 32, 34, 43, 64, 70, 140
    interstitial-cell tumor, 222
    kidney, 211, 212
    leukemia, 97, 192, 204
    lipomas, 41, 140, 187, 254
    liposarcomas, 41
    liver, 191-194
    lung, 185-187
    lymphosarcomas, 32, 52, 60, 72, 96, 97, 165, 191, 192, 211, 212, 232, 238, 252
    malignancy criteria, 16, 17
    mammary, 86, 87
    mast-cell tumors, 32, 34, 64, 165, 192, 252
    melanomas, 42, 59, 64, 71, 72, 97
    mesenchymal tumors, 40-43, 51, 59, 60, 87, 165, 212
    mesotheliomas, 165, 166
    multiple myeloma, 118
    muscle, 140
    myxomas, 43
    myxosarcomas, 43
    nasal, 51, 52
    nephroblastoma, 211
    neurofibromas, 43
    oropharyngeal, 58-60
    osteosarcoma, 138, 139
    otic, 77, 80, 81
    parathyroid, 91
    perianal-gland tumors, 39
    plasma-cell myeloma, 139
    plasmoma, 69
    prostatic, 219, 220
    pulmonary, 185-187
    renal, 211, 212
    renal-cell carcinoma, 211, 212
    respiratory, 177, 185-187
    round-cell tumors, 17, 32, 52, 59, 60
    sarcomas, 72, 86, 252
    sebaceous-cell tumors, 38, 39, 250
    seminoma, 221, 222
    Sertoli-cell tumor, 219, 221
    skin, 31-43
    spindle-cell tumors, 40-43, 51, 59, 60, 64, 87, 165, 212
    splenic, 204-206
    squamous-cell carcinomas, 38, 51, 59, 64, 71, 87, 88, 214, 216, 232, 250
    sweat-gland tumors, 39
    testicular, 221-223
    thoracic, 165, 166
    thymoma, 187
    thyroid, 90, 91
    transitional-cell carcinoma, 215, 216, 232
    transmissible venereal tumors, 32, 33, 51, 60, 72, 97, 222, 232, 252
    types, 12-17
    undifferentiated carcinomas, 40, 91
    undifferentiated sarcomas, 43, 52
    urinary tract, 215, 216
    vaginal, 232
Neorickettsia helminthoeca, 96
Nephroblastoma, 211
Neurofibromas, 43
Neutrophilic conjunctivitis, 65-68
Neutrophils, 57, 155, 172, 175, 182, 184, 208, 210, 214, 240, 244
New methylene blue stain, 9
Nictitating membrane, 68, 69
Nocardia, 27, 138

Nodular episcleritis, 70
Nose, see Nasal passages
Nucleolus, angular, 252, 254
　　large, 250, 252, 254
　　　prominent, 240, 248, 250, 252, 254
　　　variably sized, 252, 254
Nucleus, anisokaryosis, 250, 252
　　bilobed, 252
　　chromatin, 240, 250, 252, 254
　　poorly stained, 242
　　pyknotic, 240, 254

O

Orbit, 74, 75
Orchitis, 220, 221
Oropharynx and tonsils, 55-62
　　epulis, 59
　　neoplasia, 58-60
　　ranula, 56, 88
　　sample collection, 55
　　tumors, 58-60
Osteoblasts, 108, 138
Osteoclasts, 108, 138
Osteoid, 138
Osteomyelitis, 138
Osteosarcoma, 138, 139
Otic tumors, 77, 80, 81
Otitis externa, 77-81
Otobius megnini, 77
Otodectes cynotis, 79, 80

P, Q

Panniculitis, 31
Pannus, 71
Papanicolaou stain, 9, 10
Parabasal cells, 226
Parasite-induced reactions, 30
Parasitism, also see Infectious agents
　　Aelurostrongylus abstrusus, 175
　　Babesia, 199, 202
　　Balantidium coli, 238
　　Capillaria aerophila, 50, 175
　　Crenosoma vulpis, 175
　　Cytauxzoon felis, 96, 176, 185, 199, 202, 248
　　Demodex canis, 80
　　Demodex folliculorum, 63
　　Dipetalonema, 157
　　Dirofilaria immitis, 157, 177, 254
　　ear mites, 79, 80
　　Entamoeba histolytica, 238
　　Filaroides, 175
　　Hemobartonella, 199
　　Linguatula serrata, 50
　　microfilariae, 73, 157, 254
　　Otobius megnini, 77
　　Otodectes cynotis, 79, 80
　　nasal, 50
　　Paragonimus, 175
　　Pentatrichomonas hominis, 238
　　Pneumonyssus caninum, 50
　　Toxoplasma gondii, 96, 99, 108, 117, 155, 176, 185, 248
Paragonimus, 175
Parathyroid glands, 83, 91
Pasteurella, 131
Penicillium, 49
Pentatrichomonas hominis, 238
Peptococcus, 26
Perianal-gland tumors, 39
Perinuclear vacuolation, 166, 250
Peritoneal dialysis, 153
Peritoneal fluid, see Abdominal fluid
Peritonitis, 162, 163
Phycomycetes, 29
Pityrosporum pachydermatis, 78, 79
Plasma cells, 107, 118, 172, 182, 209, 211, 240
Plasma-cell myeloma, 139

Plasmacytic-lymphocytic synovitis, 133
Plasmoma, 69
Pleocytosis, 145, 146
Pleural fluid, see Thoracic fluid
Pleuritis, 162
Pneumocystis carinii, 176, 185, 248
Pneumonyssus caninum, 50
Polychromatophilic erythrocytes, 105
Polycythemia vera, 110, 112
Postenucleation orbital cyst, 75
Primary granules, 105
Proestrus, 228
Promegakaryocytes, 107
Promyelocytes, 105
Progranulocytes, 105
Prorubricytes, 104, 203
Prostate gland, 217-220
　　abscesses, 219
　　cysts, 218
　　hyperplasia, 219
　　neoplasia, 219, 220
　　prostatitis, 218, 219
　　sample collection, 217
　　Sertoli-cell tumors, 219
　　spermatozoa, 218
　　squamous cells, 218
　　squamous metaplasia, 219
　　transitional epithelial cells, 214, 218
　　tumors, 219, 220
　　urothelial cells, 214, 218
Proteus mirabilis, 79
Prototheca, 248
Prototheca wickerhami, 29
Prototheca zopfii, 29, 72, 73, 210, 237
Protozoal colitis, 237, 238
Pseudochylous effusions, 156, 160, 163-165
Pseudomonas, 70, 79
Pseudopregnancy, 232
Pulmonary tumors, 185-187
Pyelonephritis, 210

R

Ragocytes, 133
Ranula, 56, 88
Rectum, 235-239
　　eosinophilic colitis, 236, 237
　　fungal colitis, 237
　　hematochezia, 235
　　neoplasia, 238, 239
　　protozoal colitis, 237, 238
　　sample collection, 235, 236
　　tumors, 238, 239
Renal-cell carcinoma, 211, 212
Reserve cells, 39
Respiratory system, see Lungs, Tracheal washes
Reticulocytes, 105
Rhinosporidium seeberi, 26, 49, 50
Romanowsky stains, 2, 9
Round-cell tumors, 17, 32, 52, 59, 60
Rubriblasts, 104
Rubricytes, 104, 203
Russell's bodies, 94, 95, 107, 118

S

Salivary glands, 83, 87-89
　　neoplasia, 88, 89
　　ranula, 56, 88
　　sialadenitis, 88
　　sialoceles, 87, 88
　　tumors, 88, 89
Salmon disease, 96
Salmonella, 131
Sample collection, 2-5, 17-19
　　abdominal fluid, 152
　　aqueous humor, 72

　　bone, cortical, 137
　　bone, marrow, 99-103
　　cerebrospinal fluid, 143
　　cutaneous, 21-23
　　ear, 78
　　fistulous tracts, 23
　　hepatic, 189, 190
　　joint, 121-123
　　kidney, 207, 208
　　liver, 189, 190
　　lung, 179-181
　　masses, 4-9, 21-23
　　mouth, 55
　　muscle, 137
　　nasal cavity, 47, 48
　　orbit, 74
　　oropharynx, 55
　　peritoneal fluid, 152
　　pleural fluid, 151, 152
　　prostate, 217
　　pulmonary, 179-181
　　rectum, 235, 236
　　renal, 207, 208
　　semen, 223
　　skin, 21-23
　　spleen, 199-201
　　subcutaneous, 21-23
　　synovial fluid, 121-123
　　testis, 220
　　thoracic fluid, 151, 152
　　tonsils, 55
　　tracheal, 167-171
　　ulcerated lesions, 23
　　urine, 213, 214
　　vagina, 225
　　vitreous body, 73
Sample shipping, 17-19
Sarcomas, 72, 86, 252
Sclera, 69, 70
Scrapings, 2-4, 21
Sebaceous adenoma, 250
Sebaceous cells, 250
Sebaceous-cell tumors, 38, 39, 250
Secondary granules, 106
Segmented granulocytes, 106
Semen, 223, 224
　　evaluation, 223, 224
　　sample collection, 223
Seminoma, 221, 222
Seromas, 45
Sertoli-cell tumors, 219, 221
Sialadenitis, 88
Sialoceles, 87, 88
Signet-ring cells, 39, 88
Simonsiella, 48, 56, 175, 244
Skin, 21-46
　　abscesses, 44, 45
　　allergic reactions, 30
　　collagen neurosis, 31
　　cysts, 43-45
　　dermatitis, 23-31
　　eosinophilic granulomas, 30
　　epidermal cysts, 43
　　fat necrosis, 31
　　foreign bodies, 30
　　hematomas, 45
　　hygromas, 45
　　immune-mediated lesions, 30
　　infection, 27-30
　　inflammation, 23-31
　　insect bites, 31
　　neoplasia, 12-17, 31-43
　　panniculitis, 31
　　parasite-induced reactions, 30
　　sample collection, 21-23
　　seromas, 45
　　snake bites, 31
　　steatitis, 31
　　traumatic lesions, 30

259

tumors, 12-17, 31-43
   virus-induced lesions, 30
Smear preparation, 2-9, 101-103
Snake bites, 31
Sperm, 218, 223, 224
Spindle cells, 252
Spindle-cell tumors, 40-43, 51, 59, 60, 64, 87, 165, 212, 252
Spleen, 199-206
   cytologic evaluation, 201-206
   extramedullary hematopoiesis, 203
   Heinz bodies, 203
   hyperplasia, 202, 203
   lymphoproliferative disorders, 204
   myeloproliferative disorders, 204
   neoplasia, 204-206
   parasites, 199
   sample collection, 199-201
   smear preparation, 201
   splenomegaly, 199
   tumors, 204-206
Splenomegaly, 199
Sporothrix schenckii, 28, 131, 176, 185, 246
Squamous cells, 218, 250
   basal, 250
   mature, 250
   neoplastic, 250
   tadpole cells, 38, 250
Squamous epithelial cells, 56, 214, 218
Squamous metaplasia, 219
Squamous-cell carcinoma, 38, 51, 59, 64, 71, 87, 88, 214, 232, 250
Squash preparation, 6, 7, 22, 189
Stains, artifacts, 10, 11
   Diff-Quik, 2, 9
   DipStat, 9
   Giemsa, 2, 9
   hematologic, 2
   new methylene blue, 9
   Papanicolaou, 9, 10
   problems, 10, 11
   Romanowsky, 2, 9
   Wright's, 2, 9
Staphylococcus, 26, 49, 79, 84, 131, 138, 176, 184, 210
Starfish preparation, 7, 8, 22
Steatitis, 31
Streptococcus, 26, 49, 79, 84, 131, 138, 176, 184, 210
Streptopeptococcus, 26
Subcutis, see Skin
Superficial epithelial cells, 227
Superficial keratitis, 71
Swabs, 4, 21
Sweat-gland tumors, 39
Synovial fluid, 121-136
   arthritis, 130-133
   cell counts, 125
   characteristics, 123-127
   color, 123, 124
   cytologic evaluation, 126
   eosinophilic polyarthritis, 133
   hemarthrosis, 123, 127-129
   joint degeneration, 129, 130
   joint infection, 130, 131
   mucin clot test, 122, 123, 125
   plasmacytic-lymphocytic synovitis, 133
   protein content, 127
   ragocytes, 133
   sample collection, 121-123
   systemic lupus erythematosus, 133
   thixotropism, 127
   turbidity, 123, 124
   viscosity, 124
   volume, 123
   windrowing, 124
Systemic lupus erythematosus, 133

T

Tadpole cells, 38, 250
Tear gland, 69
Testis, 220-223
   epididymitis, 220, 221
   interstitial-cell tumor, 222
   orchitis, 220, 221
   neoplasia, 221-223
   sample collection, 220
   seminoma, 221, 222
   transmissible venereal tumor, 222
   tumors, 221-223
Thixotropism, 127
Thoracentesis, 151, 152
Thoracic fluid, 151-166
   cell counts, 154
   cell types, 155-162
   chylous effusions, 156, 160, 163-165
   culture, 154
   effusions, 155-166
   exudates, 160-162
   glove powder, 157
   heart disease, 163
   hemorrhagic effusions, 165
   hemothorax, 165
   mesothelial cells, 155, 156
   neoplastic effusions, 165, 166
   pleuritis, 162
   protein content, 154
   pseudochylous effusions, 156, 160, 163-165
   sample collection, 151, 152
   smear preparation, 152-154
   thoracentesis, 151, 152
   transudates, 158-160
Thrombocytes, 107
Thymus, 187
Thyroid glands, 83, 89-91
   adenomas, 90
   goiter, 89, 90
   hyperplasia, 89, 90
   neoplasia, 90, 91
   thyroiditis, 89
   tumors, 90, 91
Tingible bodies, 94, 96
Tonsils, 55-62
Toxoplasma gondii, 96, 99, 108, 117, 155, 176, 185, 248
Tracheal washes, 167-177
   allergic bronchitis, 175
   bacterial infections, 176
   cell counts, 171
   cell types, 171-174
   Charcot-Leyden crystals, 175
   contaminants, 174
   Curschmann's spirals, 171
   cytologic evaluation, 171-177
   dysplasia, 173
   eosinophilic infiltrates, 175
   glove powder, 174
   hemorrhage, 177
   inflammation, 175
   metaplasia, 173
   mucus, 171
   mycotic infections, 176
   neoplasia, 174, 177
   parasites, 175
   protozoal infections, 176
   sample collection, 167-171
   smear preparation, 171
   viral infections, 176
Transitional-cell carcinoma, 215, 216, 232
Transitional epithelial cells, 214, 218
Transmissible venereal tumor, 32, 33, 51, 60, 72, 97, 222, 232, 252
Transtracheal washes, see Tracheal washes
Transudates, 158-160
Traumatic lesions, 30
Trichophyton, 29
Triglyceride concentration, 164
Trophozoites, 238
Tumors, see Neoplasia

U

Ulcerated lesions, 23
Undifferentiated carcinomas, 40, 91
Undifferentiated sarcomas, 43, 52
Urine, 213-216
   chemotherapy, effects of, 215
   cystitis, 214, 215
   cytologic evaluation, 214-216
   neoplasia, 215, 216
   sample collection, 213, 214
   tumor cells, 215, 216
   urothelial cells, 214, 218
Uroperitoneum, 163
Urothelial cells, 214, 218
Uterus, metritis, 232
Uveitis, 72

V

Vagina, 225-233
   cell types, 225-228
   estrous cycle stages, 228-232
   metritis, 232
   neoplasia, 232
   sample collection, 225
   tumors, 232
   vaginitis, 232
Virus-induced skin lesions, 30
Vitreous body, 73, 74

W, X, Y

Windrowing, 124
Wright's stain, 2, 9

Z

Zygomatic mucocele, 68